Clinical Cosmetology:

A Medical Approach to Esthetics Procedures

Victoria Rayner

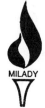

Milady Publishing Company
(A Division of Delmar Publishers Inc.)
3 Columbia Circle, Box 12519
Albany, New York 12212-2519

NOTICE TO THE READER

Credits:

Senior Administrative Editor: Catherine Frangie
Developmental Editor: Joseph Miranda
Editing Supervisor: Marlene McHugh Pratt
Project Editor: Pamela Fuller
Production Manager: John Mickelbank
Design Coordinator: Karen Kemp
Art Coordinator: Brian Yacur

10 9 8 7 6 5 4 3 2   XXX 99 98 97 96 95 94

Library of Congress Cataloging-in-Publication Data:

Rayner, Victoria
   Clinical cosmetology: a medical approach to esthetics procedures/Victoria Rayner.
      p. cm.
   includes bibliographical references and index.
   ISBN: 1-56253-056-9 (textbook)
   1. Medical rehabiliation. 2. Beauty, Personal. 3. Body image. 4. Surgery, Plastic.
   5. Cosmetics. I. Title.
   [DNLM: 1. Cicatrix — rehabilitation. 2. Cosmetics — therapeutic use. 3. Facial Injuries —
   rehabilitation. 4. Self-concept. 5. Skin Diseases — therapy. 6. Surgery, Plastic — methods.
   QT 275 R275c]
RM930.R34 1993
617.1'03—dc20
DNLM/DLC
for Library of Congress   92-22650
                                                                        CIP

Table of Contents

CHAPTER **3**

Cosmetology Therapy with Disfigured Children

CHAPTER **4**

Documentation, Medical Terminology, and Record Keeping

CHAPTER **7**   Corrective Makeup 123

CHAPTER **10** **Adaptive Grooming Techniques for the Visually Impaired** 177

CHAPTER **12**   **Camouflage Therapy and the Burn Patient** 268

CHAPTER **15**

AIDS 395

Contributors

Darrick E. Antell, M.D., D.D.S., P.C., Plastic Surgeon, New York City, New York.

Martha Beazley, President of the Alemeda Beauty College, Alemeda, California.

Richard Barboni, D.D.S., Consultant to AIDS chapter, San Francisco, California.

Timothy Berger, M.D., Chief, Department of Dermatology at San Francisco General Hospital, San Francisco, California.

K.H. Blacker, M.D., Professor and Chair Department of Psychiatry, University of California Medical Center, Davis, California

Melanie Boyd, San Francisco Women Against Rape's Services, San Francisco, California.

Joanna M. Cain, M.D., Associate Professor at the University of Washington Medical Center, Seattle, Washington.

Michael Carson, O.D., Senior Optometrist, University of California Medical Center, San Francisco, California.

Christine Cobaugh, Education and Prevention Assistant at Marin Abused Women's Services, San Rafael, California.

Jessica L. Elkins, R.N., B.S.N., Micropigmentation, San Francisco, California.

Donna R. Fox., Ph.D. in Speech and Psychology, Houston, Texas.

Chuck Frutche, Director of San Francisco AIDS Foundation, San Francisco, California.

James Groundwater, M.D., Dermatologist, San Francisco, California

Lovic Hobby, M.D., Plastic Surgeon, Instructor for the Department of Surgery, Piedmont Hospital, Atlanta, Georgia.

Charolote Jane, Consultant on hair and wig replacements, Newport Beach, California.

Jerold Kaplan, M.D., Medical Director of the Burn Center at Alta Bates Hospital, Berkeley, California.

Peggy Knight, President of Knight and Day Hair Products, San Rafael, California.

John Y.M. Koo, M.D., Psychiatry and Dermatology, University of California Medical Center, San Francisco, California.

Theodore A. Labow, M.D., Assistant Clinical Professor, Department of Dermatology, College of Physicians and Surgeons at Columbia University, New York City, New York.

Peggy Mellody, R.N., Beauty and Cancer, Los Angeles, California.

Diane Doan Noyes, Beauty and Cancer, founder of Appearance Concepts Foundation, Kirkland, Washington.

Mark Olsen, Assistant Editor, San Francisco, California.

Maurice Parecki, Certified American Board of Opticianry, San Francisco, California.

Susan R. Parecki, Certified American Board of Opticianry, San Francisco, California.

Shireen Perry, home economics instructor to the blind, Center for Independent Living, Albany, California.

Mary Smith, Coordinator of the Disabled Community Health Clinic at Alta Bates Hospital, Berkeley, California.

Stephen P. Sturges, M.D., Psychiatrist, Alta Bates Hospital, Berkeley, California.

Lewis Tannenbaum, M.D., Dermatologist, San Francisco, California.

Ronald E. Tegtmeier, M.D., Plastic Surgeon, Denver, Colorado.

Sigi Torinus, photographer and visual artist, Fine Arts Degree from universities in Germany and the United States.

Rollie Turpin, Consultant, Apple Computer.

Dr. Karen Walker, Optometrist and Medical Editor, San Francisco, California.

Rochelle B. Wolk, Ph.D., Assistant Clinical Professor, Division of Behavioral Pediatrics, Department of Pediatrics, University of California Medical Center, San Francisco, California.

Illustrators
Diana Hill
Richard Mandrachio
Fred Nin

Acknowledgments

This book is dedicated to the loving memory of Nelson N. Tunis, my attorney and close friend; had it not been for his insistence I would not have had the courage or the persistence to finish this book.

To Dr. Timothy Berger for his generous support and contributions and the endless time he spent medically editing and supervising this material and whose belief in camouflage therapy when challenged was unshakable.

Most importantly, to my husband, who stood by me and assisted me with all the major and trivial details connected with this project over the past four years.

About the Author

Over twenty years ago Victoria Rayner was badly burned. The appearance of the scars she sustained made her the subject of cruel jokes, icy stares, and the thoughtless remarks of others. Sadly, even after two decades and in a liberal society such as ours, disfigurement is still considered a social handicap. People with physical irregularities struggle desperately to be accepted and to lead normal lives. The painful memory of her own tragic experience made Victoria Rayner feel compassion for others who, like herself, have had to learn to live with both the emotional and physical scars of a temporary or permanent disfigurement.

Ms. Rayner has devoted her entire professional life to educating the public and to helping others who suffer from the stigma of disfigurement cased by birth defects, disfiguring disease, or traumatic injuries. She is credited with pioneering the first skin-care center in a medical building to provide medically supervised skin care to patients with problematic skin conditions.

After completing a basic course in paramedical makeup she went on to redefine the art of camouflage makeup by introducing cosmetic rehabilitation therapy. For years Rayner patiently volunteered her services, working closely with reconstructive surgeons and dermatologists, helping with their patients, to firmly establish cosmetic clinics in hospitals. Carefully documenting her encounters, she shared her experiences with other estheticians and nurses by writing articles in trade and medical journals. Finally, after four years, with the cooperation of physicians at the University of California Department of Dermatology, she was able to create the first salaried position for an esthetician in a hospital. Most importantly she insisted that the cosmetic therapist be given a formal title, "Dermatology Associate." It has been chiefly through her efforts that the medical community has embraced cosmetic rehabilitation therapy as a legitimate part of medical treatment. Her lectures and presentations at medical conferences and universities have expanded the awareness of the medical community of the skills and expertise of all beauty professionals. Today, Victoria Rayner is the director of five camouflage therapy clinics, all of which are located in teaching hospitals.

In 1987 Rayner expanded her skin-care clinic with the addition of a school for clinical cosmetology, offering advanced training to licensed cosmetologists, estheticians, and medical professionals. She developed the curriculum, established rigorous certification criteria, and built a unique program of educators, including dermatologists, burn survivors, psychologists, reconstructive and plastic surgeons, and anaplastologists.

To date Victoria Rayner has shared her knowledge with over 400 estheticians. Because of her emphasis on job-related training many of her graduates have been placed in physicians' offices or have established camouflage clinics on their own throughout the United States and Canada.

Ms. Rayner has devoted the last four years to writing and completing the first textbook on clinical cosmetology, entitled *Clinical Cosmetology: A Medical Approach to Esthetic Procedures*. It is to be used by estheticians and cosmetologists as a teaching guide and a working manual.

Victoria Rayner has also co-authored a medical textbook with five medical professors to be published this spring in England, entitled *Cosmetic Dermatology*. She has just released her first audio cassette to 1,500 dermatologists on cosmetic therapy.

Introduction

James Groundwater, M.D.

Esthetics and dermatology have much to share with one another, and a new, more exciting era of cooperation and mutual enrichment is not only possible but is happening. Leading the way is my good friend, Victoria Rayner, who realized early on that esthetics and dermatology had similar goals and that each had knowledge and experience that could help the other. She opened the doors by initiating a dialogue in a spirit of humility without a trace of false arrogance. She sought and received information about dermatology and freely gave of her own knowledge. Soon she was working with private dermatologists and university dermatology departments, sharing her wealth of knowledge in a spirit of good will and mutual trust.

Estheticians, cosmetologists, cosmetic scientists, dermatologists, plastic surgeons, and, indeed, pharmaceutical companies can all contribute their expertise to the effective creation and utilization of what many now call cosmeceuticals. Although cosmetics and skin-care products have usually had a scientific basis, marketing and professional interests have sometimes led to pseudoscientific jargon and, indeed, pseudoscientific products. Often bewildered and confused by claims and counterclaims, the general public has sometimes succumbed to the most seductive slogans and attractive packaging.

Informed practitioners are in a position to work with each other or independently to provide the public with the knowledge it needs to choose and use effective and, indeed, esthetic cosmetics and skin-care products. By bringing together related disciplines in a spirit of cooperation, Victoria Rayner has facilitated this development.

Dermatologists see many irritant and allergic reactions from cosmetics and skin-care products. Furthermore, follicular occlusion (pore blockage) can occur, leading to blackheads, whiteheads, pimples, and pustules. This is often secondary to topical product usage. Dryness and oiliness are important factors in many conditions involving the skin, hair, and nails.

Many topical products can alleviate or exacerbate dryness and/or oiliness. Consequently, they may influence those conditions profoundly. Esthetic techniques can be very helpful to relieve occlusive follicular processes in a relaxing, supportive environment. Appropriate selection and instruction in the usage of cosmetic and skin-care products can prevent or alleviate many allergic and irritant reactions, dry and/or oily skin conditions, and even neoplastic (new growths) processes.

Estheticians can learn to recognize many infectious, congenital, and even neoplastic conditions of the skin, hair, and nails. In so doing, they can protect themselves and their clients from such infectious processes as boils, impetigo, warts, molluscum contagiosum, herpes, mites, and lice. Such congenital states as portwine stains and giant pigmented and epidermal nevi can be concealed until such time as they can be removed or treated appropriately. Pre-malignant and malignant conditions can be recognized and referred for dermatologic management. Melanoma in particular is nearly 100 percent curable if recognized early but rapidly fatal if allowed to progress. This pigmented lesion now occurs in one in one hundred Caucasians and can be recognized and referred early, thus saving lives. Gross disfigurement can be prevented by early management as well as basal and squamous cell carcinomas, commonly occurring in sun-exposed individuals. Appropriate counseling in measures for protection from the sun can be extremely helpful.

In conclusion, estheticians, dermatologists, and others can work together to serve the needs of a public that deserves and demands healthy, vibrant, and attractive skin, hair, and nails. This book is a great step in that direction.

Letter to the Reader

This book, by Victoria Rayner, is certain to achieve its stated goal. The contributing authors represent a broad spectrum of professionals involved in the teaching as well as the development of concepts related to this expanding field.

I have had the personal pleasure of seeing Ms. Rayner spearhead the development of clinical cosmetology through her tireless efforts at lecturing, teaching, and now publishing.

Whether dealing with birth defects or acquired traumatic defects, Ms. Rayner has confirmed the need for cosmetic camouflage within the medical setting. Both the physical need as well as the psychological importance to the patient make the clinical cosmetologist an integral part of the health-care team.

Despite the remarkable recent advances in medicine, we should never forget the oldest medical treatment of all, which is "laying on the hands." By caring for and physically touching patients, estheticians and cosmetologists reinforce the oldest of medical treatments. Both the appearance as well as the attitude of our patients can be elevated through clinical cosmetology.

"Efforts encouraged are not enough without purpose and direction." (John F. Kennedy) The purpose of this textbook is well stated in its title, and direction is provided by an outstanding collection of authorities in their respective fields.

Darrick E. Antell, M.D., D.D.S.
Board Certified Plastic Surgeon
New York, New York

1 Cosmetology and Medicine

From the beginning of time a small group of people were particularly interested in mankind's ills and sought the knowledge and skills to treat them. Because of their ability to help the afflicted and the injured, those few individuals acquired a position of respect and honor among their fellow people.

Comparatively modern compared with other medically affiliated specialties, clinical cosmetology nonetheless has roots buried deep in history. Cosmetic techniques and camouflage alternatives were offered to war veterans in hospitals by cosmetologists over sixty years ago. According to *The Psychology of Cosmetic Treatments,* the British Red Cross has successfully used this kind of beauty care for the hospitalized for the last twenty-five years.

When a patient with a disfigurement who has undergone camouflage therapy feels an enhanced sense of self-improvement and self-sufficiency, it is clear to all, including health-care professionals, that progress has been made. Medical care is not complete until the patient has been trained to work and live with what he or she has left.

A therapeutic camouflage program focuses on all aspects of the patient's appearance. It includes cosmetic procedures, facial and hair prostheses, and hairstyling.

GOALS AND CONSIDERATIONS OF CLINICAL COSMETOLOGY

The term *clinical* is defined as the practical, experimental method of medical education resulting from the observation and treatment of patients. *Cosmetology* refers to the scientific study of beauty. A professional career as a clinical esthetician/cosmetologist offers many opportunities and rewards to those who become experts through training in cosmetically camouflaging and normalizing a disfigured patient's appearance.

A clinical esthetician/cosmetologist collaborates with a patient's physician and other health-care providers to assist the patient in normalizing his or her appearance. The role of the medically affiliated beauty professional is that of a camouflage therapist. He or she describes the type of camouflage options available, along with their advantages and disadvantages, to the patient.

Cosmetically, the camouflage therapist plans for and assists the patient in obtaining a normalized cosmetic result that can be achieved by disguising undesirable features and physical irregularities with the skillful art of illusion.

Camouflage makeup techniques are an important adjunct to the field of medicine. Cosmetic therapy is often the last hope for patients for whom no further medical or surgical treatments can provide benefit. It is then that a patient can be referred by a medical specialist to a clinical esthetician/cosmetologist for cosmetic therapy. Many patients, especially accident victims with severe scarring, benefit greatly from the psychological support cosmetic treatment promises. Camouflage therapy provides the patient with a choice and a degree of control that would not otherwise be there.

However, merely having the skills of a makeup artist and using that ability to conceal a burn, laceration, or lesion is not what camouflage therapy is about. A beauty professional faces specific challenges when caring for scarred patients.

CAMOUFLAGE THERAPY

Camouflage therapy is a specialty that helps people with disfigurements help themselves. In therapy, patients solve some of the major emotional problems associated with the disfigurement that prevent them from leading happy, normal, and productive lives.

When working with disfigured patients, camouflage therapists are brought face to face with people who have undergone immense personal tragedies. Not only do these individuals suffer from their physical traumas, but they endure emotional trauma as well.

Because of their altered physical appearance, many patients also experience a loss of identity. People who provide camouflage therapy to patients are always a little surprised to find that those with slight disfigurements have a greater desire to conceal their disabilities than patients whose disabilities are undeniable. The evidence shows that our culture is indifferent toward persons with any type of physical disabilities. These negative attitudes are apt to disturb anyone who is suffering from a disfigurement, regardless of its severity, and as a result can affect such a person's sense of what he or she "ought to be." Patients with disfigurements believe that they are terribly flawed, and as a result they cannot judge the appearance of their scars in proportion to their physical image as a whole. This poor self-concept leads to low self-esteem and a strong feeling of inadequacy. Helping the patient to identify those distortions becomes a major component of camouflage therapy.

This introspection allows patients to acknowledge their disfigurements as a part of their new physical image. This new image should include awareness of their personal assets that are also undeniably a part of their physical identity. Through exploration of themselves, patients can eventually reach a more accurate self-evaluation. A camouflage therapist can intervene by offering a method of treatment that assists patients in seeing their entire image, which includes their positive physical aspects.

A drastic or severe physical change requires a new self-definition. When people suffer a severe enough trauma to cause them to lose all sense of self, they are forced to redevelop the entire personality before a new self-image can be fully established. Much of this psychological rehabilitation transpires during the time they are seeking camouflage alternatives. Patients will cling to the past until a new self is established.

The goal, therefore, of the paramedical consultant should be not only to support the patients' efforts to restore physical appearance with the use of cosmetics, but also to offer them an open forum for personal discovery.

Most makeup artists who practice paramedical camouflage do so because they enjoy feeling needed. When they design a camouflage plan for a patient with a disfigurement, they always hope that they will come up with the perfect solution to make the patient look and feel normal again. This very rarely happens.

In reality, the most extremely disfigured patients can hope for is slight improvement, with scarring not as obvious. From the beginning, patients should understand that the cosmetic procedure will not transform their appearance beyond recognition. They can expect to look better, but not totally changed. Therefore, a successful outcome will depend more on patients' acceptance of cosmetic treatment than on the actual physical result achieved by the makeup artist.

Paramedical makeup consultants are highly trained makeup artists who devise innovative ways to cover temporary or permanent scarring using makeup. Many of these individuals have attended courses given by the manufacturers or distributors of cover creams, which are limited to the physical aspects of this specialty. Because much of the training is highly technical, most students focus their attention primarily on learning the "how to's" of cosmetic application and as a result fail to develop the patient management skills required to work effectively with emotionally traumatized people.

Many paramedical consultants feel that as graduates of these cosmetic training programs they possess all the knowledge and skills required to camouflage scars with cosmetics. Some even leave the seminars believing that applying cover creams is all they will ever really need to know in order to work with physically challenged patients.

Confident that they will devise the most appropriate camouflage solutions for patients, they set up a practice and begin to give cosmetic recommendations. Unaware of the underlying emotions affecting the sessions, many continue despite patients' protests that the makeup process is too complicated for them to grasp. Sometimes they even offer makeup consultations when it is obvious that the patient is psychologically unprepared for a new physical image.

This accounts for some of the negative feedback that doctors receive from patients who have had paramedical makeup treatments. The major complaint is that the camouflage makeup sessions are too technical. Many patients feel frustrated because after one session they are not able to perform the color blending techniques required to match their skin tone and to camouflage their scars.

It is interesting that many patients actually go back to their physicians and speak highly of the esthetician's skill as a makeup artist, complimenting the esthetician's ability to disguise flaws during the session. But later, they claim that the paramedical consultant's treatment is too complicated and that their real needs are not met.

Whether it is our intention to work to provide corrective makeup services in salons or inside a hospital, we must first ask ourselves exactly what will be required of us and how we can truly help these patients to make a difference in their lives. An old saying has relevance here: "If you give a man a fish to eat, you can feed him for one night, but if you teach a man how to fish, you can feed him for a lifetime."

On the other hand, camouflage therapists differ from paramedical makeup consultants. The focus of their training, from the beginning, is on patient management. They know that they are dealing with individuals who are feeling temporarily vulnerable because they have been physically challenged. They also recognize that their patients are not emotionally weak and that they do not think of themselves as victims. They know full well that these individuals are extremely strong because they have had to come to terms with what has happened to them. Through the patients' emotional struggles, they have become more aware of their inner strengths. Camouflage therapists recognize that what these patients are trying to do is develop a new sense of identity; therefore, they consider their role as a makeup artist secondary in the treatment. Much of the time that they spend with patients is devoted to helping them work through the identity process. They realize that they must be careful not to introduce their own opinions into the therapy unless they are needed.

Camouflage therapists use their communication skills to empower patients by giving them the confidence necessary to perform the makeup techniques themselves. Camouflage therapists outline a specific method of treatment for a patient based on his or her intellectual ability. They realize that each patient is different and that it takes longer for some to learn than others. They may even extend the therapy to do more than they are intellectually, emotionally, or physically capable of in one session. This allows patients the opportunity to slowly master the more technical aspects of the therapy until they can successfully apply the corrective makeup themselves. During this time, patients' confidence in their own ability begins to increase.

Most of us magnify, in our minds, the appearance of our physical flaws to begin with. These blind spots interfere with an accurate physical assessment of ourselves. People as a rule are constantly comparing their physical image to that of others. This abstract self-definition prevents us from celebrating the uniqueness of our being.

Patients with disfigurements are automatically considered different because of their appearance. Once patients begin to understand this difference they are on their way to accepting it. In a national best seller written by Ann Kaiser Stearns, *Living Through Personal Crisis*, she writes, "Our scars, even those representing permanent injury, are the 'war ribbons' that indicate where we've been. They are a part of our personal histories and present strengths. Why should we disclaim them?" Patients learn in therapy to redefine their previous definitions of beauty to include the awe-inspiring physical appeal of self-acceptance and individuality.

The major difference between a paramedical makeup consultant and a camouflage therapist is that at the end of the session, the therapist hopes that patients will feel confident enough about themselves that they will not need to feel as if they have to cover their scars. Camouflage therapists only consider their treatments successful if patients become enlightened with the understanding that their scars are only physical aspects of their individuality and just another form of personal identification. They also believe that it is important for patients by the end of their sessions to be able to acknowledge that these differences are now a part of their physical character.

Most significantly, camouflage therapists recognize that the most important measure of success of the treatment is the way patients perceive their physical images in the future and the importance they will place on their scars in relationship to their overall appearances.

DUTIES OF THE CAMOUFLAGE THERAPIST

To assist the physician in providing patients, with both permanent and temporary disfigurements, personal appearance counseling.

To provide patients with a variety of esthetic suggestions that can be used to normalize his or her appearance.

To monitor feelings and, based on the patient's response, individualize a camouflage plan that incorporates ideas and strategies that specifically appeal to the patient.

To encourage patient involvement by actively listening to the patient's contributions to assure his or her full participation in the therapy.

To consult with the patient's family if necessary, and to instruct them on camouflage or esthetic procedures with which to assist the patient.

To prepare the patient for the camouflage session by recording the medical history and condition, systematically reviewing the information, making an assessment, devising a treatment plan, and together with the patient following it through.

To perform professional skin-care treatment and to instruct patients on follow-up skin-care and basic grooming procedures.

To refer the patient back to a physician or to other specialists in health care if the patient's condition requires additional medical attention.

REVIEW

You should now be familiar with:

- the goals and considerations of clinical cosmetology.
- how camouflage therapists differ from paramedical makeup consultants.

2 Patient Management

Psychological Aspects of Working with Disfigured Patients

Stephen P. Sturges, M.D.

Health-care personnel have a role as confidants and psychological healers for patients. This is true even if patients do not confide in them directly. People sometimes find it easier to confide in strangers than in their friends and families, particularly if they believe that the stranger has some special skill, experience, or knowledge gained through working with others with similar afflictions.

Given this phenomenon, it is not surprising that we find ourselves unexpectedly listening to patients tell us about psychological and emotional problems when we are attending to physical concerns. This offers us an important opportunity to help by being understanding and supportive.

Often we can be of the most assistance to the patient not through directly discussing their difficulties but by understanding the nature of their problems and knowing what will be most helpful.

In some settings where patients are treated for disfigurements resulting from injuries, there is no one with extensive for-

mal training available to talk with them, even though this is the time when their psychological and emotional needs are the greatest.

The trend in this country has been to focus on technological solutions to medical problems (rather than on the emotional needs of the individual) to the point of losing sight of the healing powers in human relationships. This power tends to be devalued while we focus on the use of new medicines and technology.

As a culture, we are largely deprived of the salve of human contact. This becomes very obvious when working with a patient who has recently suffered a physical disfigurement. In a very real way, these people have lost their own identity. Not only do others see them differently, but they see themselves as changed, less than they were. They may have experienced or fear that others will react to them differently than before their appearance was physically altered.

Attempts to re-establish their self-image

Dr. Stephen Sturges is board certified in psychiatry. He received his medical training at Columbia University. Dr. Sturges received his psychiatric training at the University of California, San Francisco; Stanford University; and Napa State Hospital. He is currently practicing at Alta Bates Hospital in Berkeley, California.

are influenced by changes in their appearance and their ability to function normally. They watch closely to see how people react to them, much the way they did when they first developed a sense of self as children. If their personal loss is too painful to handle, they avoid conscious awareness of rejection by refusing to care about how others respond to them. However, they continue to notice the reactions of others on an unconscious level. Often they expect that others will be horrified by their injuries and their appearance and find ways of avoiding human contact.

Many people suffering from a recent disfigurement are in emotional shock and fearful of interaction with others. These persons are unable to think or talk about events of their injuries because it reminds them of their painful loss. Their reactions are very individual, however, because some people start to make an adjustment immediately while others remain unable to think or talk about the events that resulted in their injuries even many years later.

When I worked in the burn unit of a general hospital there was a patient, an attractive 16-year-old girl whose face had been burned in a fire after a truck in which she was riding collided with another vehicle. Her face had severe scarring, with keloid formation and red discoloration. For many weeks, she was unable to grasp just what had happened to her. She was distraught, withdrawn, and angry. She involved herself only superficially with family and friends.

During the first several months following her accident, she had to undergo the painful process of debridement and skin grafting, which needed to be repeated every few days. Just when she would start to experience some decrease in pain, she would have to begin the process all over again. She felt isolated and was unable to confide in the staff who had to perform the unpleasant but necessary task of the painful debridement.

When this process was finally over and skin grafting was complete, she was left with disfiguring scars. Once she was past the physical pain of recovery, she was then forced to deal with re-establishing a new self-image.

The rest of the burn unit staff and I were surprised when she began to talk meaningfully about her sadness over losing her facial beauty. Patients generally are unable to face these issues so directly so soon after the debridement and grafting phase.

Underneath she felt she was the same person as before, but now she would have to cope with the new way in which other people responded to her. She showed some uncertainty about this at first.

Even though the efforts of the staff to reflect back to her and to recognize her underlying feelings of strength encouraged her, she rejected meeting with me as the psychiatrist, and rejected using cosmetics to make her scars less noticeable. This was her way of declaring herself strong, independent, and able to cope.

At first, I felt rejected and hurt by her expressed lack of need for my help and angry at her for rejecting me. Didn't she realize she had serious psychological injuries and needed my counseling as well as cosmetic camouflage therapy in order to be able to function normally again?

Slowly I began to realize that she was rejecting me as a symbolic way of showing her inner strength. She likewise rejected the idea of covering her scars and decided instead to include them in her new sense of self.

In retrospect I think she trusted me not to be overly injured by her rejection and to support her need to feel independent. She was "turning the tables" on her fate by actively controlling the intervention of others (the camouflage therapist and me in this case) and was no longer at the mercy of what others did to her or thought about her.

It was important that I did not get angry with her or become rejecting of her as a way of dealing with her "rejection" of me. Much later she confided in me that my continued support in the face of her rejection helped her adjust to her new identity. This illustrates how being helpful often involves "listening" to nonverbal messages as well as spoken ones. She re-entered social life with friends her own age with a strong sense of self and of renewed confidence.

I have had some patients who recover from their psychological injuries slowly or sometimes not at all. This often happens when a person's self-image is based on superficial concerns to begin with. These patients are at greater risk of lasting psychological injury, and quite frequently are slow to heal emotionally or will not recover completely. Nevertheless, the treatment is much the same, except that younger persons are more able to adapt because their sense of self is not as complete. Older persons usually have more trouble adjusting to a new self-image that includes their injuries and disfigurements because they have become accustomed to experiencing themselves as they were prior to their disfigurements.

SELF-IMAGE

Physically challenged patients have many problems that are associated with their altered appearance. Understanding these problems and the psychological influence they have on the patient will aid the clinical cosmetician in providing quality professional care. To further explore how the impact of physical disfigurement can affect an individual's self-ideal, we must first examine how self-image develops.

Since the size, function, and appearance of our body is the most visible and material part of ourselves, it is the major component of the way we perceive ourselves. As we grow we slowly develop an awareness of our physical selves through examination of the physical aspects of our bodies. Later we become aware of our physical limitations. During adolescence we begin to feel awkward as our bodies physically change. When we reach middle age we begin to realize our bodies are not functioning as well as they did when we were younger. This is because metabolism slows down and muscle tone decreases. We first notice signs of aging as we gain weight and our skin loses elasticity. Complexion becomes coarse, and fine lines or wrinkles start to appear. In later years physical abilities decrease. Hair loses its color and becomes gray or white; we may even lose hair. Our senses become dull; our hearing, vision, and sense of taste diminish. These changes are all part of a natural process of aging. However, the way we respond to these physical changes can greatly affect our self-esteem. All through the course of life our awareness and acceptance of our appearance is an integral part of self-esteem. To maintain what we feel is an acceptable body image we camouflage our physical faults by dying the color of our hair, wearing cosmetics, dressing in certain clothing, and in some cases even undergoing cosmetic surgery.

It is a popular belief that individuals who are concerned about the physical aspects of their appearance are vain and superficial. But research has revealed that the closer the resemblance between a person's physical appearance and his or her ideal concept of what he or she should look like, the more successful an individual will be at balancing both physical and non-physical components of the personality.

In working with patients who have lost their physical identities, the camouflage therapist will encounter a variety of different body perceptions. The altered appearance of these individuals can lead to serious body image disturbances. Some patients may have a clear and realistic understanding of their new self, while others may have a vague, unrealistic, and demanding idea of what they feel their physical image should be. The camouflage therapist must keep in mind that many patients may be resistant at first to changing their self-ideal (image). The process of accepting the new physical aspects of their altered appearance may be slow. In the psychological aspects of this transition, a patient may appear resentful at first. But if the camouflage therapist is patient, he or she can eventually assist the individual in re-establishing a new self-concept by helping the patient to picture him or herself more realistically.

Helping the patient achieve a positive self-concept is what camouflage therapy is all about. The plan for providing camouflage therapy begins with determining what can be done to assist the patient; this involves setting goals and objectives with the patient, judging his or her priorities, and designing methods to resolve problems. In order to accomplish the patient's goals, the cosmetician must recognize subtle clues when conversing with the patient to pick up on emotional messages that the patient is sending.

Being professional does not mean being impersonal. Because of the motivation to integrate effectively with the members of the medical profession, cosmeticians must be careful not to become too detached from patients during therapy. The way in which the camouflage process is implemented should reflect the intellectual, interpersonal, and technical skills of the cosmetician. Camouflage therapists, therefore, should be encouraged to be themselves and to freely express their personalities by using their own unique and imaginative ways to relate to their patients. If the the camouflage therapist is afraid or unaware of his or her own self, he or she may be apprehensive if the patient is unresponsive to his or her approach.

CLEAR COMMUNICATION

Clear communication is the first step to successful patient management. It involves an exchange of information between the camouflage therapist and the patient.

The Elements of Good Listening

The elements of good listening are vital to interpersonal communication. To be most helpful those of us who work with patients will need to identify exactly what those patients' real needs are. Only then will we be able to determine what we can or cannot do to help.

There is more to listening than nodding your head in agreement or politely gazing at another while he or she is speaking. Most of us are poor listeners because we have never been taught how to receive verbal messages correctly. We may be thinking of something else when someone is speaking to us, or we may become bored with what we are hearing. We may even feel as if we have heard what is being said before. Whatever the reasons, the significant fact is that we simply tune out what we don't wish to hear. We often focus only on words or phrases that interest us. This form of selective listening limits communication. The average person is capable of understanding speech at a rate of 600 words per minute, and yet we only speak between 100 and 140 words

PATIENT MANAGEMENT **13**

per minute. As a result, our minds tend to wander when someone else is talking. It is very easy for us to become distracted. The sounds of traffic, music, others speaking, and ordinary day-dreaming can all interfere with our ability to hear well.

Concentrating solely on what the speaker is saying will help you to be an accurate receiver of verbal messages. Concentration requires the following:

1. Listening without judging or analyzing what is being said.
2. Refraining from offering advice or moralizing.
3. Questioning the speaker only if you are unclear about what is being said.

Actively listening takes time and patience. As with any new skill, you will have to practice being an active listener. It involves allowing the patient to express thoughts freely. By interrupting and trying to relate what is being said to your own life experience you can interfere with this process. If you show a sincere interest in what the patient is saying, it will encourage him or her to share more.

Body Language

Body language is another powerful form of communication. Posture, body movements, and facial expressions can provide nonverbal clues about the patient's emotional reaction to the treatment. By learning how to recognize these actions, you can gain a better perspective on how patients are responding to your camouflage instruction. Actors, models, speakers, and politicians all rely on body language to project their emotions. These professionals have mastered this fine science and have come to realize the importance of it as a powerful communication tool.

Our gestures and expressions all indicate our feelings before we verbally express our thoughts. People may hear our words, but the messages we most successfully communicate to others originate from a more visual form of communication — body language. We can stop speaking, but we cannot stop communicating through our body movements. Nonverbal communication consists of a mixture of body gestures and facial expressions, which we are unconscious of most of the time. Being alert to these physical signals can lead to better patient management.

Words can be deceptive. We may listen to a patient express something verbally, yet body language may convey a totally different message. By tuning into these signals, you will become more aware of patient's true emotions, and you will be better equipped to respond to their behavior.

For example, a smile can indicate a general feeling of friendliness. But a smile that is too long or too obvious can be interpreted as more than merely a friendly gesture. It can be irritating and haunting. Combine that same smile with a wink, and the meaning again changes. The smile and the wink suggest an invitation to a flirtation.

To thoroughly study body language, we must take into account the mixture of all the body movements, those that are deliberate and those that are involuntary. We must also consider who is sending the nonverbal messages as well as who will be receiving them.

Gestures That Have Particular Meanings
Puzzlement or confusion (See Figure 2-1.):

1. Scratching the head can be an expression of puzzlement.

2. Signals that indicate confusion are hand or fingers raised to the lips, hand on the forehead, furrowed eyebrows, or a down-turned mouth.

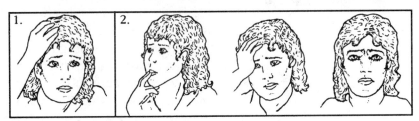

Figure 2-1. Puzzlement or confusion

Refusal or reluctance (See Figure 2-2.):

1. Knitting the forehead.

2. Wrinkled or lowered eyebrows.

3. Pulling away.

4. Raising both hands in despair.

5. Tight-mouthed expression.

6. Covering eyes or ears.

Anxiety or fearfulness (See Figure 2-3.):

1. Biting the lip.

2. Fully opened eyelids.
3. Muscular tenseness.
4. Holding onto an object for support.
5. Staring or a fixed gaze.
6. Nervous laughter.

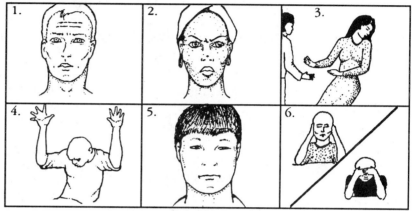

Figure 2-2. Refusal or reluctance

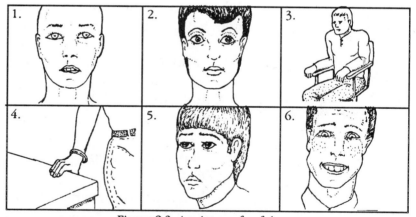

Figure 2-3. Anxiety or fearfulness

You can establish a better rapport immediately with patients and set the tone of the visit by being alert to their body movements. Identifying certain gestures patients make during treatment sessions can be helpful in accessing the emotional state at the time of their appointment. Open body posture, uncrossed legs or arms, for example, may signify a relaxed and comfortable emotional state. Generally, patients whose body movements appear less rigid are more trusting and therefore more approachable.

Body language also sends nonverbal messages to our patients. Improper nonverbal communication from the therapist not only complicates the communication process, it can also have a negative effect on the healing environment because it discourages positive interaction. For instance, leaning forward toward patients while conversing lets the patient know that you are attentive and taking in their information; if you pull your shoulders back slightly, the patient feels that you are distracted and are withdrawing from the conversation. Nail biting, rapid gum chewing, and foot tapping are all signs of destructive and anxiety-induced behavior. When instructing patients, be careful not to make any rapid, exaggerated, or abrupt movements that can easily be misinterpreted as impatience or intolerance.

Proxemics

Proxemics is the term used to define appropriate distance in the field of nonverbal communication. People's need for this personal space is a very primitive one. The way a patient reacts to the invasion of his or her private space can affect his or her behavior and pose intercommunication problems during treatment. When working with patients, always maintain enough distance so the patient appears comfortable and non-threatened by your physical presence.

Four distinct measurements define distance in relationship to others. See Figure 2-4.

1. Intimate space: The distance between those who are romantically or intimately involved; 6 to 18 inches.

2. Personal distance: The comfortable span between individuals engaging in casual conversation; 1 ½ to 2 ½ feet.

3. Impersonal distance: A wider division of space of 3 to 7 feet. Such a distance would be appropriate when conversing with someone on a more formal basis.

4. Public distance: The range of 12–25 feet; the general distance observed between a speaker and audience.

When working with a patient, you should stand or sit at a distance of at least 2 to 2 ½ feet for casual conversation. Always face the patient shoulder to shoulder. Initial physical contact should be made by shaking hands. A firm handshake will convey confidence and put the patient at ease. Direct eye contact should always be maintained. It has been said that eye contact is the single most important clue to a person's attitude. Observe the patient's eyes to see if they are focused on yours or if they are wandering and avoiding eye contact. Lack of eye contact could mean that the patient is distracted or feeling uncomfortable.

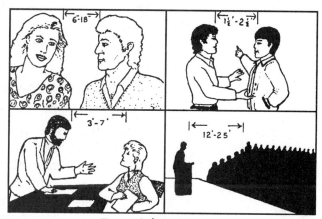

Figure 2-4. Proxemics

Kinesics

Kinesics is a term that refers to body movement and posture. Our emotions can cause our body to settle into set physical patterns. A patient who slumps in a chair or slouches may feel that he or she is carrying the weight of the world on his or her shoulders. This posture might indicate depression and may indicate a feeling of helplessness. Such a patient could be a poor candidate for camouflage rehabilitation, because he or she may feel more like a victim than a survivor. Patience will be required to work with these individuals. On the other hand, the patient with very rigid posture may be less flexible and may offer even more resistance to treatment. Introverted patients who tend to be defensive will sit closed off from nonverbal communication by crossing their arms or legs in an effort to shield themselves from others.

The way a patient's body is positioned will indicate the level of his or her involvement in your therapy. You should be particularly aware of the way in which your patient controls his or her body structure. Gestures and expressions can speak louder than words if they are properly interpreted.

It is very easy for those of us who work with patients to become manipulative and overprotective. We can safeguard against this by remembering that the patient must be given every opportunity to express concerns freely. This can be achieved by concentrating on what the patient is saying and observing body language to properly assess the patient's emotional and physical state at the time of the appointment.

The elements of good listening require that we respond to the patient appropriately and that we ask only relevant questions during treatment. In order to assure proper communication at all times we must follow some guidelines in our social contact with others until they become second nature.

1. Suspending judgment.
2. Isolating key words and phrases.
3. Identifying the patient's intensity.
4. Determining the patient's mood.

The Power of the Spoken Word

Our words communicate our thoughts and ideas to others. There is an art to self-expression. The way in which we color our sentences can excite, anger, impress, disappoint, and hurt. Words have an overwhelming power; we can use speech to command others to fulfill our wishes. For this reason it is important that you weigh your words carefully before you speak, to insure that your meaning is clear. The way in which you verbally express yourself to the patient should communicate your self-confidence and your commitment to helping. The following guidelines will assist you in acquiring the basic skills necessary in assuring positive verbal communication with patients.

Proper Verbal Communication

Your ability to effectively communicate with patients will win their trust and co-operation.

The first step to instilling confidence is to believe what you say. Before you communicate with the patient, ask yourself how your knowledge can help this person solve his or her problems and achieve his or her goals. If you focus on your inner resources and how your skills can help the patient, you will gain a feeling of strength and power. Your self-assurance will become evident to the patient as you express your ideas. By concentrating first on what you are trying to say and then on the best way to get your point across to the patient you will easily find the proper words to articulate your thoughts.

Always be sincere when you speak. Whenever possible, practice using words to let others see what is in your mind and your heart. As you do, you will find that your words will soon create a powerful impact on others.

Establish a direct relationship with your patient. You can do this by using the patient's name. Let the patient know right away that you appreciate the fact that he or she has come to see you for treatment and give assurance that you will do whatever you can to help.

Do not lecture or preach. Always leave room for open dialogue. Encourage the patient to express any feelings about what he or she is hearing. As you talk, watch the patient's reactions and listen carefully to his or her responses. The patient might have an interesting idea that could prove useful to the treatment.

When you speak, state simply a few of your points at time. If what you are trying to say becomes too cluttered with irrelevant remarks, you could end up confusing or boring the patient. To gain the patient's respectful attention, begin by offering general information about your topic and then narrow down your thoughts by being more specific. This will help the patient to understand your message more clearly.

While speaking, pause occasionally and ask the patient a question that requires a response. This will maintain his or her attention and encourage him or her to participate in the conversation.

Speaking is a visual as well as an auditory art. To make your phrases stand out, use words to paint vivid pictures in the patient's mind. Since so much of camouflage therapy is based on patient instruction, this visual speaking technique will prove quite useful in giving directions or dispensing information.

Use comparisons that the patient can relate to in order to further stress your point.

When you give instructions to the patient, enumerate your points. Arrange your steps in logical sequence; step 1, step 2, and so forth. Make sure that the patient understands each step before moving on to the next one.

Avoid using technical terms when conversing with the patient. Such terms may be meaningless and will confuse the patient. If you must use a technical term, explain it first.

MANAGING DIFFICULT PATIENTS

Sarcastic Patients

Sarcasm is usually a response to an unresolved problem. Sarcastic patients usually are trying to prove to others and to themselves that their ideas are right.

1. Always try to deal with sarcastic patients alone.
2. Ask what was meant by a sarcastic remark (surface the attack).
3. Let the patient know you won't be intimidated.
4. Try to identify underlying problems.

Complaining Patients

Chronic complainers find fault with everything and everyone. Complainers consider themselves victims.

Dealing with complaining patients:

1. Acknowledge what the patient is saying.
2. Repeat what was said back to him or her.
3. Do not agree with complaining patients.
4. Try to get complainers to concentrate on problem solving.

Negative Patients

This personality type expects the worst; they are pessimists. They believe that they cannot trust others. They are disheartened and discouraged.

1. Acknowledge what negative patients say but never argue.
2. Be realistic; don't make false promises.
3. Completely think through all possible solutions before offering possible camouflage alternatives.
4. If a negative patient is reluctant to problem solve, ask what is the worst that can happen if he or she takes a risk.

Silent, Withdrawn Patients

A patient's unresponsiveness can mean any number of things. Silence can represent anger, lack of commitment, or a wish to maintain control.

1. Relax the patient by starting up a casual conversation.
2. Ask questions that require more than just a simple yes or no answer to draw the patient out.
3. After you have asked a question, wait expectantly with eyebrows raised and eyes wide open and a slight smile on your face until the patient responds. Lean forward and maintain eye contact; patiently wait for a response.
4. Allow a little more time for this patient to open up.

5. When the patient does talk, be attentive and repeat back what you think he or she meant to say.

Overly Agreeable Patients

This type of patient has a strong need to be liked. In order to gain your acceptance he or she will commit to actions and not follow through on them.

1. Let the patient know you want him or her to honestly express feelings.
2. Do not place the patient in a situation where he or she will be forced to make a commitment that can't be kept.
3. This personality type often communicates true feelings through humor. Listen carefully for hidden emotional messages. The way you react to this patient's teasing will indicate how open he or she can be with you.

Psychiatric Aspects of Camouflage Therapy

John Y.M. Koo, M.D.

DELUSIONAL PATIENTS

Patients with primary psychiatric disorders are patients who have no significant cosmetic defect but are mentally fixated on the idea of having one. This type of patient perceives a specific defect on his or her body that cannot be perceived by others. The validity by which those false beliefs are held varies from patient to patient. Some patients who suffer from a psychiatric disorder may be mildly aware of their fixation and may even apologize for their "vanity" or acknowledge the possibility that their complaints may be exaggerated. Other patients who are truly delusional will not respond to any argument that conflicts with their deranged perception. This type of patient is often so defensive that he or she is easily offended by any suggestion that the perception is not shared. Such a patient may, for example, demand that a plastic surgeon alter the shape or size of his nose because he is convinced that his nose is "ugly," or he may demand a dermabrasion for "unsightly scars," which in fact are normal sized pores; or the patient may complain of severe "hair loss" when no loss can be substantiated.

ANOREXIA NERVOSA AND BULIMA

Anorexia nervosa and bulimia refer to a subtype of patients with distorted belief systems regarding body image. See Figure 2-5. Anorexia nervosa is characterized by a delusional belief that one is overweight; consequently, these patients engage in extreme, at times life-threatening, forms of diet, exercise, and use of laxatives and other materials to reduce weight. Bulimic patients

Dr. Koo is board-certified in both psychiatry and dermatology. He received his medical training at Harvard Medical School, his psychiatric training at the University of California, Los Angeles, and his neuropsychiatric and dermatology training at the University of California, San Francisco Medical Center. He is currently a full-time faculty member at the University of California Medical Center and director of the Psoriasis and Skin Treatment Center.

also hold extreme concerns about the shape and weight of their bodies but they are different from purely anorexic patients in that they engage in recurrent episodes of overeating ("binges") followed by self-induced vomiting and the use of laxatives to lose weight. The treatment of both conditions is individual psychotherapy and group therapy directed at the underlying personality disorder, family therapy, behavioral therapy designed to restrict destructive behavior and reward healthy food intake, and judicious use of medications as well as close monitoring of the physical condition to avoid serious complications from extreme eating behaviors.

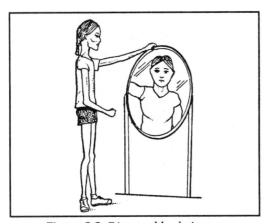

Figure 2-5. Distorted body image

The risk in treating these delusional patients by physical means, such as camouflage therapy, is that they are likely to never be satisfied with the cosmetic treatment. Since the fundamental problem is psychiatric, even if some improvements were made on mild "blemishes," the patient would still find other ways to distort reality and claim therapeutic failure.

In terms of managing patients with psychiatric disorders, the ideal situation would be for the camouflage therapist to refer them to a psychiatrist. Unfortunately, most of these patients will not only refuse such a referral but could become infuriated by the cosmetician's suggestion that their problems may not be physical. Therefore, the camouflage therapist should be diplomatic in his or her approach. A limited period of cosmetic treatment might be necessary to first build a rapport with the patient so eventually a referral to a psychiatrist can be made.

One suggestion to the therapist is to avoid agreeing with any of the patient's comments that might reinforce his or her delusional belief system. Instead, the camouflage therapist should remain neutral while trying to build a rapport. This may present a challenge since these patients often seek confirmation from others. Once a good rapport with the patient has been made, a suggestion for psychiatric referral can be attempted. If the therapist acknowledges the patient's emotional distress, he or she can recommend that the patient see a psychiatrist as a way to relieve some of that distress rather than suggesting that the patient need counseling because he or she is delusional.

PATIENTS WITH REAL COSMETIC DISFIGUREMENT

In contrast, camouflage therapists are in an excellent position to help patients with mild psychiatric problems caused by real disfigurements, because generally a patient's psychological status will improve if he or she can successfully conceal a disfigurement. However, the clinical cosmetologist must also be aware that not every patient will respond to cosmetic therapy. If a patient begins to experience serious social or occupational dysfunction as a result of a physical disfigurement, a psychiatic referral should be considered. Some patients may be so emotionally traumatized by their disfigurement that, even though they can learn to superficially normalize their appearance with the use of cosmetics or camouflage procedures, this form of therapy will do little to ease the emotional pain of dealing with the disfigurement. For these patients, no amount of cosmetic cover-up will eliminate the suffering that accompanies the loss of their physical image, and they should be referred to a professional for psychriatic treatment.

Four of the most common psychiatric disorders seen in disfigured patients are: depression, social phobia, anxiety disorders, and agoraphobia. These disorders are outlined below to facilitate their recognition by the clinical cosmetician or cosmetologist.

DEPRESSION

A devastation to self-esteem frequently results in clinical depression. *Depression* in psychiatric usage refers to a condition more serious than usual variations in mood. It is characterized by a loss of capacity to feel pleasure, loss of appetite, difficulty with sleep, and at times suicidal thoughts. Most cases of depression are treatable with the use of medication, psychotherapy, or a combination. However, if depression is not diagnosed and remains untreated, it can linger on for years and may result in suicide.

SOCIAL PHOBIA

Social phobia is experienced as signifi-

cant distress that the patient feels when he or she encounters a social setting. The patient frequently recognizes this fear as excessive or unreasonable, but simple recognition does little to stop this undesirable reaction. Social phobia can be treated with psychotherapy. Group sessions can provide the patient with realistic feedback regarding his or her social interactions. Medication may also be prescribed to reduce anxiety, and patients can learn a variety of behavioral methods to "desensitize" themselves in social situations.

ANXIETY DISORDERS

The manifestations of anxiety can be psychological, physiological, or both. Psychologically, patients often experience feelings such as worry or fear. Physiologically, anxiety can be manifested by numerous symptoms such as shortness of breath, tension headaches, abdominal discomfort, heart pounding, sweating, frequent urination, trembling, or diarrhea. Anxiety attacks cause patients to avoid social and occupational settings in which the last anxiety attack was experienced. In extreme cases this avoidance can result in complete isolation.

AGORAPHOBIA

Agoraphobia can be defined as a "fear of open places." It is a phobic disorder characterized by fear of leaving ones's home. Treatment of agoraphobia requires the use of specific medications that diminish the intensity of the fear or decrease the frequency of the anxiety attacks in conjunction with individual psychotherapy.

SPECIAL PATIENTS

Foreign Language Speaking Patients

If a patient speaks only a foreign language or has difficulty expressing him- or herself in English, try to find someone at a local community college or university who can translate for you. Position the interpreter next to you. Speak directly to the patient, and only turn to the interpreter when you need to convey detailed descriptions. If the patient speaks limited English, try observing the patient's facial expressions and body language to determine if you are communicating with him or her effectively. Speak slowly and clearly. Be sure to plan your treatment carefully. Keep instructions simple. Do not give the patient unnecessary information or more instruction than is required. If additional instruction is necessary, do not condense it; instead schedule another session rather than complicate and confuse the patient with too much instruction in one visit. You can also use body language or pictures to explain the camouflage process to the patient. To determine if the patient understands you ask him or her to mimic your gestures. Answers to questions should require more than just a simple yes or no since those are words easily learned by foreign patients and can be misinterpreted by you.

Children   Children are much stronger and more courageous than we imagine. Each child will require a special approach that will depend on the special set of circumstances that caused the disfigurement (see Chapter 3 on children).

THE PHYSICALLY DISABLED

Physically disabled people are men, women, and children who were either born with a physical limitation or developed one as a result of an injury, illness, age, or an accident. A physical disability is any physical impairment that lasts for at least six months or more and interferes with major life tasks such as walking, seeing, hearing, or talking. Very few people are completely handicapped. Most individuals who are disabled find unique solutions to compensate for their physical limitations.

Since the words we use reflect our attitudes, using the term "the handicapped" stereotypes individuals with disabilities. It groups all persons with physical limitations, regardless of their impairment. Each person with a disability has different limitations, depending on how extensive the disability is. All people with physical limitations cannot be considered "handicapped."

The way a person with a disability looks strongly influences the impression that he or she makes on others. A well-trained camouflage therapist can help persons with disabilities learn how to improve their outward appearances. Regardless of the physical limitation, when a person looks better he or she feels better psychologically. A well-groomed appearance can boost patients' morale and enhance self-esteem.

Understanding the causes of the patient's disability and recognizing his or her capabilities will help the camouflage therapist assist the patient with difficulties encountered in treatment. How much a patient can actually do will depend not only on the patient's physical capacities, but also on his or her age and general state of mental and physical health at the time of the camouflage session. The extent to which a person is actually handicapped will also largely depend on his or her attitude about the disability. The most important thing is that the patient views him- or herself realistically. Some patients will over-identify with their disability by believing they are more physically restricted than they actually are, while others may play down their limitations and force themselves to do things they can't actually do. Once a person acknowledges his or her limitations, he or she can learn how to cope with them.

No matter how independent a patient appears, inevitably situations will arise where your assistance will be needed. The patient's requirements for your help will vary depending on the extent of his or her condition and emotional needs. Patients who are severely disabled may need someone to assist them with every aspect of the therapy, while those with less extensive disabilities will need little or no assistance.

People with disabilities go through most days like the rest of us, balancing what they know they can achieve with what they can actually manage; but for someone with a limitation, one miscalculation has greater consequences: exhaustion sets in, defenses are down, and suddenly even the slightest challenge might appear impossible. The camouflage therapist can help prevent the patient from becoming discouraged by developing an organized plan for the camouflage treatment and by discussing this plan in detail with the patient beforehand to let the patient know what will be required to perform the process independently. A schedule should also be set up that will allow periodic intervals for the patient to rest or review the camouflage procedures so as not to become overwhelmed or fatigued.

Working with the Disabled

Mary Smith

It is estimated that today persons with disabilities comprise about 13 percent of the entire U.S. (and world) population. Some are born with such conditions, while others acquire them during their lives. Ironically, perhaps, they are often more seriously impeded by barriers created through myths, prejudices, stereotypes, fears, and ignorance than by the effects of their disabilities. This section attempts to address these barriers with facts, understanding, and common sense.

Simply put, *disability* means that one or more things most people can do, a disabled person cannot do as easily, or, sometimes, at all. It is important to remember that disability is almost never "total," and disabilities usually affect a surprisingly narrow range of activity. Disabilities can be visual, aural, physical, communicative, or developmental. One person may have a combination of disabilities. Disabilities can be caused by birth defects, illnesses, or injuries. But a disability is always a residual effect, not the birth defect, illness, or injury itself.

Meeting a disabled person is meeting a person. Yet, many non-disabled people find themselves feeling awkward, fearful, or self-conscious, without really knowing why. Disabilities — and the people who have them — are as varied as social situations. Interacting with disabled people will, like social situations, emphasize your (and our) courtesy, caring, and common sense, far more than an ability to quote from a rulebook.

I think it might be good at this point to introduce some facts:

1. Disabilities are not contagious.

2. Disabled people know they are disabled and know that you know.

3. Disabilities are frequently permanent; miracles sometimes happen, but most disabled people are not waiting around for them.

4. Disabled people prefer to emphasize what they can do, rather than what they cannot do, just like you.

5. Disabled people have the same range of personality traits that non-disabled people do, and disability is not one of them.

Mary Smith is the Coordinator of the Disabled Community Health Clinic at Alta Bates Hospital at Berkeley, California. Born with arthrogryposis multiplex congenita (AMC), she has intimate experience of physical disability.

Ms. Smith spent the first nine months of her life in the hospital, as only her involuntary muscle groups worked at birth, enabling her only to move her eyes, suckle, swallow, and wet her diapers. Throughout her childhood, she worked through an intensified regime of physical, occupational, and speech therapies along with numerous corrective orthopedic surgeries. As a result of her disability, she received her elementary and high school education at a boarding school for orthopedically handicapped children. She received her undergraduate degree in social work and returned to graduate school for a master's degree in rehabilitation counseling. Currently she lives in Oakland, California, without the need for outside assistance or attendants.

Ms. Smith has worked as a social worker, a rehabilitation counselor and counseling supervisor for a state agency, and a program manager for an independent living center. Over the years, she has been involved in groups and organizations that promote the rights of the disabled.

6. Disability is not the sum total of a disabled person's life, any more than having a certain hair color is yours.

7. Disabled people can — and do — engage in sex.

A most important difference between disabled and non-disabled people is that people with disabilities have to adapt to an environment designed for the non-disabled. If the environment were designed to accommodate us, our disabilities would be comparatively unimportant. A few special guidelines for interacting with disabled people will be helpful; otherwise, the rules are the same as for anyone else.

- If you would like to help a disabled person, say so. But wait until the offer is accepted before you move. Even then, it is wise to discuss the best way to approach the problem at hand.

- Talk to the disabled person, not to a companion or an attendant. This is true even if the conversation is carried on through an interpreter.

- Do not try to filter your conversation of common expressions. "I've got to run," and "See what I mean?" are not puns unless you make them so.

IMPAIRED MOBILITY

To the non-disabled, wheelchairs can be an emotionally-loaded symbol of disability. To the person in the wheelchair, the chair is a means of mobility and freedom, nothing less or more. Some pointers:

- Remember that to a person in a wheelchair, the chair is part of personal space, as intimate as your belt buckle is to you.

- Do not push a person in a wheelchair without first asking. A sudden jerk or movement can upset the person's balance and may cause injury.

- Many people in wheelchairs can transfer themselves to cars, bathtubs, toilets, etc., usually with little or no help. If they do so, do not move the chair out of their reach.

- Architectural barriers, such as narrow doorways, stairs, and curbings, present special problems to people in wheelchairs. They can overcome some of these problems by themselves. Others require some help. Again, the rule is: "Before you try to help, find out what to do and how."

- Some people in wheelchairs can walk with crutches, braces, canes, and other aids, usually slowly. A wheelchair is not an act: it may be faster or a way of conserving energy.

- Unless they are five years old or younger, most people in wheelchairs hate to be patted on the head, even though the height is right.

- People in wheelchairs are not contortionists. If your conversation looks like it is going to last, sit down and make yourself (and the other's neck muscles) comfortable.

VISUAL IMPAIRMENT

In their own way, the white cane and the guide dog are just as symbolic as wheelchairs. All the groundrules apply for interacting with people who have visual impairments (see chapter on adaptive blind techniques). Keep in mind a few specific points:

- Remember that there are many kinds of visual impairments and that many visually-impaired people are not totally blind.

- Not all visually-impaired people can hear better than you or have ultra-developed senses of touch. They may, but don't assume it.

- Not all visually-impaired people read braille; they may rely on tape recordings or read with special equipment.

- When talking to a visually-impaired person, start out by announcing yourself and to whom you are speaking; otherwise, you may sound like you are just talking to yourself.

- If a visually-impaired person seems to need help, do not be afraid to offer. "Hi there. Need some help?" is just fine.

- Guide dogs should not be petted, especially when they are working. They know what they are doing and need to concentrate on it.

HEARING IMPAIRMENT

Hearing is one of our most vital senses. It allows us to communicate with and learn from the people around us. Hearing also keeps us in constant contact with our surrounding environment, even when we are asleep. The ramifications of a hearing impairment can be devastating psychologically, educationally, and socially.

Hearing loss has been labeled a "hidden disability" because there are no obvious markers such as white canes or wheelchairs to indicate a special need. Even

hearing aids can be very inconspicuous. Furthermore, hearing aids do not completely correct a hearing deficit. Even when amplified, sounds may seem distorted and unnatural to the hearing-impaired listener. Here again are some facts:

- Remember that there are different types and degrees of hearing impairment, and that many hearing-impaired people are not totally deaf.

- Some people acquire their hearing losses long after they have learned to speak their native language. However, people who have been deaf or hearing impaired since birth may never have the chance to learn speech and language in the usual way ... by listening. The latter group of individuals may sound odd as they speak and may even need to rely on visual or manual forms of communication.

- Many hearing impaired people who have normal or near-normal vision will try to supplement their residual hearing by using speech-reading cues. Make sure when speaking to someone with a hearing loss that you are face to face and enunciate clearly. Do not assume they can read all of what you say.

- Yelling, screaming, or exaggerating your articulation will not help a hearing-impaired listener. Speak from a close proximity and make a point of speaking clearly.

SPEECH DISABILITIES

Speech disabilities range from a slight lisp to inability to speak. Much research is being put into speech alternatives such as synthesized voices, special typewriters, and other assistive devices. Many of these are not yet on the market or may be unsuitable for certain people, who must adapt vocally to their disability. In almost all cases, people with speech impairments can communicate; but it is usually a partnership: whether they can do so successfully depends on you.

- Speech impairments do not imply reduced intelligence. People with speech impairments have things to say worth listening to.

- Be alert to the presence of an alternate form of communication, such as a typewriter or computer device.

- If the person with whom you are talking can speak only with difficulty, do not be afraid to ask for a repeat, even three or four times. Repeating is less difficult for the speech-impaired individual than knowing that you do not understand or do not care enough to.

- Do not simplify your own speech, use "baby talk," or raise your voice.

Most speech-impaired people can hear and understand.

DEVELOPMENTALLY DISABLED

People who are developmentally disabled are often confused with people who are mentally ill, which is probably the source of many myths and prejudices. Some facts:

- Only about 15 percent of developmentally disabled people are "profoundly" retarded. The remaining 85 percent can read, write, work, drive, think, and live productive, independent lives.

- Developmentally disabled people are responsible, industrious, and reliable to the same degree as non-disabled people are.

- A man and a woman who are developmentally disabled will not necessarily have developmentally disabled children.

- Cerebral palsy and developmentally disabled are two different disabilities. They may, but not necessarilly will, occur in combination.

INTERACTING WITH DISABLED PEOPLE

As service providers, health-care professionals, and clinicians with specialized skills and services that an individual with a disability may purchase, the following are a few more facts and pointers that may assist you in successfully interacting with people who have disabilities.

- Many people with disabilities employ attendants to assist them with their grooming, dressing, and personal hygiene. The disabled person may wish to have his/her employee present when receiving instructions from you.

- Likewise, some people with disabilities use adaptive living devices to accomplish many daily tasks such as applying makeup, dressing, etc. It may be advisable to consult with an occupational therapist should it appear that your patient with a disability may need to use a device to follow your instructions.

- Do not be overly sensitive about using everyday expressions.

- Be extremely careful about using any reference to "normal" people. Other than experiencing certain unique inconveniences accompanying a disablement, people with disabilities lead normal lives; any comparison of the disabled to "normal" people disregards that fact.

- Do not be afraid to admit ignorance on a topic or subject when it seems necessary to understand the gist of a conversation.

- When in doubt, use everyday language.

People with disabilities live, breathe, learn, teach, eat, work, get parking tickets, aspire, loaf, make love, raise families, laugh, celebrate, mourn, cry, pay taxes, and die. Disabilities should be neither focused upon nor ignored. They are facts of life, which each disabled person deals with and adapts to.

Working with Communication Disorders

Dr. Donna Fox, Ph.D.

Communicating is one of our most human activities. When something goes wrong with the process of hearing, understanding, and speaking, the interchange between humans breaks down, and the process may become discontinuous or disordered. This section will explore some of the reasons for speech and language breakdown and then some of the ways to keep the process going forward. This may appear to be, in

Donna R. Fox, Ph.D., received her B.A. from the University of Washington in Seattle, her M.A. from the University of Iowa, and her Ph.D. in Speech and Psychology at the University of Missouri. She has taught at William Jewel College, at the University of Nebraska, and at the University of Houston, where she is presently Professor of Communication Disorders. She has been both Area Head and Director of Graduate Studies for Communication Disorders at the University of Houston. She has published texts in voice disorders, cleft palate, and private practice along with numerous articles in these areas. She is a member and fellow of the American Speech, Hearing, and Language Association, the American Psychological Association, the International Association of Logopedics and Phoniatrics, and the American Cleft Palate Association, where she has served as a board member. Dr. Fox has served as secretary to the Cleft Palate Foundation and as President of the American Academy of Private Practice. In addition she is a member of various state and local professional organizations.

some instances, a laborious task.

When performing camouflage makeup on a patient, you are dealing with an individual who may have some outward sign of trauma or birth defect; but in cases of communication problems, the problem may be hidden, invisible to the eye. The camouflage therapist communicates in some meaningful way in order to serve the patient's esthetic needs. The more you know and understand the specific aspects of communication disorders, the more creative you can be in helping to solve a patient's difficulties. We all realize how much emphasis is placed on appearance. How devastating it is to realize that our appearance can be so altered by trauma, disease, or birth defect that it diminishes our ability to function.

The field of communication disorders developed in the 1930s as Speech Correction. In the 1950s it became Speech Pathology; in the 1970s it changed to Speech Language Pathology and Audiology; and finally, in the 1980s, it emerged as Communication Disorders. This metamorphosis occurred because clinicians realized that speech, language, and hearing are a continuous loop. An understanding of the interrelationships between these areas was crucial in the effort to recognize and remediate a break in that communication loop.

We begin life by vocalizing our discomfort, pain, and joy. As we become aware of our environments, through hearing and sight, we learn to respond to faces, noises, and sounds. We begin to recognize friends, fear strangers, and attach meaning to words. Those words begin to emerge from us as simple sounds, "Ah" for hot, "Ma" for mama, "Dah" for dog, and finally are strung together like beads on a string to form sentences. In our first three years, we learn the

rules of the language, how to make sounds, form sounds into words, words into sentences, and finally to use sentences in a meaningful way. Further, we learn the social effect of speaking. Our voice changes from a mechanism for crying to a well-controlled instrument that produces inflections for speaking and music for singing. This process is based upon the assumption that the person develops speech in a predictable progression of stages; but what happens if something goes wrong? Something can go wrong at any time in our embryonic stage, through childhood, puberty, adulthood, and finally old age. When and what can go wrong is considered the etiology, or cause, of the communication disorder, while the results of that problem are considered to be the symptoms of the problem. The symptoms of communication disorders can be classified in four categories: articulation, voice, language, and fluency.

Disorders of articulation are thought of as deviation in the way we produce speech sounds. In English there are forty-three consonant sounds, along with approximately fifteen vowel sounds. These form the basis of our sound learning, and these sounds are strung together to make words and sentences. If we make speech sounds too different from others, others will have difficulty understanding us.

Voice disorders are any abnormalities in the tone that originate at the level of the larynx, or vocal cords. The tone can be modified by the cavities above the vocal cords, which include the throat (pharyngeal area), the mouth (oral area), and the nose (nasal resonating chambers).

Language disorders are difficulties in the use or interpretation of the symbols of speech. Language disorders can be classified into two major areas: first, the disorders that come as part of the development of language (sometimes called delayed language development or language retardation), in which a child does not develop language or develops defective language; second, the language that is lost. In this case, an adult or older child has developed language, but the language is lost due to some injury or disease process. This kind of language disorder is usually called *aphasia*.

In aphasia, the association pathways of the brain are altered, and their functions may become disordered. These functions include knowledge, learning, cognition, memory, comprehension, concept formation, perception, recognition, interpretation, and many others. These functions are the way the brain integrates and forms the relationships between different aspects of our inner experience, the language with which we talk to ourselves. We have basically three types of language: the language that we understand with when other people write or speak to us, the language with which we talk to ourselves, and the language that we use to write or to speak to other people. Any of these "languages" can become disordered at any time.

The final category is fluency disorders. Disorders of fluency affect timing of speech (the speed and phrasing of speech). It is what we think of as the rhythm of our language. An example of a disorder in fluency would be stuttering in which the flow and the pattern of speech is rapid, jerky, and indistinct, with hesitations and repetitions.

Etiologies can be divided into functional and organic categories. When a person has trouble communicating and there is no apparent organic cause for the disorder, the cause, or etiology, is said to be functional in nature. Faulty learning and faulty

motivation are both considered functional etiologies. A child who originally does not learn to make a speech sound correctly, but learns through treatment how to make the sound correctly and without interference, previously had faulty learning. If the child were to hang on to an infantile voice pattern or way of articulating for the sake of attention, faulty motivation would be the functional etiology. Most often, though, the etiologies for speech disorders are not functional but organic.

The organic causes for speech disorders fall into a number of general disorder classifications, including structural, neurological, auditory, myogenic (muscle) disorders, and endocrinologic disorders.

Examples of some structural disorders that could affect the speech, hearing, and language of an individual would be diseases such as Crouzons, or other disorders that lead to abnormalities in the head and neck. In Crouzons, for example, the head is enlarged; the eyes and the facial bones are deformed. This kind of facial deformity leads to problems with the voice, with articulation, and with language. A person with this kind of facial disorder may be difficult to understand and communication may be disordered. Very often extensive surgery is needed to correct this disorder. The same would be true of an individual with a cleft lip and palate. (These are openings in the lip and mouth where tissue has not grown together.) A cleft palate can be defined as the failure of the bones in the jaw and the top of the mouth to form properly so that an opening is left from the mouth into the nose. This opening may include the lip as well as the top of the mouth; and in this case it is called a complete cleft of the lip and palate. It may also extend so far forward that both sides of the nose and lip are affected. If these defects are repaired adequately and there is sufficient tissue to form a nearly normal closure, the patient can look forward to almost normal speech.

The appearance can be so altered with some birth defects that the individual needs years of surgical intervention. The cleft may be as mild as a cleft of the lip to a cleft of the palate only. In the case of a cleft of the lip, repair work is done when the child is only two or three months of age. For a palate, however, the surgeon may need to wait until the child is one, two, or even three years of age. The sound of the voice in this case may be very abnormal and "nasal."

Many of these syndromes can affect the hands, feet, heart, liver, and brain; but our major concern will be facial and cranial defects. A cleft of the palate may not be visible, but its presence may be signaled by the sound of the voice. Many times surgery is indicated, or a prosthesis (a false palate) may be made to help the speech, and speech therapy can help to improve the voice quality. The treatment protocol may take anywhere from several months to several years. The outcome of such treatment is often close to normal speech.

An individual can experience neurological disorders at any time in life — from cerebral palsy at birth to strokes in the older adult; or trauma from motorcycle or automobile accidents at any time during life. Very often these will leave a patient with what we call dysarthria; that is, the movement for speech may be there, but it is very slow, and it is not accurate. That slowness and inaccuracy can lead to problems in all areas of speech and language.

Auditory disorders may be due to damage to the sensitivity of the auditory mecha-nism, usually referred to as "hearing impaired." Hearing impairment is the general term used to describe all types of hearing disabilities, ranging from minute losses to profound deafness. It is the most prevalent physical disability in this country. An estimated fourteen million Americans are affected to some degree.

Not all deaf patients will communicate the same way; some may speak intelligibly and read lips, while others cannot. Lip reading is a limited source of communication because only 30 percent of normal speech is visible on the lip, and approximately 50 percent of English sounds look alike on the lips. For this reason, most deaf people use more than one form of communication.

Not only may the sensitivity to sounds be diminished, but the ability to process sound and to comprehend its meaning may be diminished. These are often referred to as auditory processing problems. We see these occasionally in the learning disabled and in the developmentally disabled as well as in the normal person with a specific learning disability.

Myogenic disorders are disorders of the muscles. This can be enervation (sapping the strength) to the muscle itself. Again, these kinds of disorders may give rise to disorders in communication, of articulation and resonance. An example of this would be myastenia gravis, in which the muscle becomes fatigued, and articulate sound production becomes diminished, the voice becomes more nasal, and the articulation becomes slovenly and unintelligible.

Endocrinological disorders are those that develop because of lack of correct production of the endocrine glands. Examples of this would be cretinism, dwarfism, or lack of growth hormone so that the individual does not develop normally. The disorders may lead to any number of problems with speech and language.

For the most part, we have been discussing logical ways to classify speech disorders in terms of both symptoms and causes. Generally, these are not widely used for everyday clinical work, but they give us a theoretical framework within which to place disorders of communication. For the most part, you will hear speech pathologists talk about disorders of language development or disorders of language loss, disorders of articulation (production of speech sounds), voice disorders, and stuttering.

The etiological categories most often used are cleft palate, cerebral palsy, aphasia, apraxia, dysarthria, and hearing loss. They are not strictly logical, but they contain the common types of clinical problems that present themselves to the speech pathologist; and they are the classifications that you will most often encounter in your work. Regardless of the system used, speech output of the individual is always compared to normal; and in order to establish it as normal, we have to classify it in relationship to what is expected in the environment as ordinary, accepted, speech patterns. If one of your patients is unable to communicate in the normal way, there are a number of alternative communication systems available.

One of the most often used modern technologies is augmentative communication. This can be accomplished by using a computer, with a communication board on which the patient can press keys, and the computer will either speak for him or her in a complete sentence or will write it on a board or screen. For the hearing-impaired or deaf person, sign language is a communication system. This involves the use of hand shapes and movements, finger spelling, facial expression, and body language to express words and ideas. Finger spelling is the use of hand signs that represent all twenty-six letters of the alphabet.

Finger spelling is used alone or with signing to express technical words for which there are no signs and for names and places. Sign language and finger spelling, however, are not universal, and patients will communicate in their own language, sometimes depending on the country they are from or the way they have learned their finger spelling and signing. The way patients with a hearing impairment will communicate will depend on where they were taught, the extent of their deafness, their preference, and how long they have been deaf. The same can be said for the trauma patient who has had to re-learn language or the stroke patient who has lost language and re-learned it. Speech may be telegraphic; i.e., it uses only short phrases to convey an entire meaning.

One of the things to ask yourself is "What can I do to help understand this person?" If something is going wrong in your understanding of the message that you are sending or receiving, ask yourself, "What are some of the things that I can do that will help?"

The first question, "Can I understand this person?" is important. If you cannot understand, ask yourself "What's going wrong?" Is it that the sounds are not being made right; or is it that the sound of the voice is so distracting that you cannot understand what is being said? Or is it because the sentences and words are put together in such a manner that the message is not clear? Perhaps the sound of the voice, the stringing together of the words, and the pauses are at the wrong places; words are repeated inappropriately and the flow is disrupted to such an extent that the message is lost. By analyzing what's going wrong, you can begin to find ways to help the patient understand you as well as for you to understand him or her.

In addition to the above question, you need to ask yourself, "What can I do to improve the communication between myself and this patient?" Several general principles will help your overall communication, and some specific techniques for specific disorders are found to be helpful. These suggestions should improve the overall communication between therapist and patient.

1. Speak to the patient directly; maintain eye contact, even when you are talking through a communication board or through signs and interpreters. Do not make this a steady gaze, a constant eye contact, but rather the kind of contact that you would have with your friends as you speak with them, looking at the face, looking at the upper part of the body, and maintaining a relaxed feeling of listening.

2. If you need to get a patient's attention, tap her or him on the shoulder lightly but firmly, or touch gently, or ask the patient to watch as you demonstrate some activity, providing some kind of clue that what you are about to do next is important, helps structure the situation and gives the patient some cues about the importance of an activity.

3. Make sure that the light is in front of you and shining on your face, and as you work in your studio, try to keep your face from being in the shadow. The person who has difficulty hearing, or has difficulty paying attention

and attending to directions, needs the advantage of a well-lit face.

4. Speak normally but distinctly. Do not exaggerate your lip movements but slow your speech to a steady and precise rhythm, with repetition of steps or instructions, followed by the patient's demonstration of the activity or repetition of the instructions. When giving instructions, use as many visual teaching aids as possible. Always write down the procedures step-by-step for the patient to take home. This provides the patient again with the structure and repetition needed to follow through.

5. Try not to walk around your treatment room or turn your back on the patient when you are speaking, but be sure that you are always standing directly in her or his line of vision with no interference.

6. Be careful not to cover your mouth or use detracting hand movements while speaking. Using hands for inflection and definition is very helpful and useful; but be careful not to use your hands directly in front of your face.

7. Have the patient repeat your instructions and demonstrate for you step by step any procedure that you have taught her or him.

8. Listen carefully. If you do not understand the patient, ask her or him to repeat or to show you, or to write the message down for you. Try to interpret the patient's message and repeat it back in order to verify that you have gotten it correctly.

You will be able to think of many other

ways to help patients, but these guidelines will provide you with some general approaches to increase your ability to communicate with patients with speech and hearing disabilities. There are some specific conditions and instructions that may be helpful for special problems. For example, if you are working with children, your attitude indicating acceptance of them is extremely important. If you do not understand, indicate that it's you who cannot listen that fast or that well. You must ask the child to help you by repeating for you, or showing you, what he or she wants. This concept — that there is not something wrong with her or him, but rather that this is something you are doing together — relieves the child of the burden of the concept that the communication breakdown is his or her fault, and indicates that you are trying to help each other.

For the patient who is hearing-impaired and is using an interpreter, it is important to permit time for the interpreter and the patient to exchange messages before the interpreter gets back to you. Try not to increase your speed beyond the time required for all of this to take place. Make your sentences short but functional. Try to keep explanations at a minimum, but clear and precise.

These same instructions are important for the patient who has aphasia, a learning disability with difficulty in processing. The aphasic may be able to understand a great deal more that she or he is able to express. Even though an aphasic person's expression may be in short words or phrases, much of what you say can be understood. You will, however, need to be certain by confirming with the patient through show-

ing or telling how much of what you have said was understood. The most important thing to remember in dealing with learning disabilities is that complex instructions must be broken down into very simple steps, or simple instructions with lots of demonstration. Always make sure through repetition or demonstration that the patient has understood what you have explained or demonstrated.

Dealing with individuals with communication disorders can be a challenging aspect of camouflage therapy. You are faced with people who have difficulty communicating their needs, desires, and ideas. As a clinician, you are asked to understand and interpret the discontinuous, broken message while providing patients with new ways of managing their appearances. As a therapist, you must find creative ways to help patients and yourself to communicate to the best of your ability. Be creative in managing the communication loop, just as you are creative in managing camouflage makeup.

Dr. Wendell Johnson was a pioneer in the field of communication disorders, and I am going to paraphrase a quote from him:

"Listen to the patient well — to what he is saying and almost saying, and not saying at all. He has something he wants to tell you — something that has meaning for him, that is important to him. He is not just being verbally frisky. Respect him as a speaker. Listen to him enough to hear him out. It is wonderful for him as a person to feel that he is being heard, that others care about what he is saying. Assume that he is doing the best he can, and that it is more important for him to want to talk to you than to sound correct."

Rape Survivors

Melanie Boyd

A camouflage therapist may be asked by a physician, a psychologist, a social worker, or a counselor at a rape-crisis center to help a rape survivor conceal some of the outward signs of the attack. Most women who have been assaulted are extremely sensitive to the reactions of people around them; the support she receives may be critical for a rape survivor to normalize her appearance so that she can resume her normal activities without feeling conspicuous due to bruises, cuts, or scratches. In order to most effectively respond to a survivor's physical and emotional needs, the camouflage therapist needs to have basic information about the dynamics of rape and its impact on the women who experience it.

Recent studies, combined with the information pouring into rape crisis centers across the country, have lead to an increasingly accurate picture of rape. The statistics are grim: one in five (some estimate one in three) women and one in ten men will experience rape in her/his adult lifetime. Of these rapes, the vast majority (70–80 percent) of the assailants are known to the victim; women are raped by their husbands, boyfriends, employers, classmates, etc.; NOT by strangers. Contrary to popular belief, these acquaintance, or "date," rapes are just as terrifying as the stereotypic rape by a stranger. In fact, many women find the betrayal involved in an acquaintance rape to be a major source of trauma.

Rape, despite its mythology, is an act of violence, not of sexuality. Almost every rape survivor fears for her life during the assault; many women are seriously injured or killed. In many ways, it is this fear that produces the most lasting effect on survivors. For this reason, survivors of attempted rape tend to experience very similar reactions to those of women who are actually raped. Survivors generally go through a process known as "Rape Trauma Syndrome," a form of Post-Traumatic Stress Disorder. Symptomatic of the initial stage of this process are fear, anxiety, lack of trust, and sleeplessness; emotional reactions range from hysteria to completely controlled calmness.

The lack of support a survivor is likely to encounter makes it doubly important that a camouflage therapist and all other professionals respond in a non-intrusive, yet supportive fashion. The experiences a survivor has after a rape can be crucial in assisting recovery.

SUGGESTIONS ON HOW TO WORK WITH A RAPE SURVIVOR

1. The manner in which you handle the appointment is crucial — you MUST let the survivor be in control of the event. Remember, she has just had a terrifying experience in which she lost

Melanie Boyd has been working with victims of violent crime for over three years. She received her undergraduate degree in Women's Studies from Yale University. She is currently responsible for San Francisco Women Against Rape's direct services, including survivor counseling, volunteer training, and support group facilitation. San Francisco Women Against Rape is a non-profit, grassroots counseling organization that was founded in 1973.

ultimate control over her body and her life; you do not want to re-victimize her by controlling any more of the situation than is absolutely necessary.

2. When the patient arrives she may be very apprehensive — it is often difficult to walk into a situation where one is immediately identified as a rape victim. She may feel embarrassed or depressed; she may or may not want to talk about it. Be willing to listen in a supportive and caring fashion if she does want to talk; don't press her to discuss any more than she desires. Let her know that you are concerned about her, not about what you want her to do. Do not touch her without asking her permission first.

3. Many survivors are burdened with guilt and self-blame; they believe (and are often told) that they must have somehow deserved it, or done something to provoke the attack. If the woman knew and trusted the rapist, she may be angry at herself for not having realized that he was dangerous. Allow her to express these feelings of self-blame if she wants to, but let her know that you do not think that the rape was her fault. Try to place the blame on the rapist.

4. If the patient brings a friend or family member for support, allow her to choose whether or not she wants to have that person in your office with her.

5. Be clear that you see camouflage therapy as a way to allow the survivor her privacy and to enable her to reveal her rape experience only when and to whom she chooses. Do not under any circumstances hint that she should conceal the injuries because rape is shameful — the only person who should be ashamed is the rapist.

6. Many women who have been raped feel extremely conspicuous, as if anyone can look at them and see what happened. A patient may therefore wish to camouflage injuries that you don't feel are obvious; you may put forth your opinion, but accept the decisions of what to camouflage or not without debate.

7. Suggest counseling; provide the survivor with the number of the local rape crisis center. Let her know that all calls to such a center are confidential, and that most centers provide free counseling. While it's important to pass this information on, do not try to force her into counseling — let the survivor make the decisions.

8. Read materials on rape and rape survivors, and/or visit a rape crisis center to get more information.

9. If you are a man, your gender may make a person who has been raped by a man uncomfortable. If this is true, you need to be willing to accommodate the survivor's need to feel safe — avoid being alone with her, or refer her to a female camouflage therapist.

Working with Battered Women

Christine Cobaugh

According to an article published in the *New England Journal of Medicine*, the most prevalent cause of injury to women treated in emergency rooms is domestic violence. Statistics show that between 20 and 50 percent of all women will be hit at least once by a partner. However, physical battering is not just one hit; it is a continuous pattern of assaults that includes black eyes, cut lips, broken teeth, bruises, and burns. Victims are often choked, kicked, or severely beaten. Some women who have been physically abused have had to stay in bed for several days or even weeks because they were too weak physically to work or too ashamed to be seen in public.

Battering is a learned behavior and crosses all socioeconomic, racial, and ethnic boundaries. Ninety-five percent of all spousal assaults are committed by men. There are many reasons why a woman stays with a man who beats her. The physical abuse is usually accompanied by verbal, emotional, and psychological attacks that keep a woman confused, feeling powerless, and doubting her own experience and perceptions. She may be afraid of what he may do to her if she leaves, or she may be fearful that she cannot support herself or her children financially. Often a woman's ethnic or religious background will interfere with her decision to divorce or separate from her partner.

Frequently, the acts of physical (and/or sexual) assault are so severe that a woman has to be hospitalized. This kind of abuse in an intimate relationship is an act of violence used by one partner to create dominance and control over the other. The pattern of imposing physical violence to maintain control over a woman is reinforced by threats, brainwashing, and coercion. Many health-care professionals overlook the most obvious signs of domestic violence, physical injuries, according to a study published in the *New England Journal of Medicine*. Most physicians do not question female patients with suspicious injuries. This can be extremely dangerous for the patient's well-being because physical violence tends to escalate. In fact, the patient's health and well-being could ultimately depend upon a conscientious health-care professional eliciting the source of her injury.

The camouflage therapist may be consulted by a patient who has been a victim of physical abuse to conceal the outward signs of this domestic violence. She may have bruises, scratches, cuts, or burns from the assault. She may be referred to the therapist by a medical social worker, physician, nurse, or psychologist. If the patient brings up the cause of her injury, it is important for the camouflage therapist to express his or her concern and refer her to an agency that helps battered women. In some

Christine Cobaugh is currently the Education and Prevention Assistant at the Marin Abused Women's Services in San Rafael, California. She has extensive experience as a volunteer and staff member in battered women's programs, as a group facilitator, hotline worker, media spokesperson, and prevention specialist. Ms. Cobaugh has implemented the Relationship Abuse Prevention Project, a model teen dating violence prevention curriculum, in over 100 classrooms in Marin County. As a member of the Formerly Battered Women's Task Force of California she organized retreats and conferences for formerly battered women and has facilitated various conference trainings for diverse groups of professionals.

instances, the patient may even be afraid to return home. A woman who has been battered is not unlike a rape survivor; both are victims of violence and should be treated in much the same manner.

You should have on hand the telephone number for the National Coalition Against Domestic Violence, (800) 333-7233. You should also familiarize yourself with local emergency resources for battered women so that you will be able to help the patient to obtain emergency telephone numbers if necessary for medical, housing, consulting, and legal counseling services. If you should suspect physical violence and emotional battering, try to question the patient to determine the source of her injury. If the patient is over 65 years old, you are required by law to report any signs of physical abuse.

Treatment of the Terminally Ill Patient

K.H. Blacker, M.D.

Thoughts of death and dying frighten many of us. Death and dying are alien to twentieth-century Americans. Our life experiences and culture do not prepare us for this natural life event. As a consequence, we may tend to avoid and withdraw from those who are seriously ill. Professionals who may become involved in the care of terminally ill individuals need to understand and change this reaction. Surprisingly, once initial fears are understood and mastered, many professionals find work with dying patients to be among the most rewarding and gratifying professional experiences.

Most people are not frightened by death, but are horrified by the thought of dying. The scarring, the odors, the pain, and the incapacities that may accompany a terminal illness are frightening. The humiliation when we are not able to attend to our personal needs and a loss of self-esteem caused by disfigurement are most troubling.

Camouflage therapists may play a pivotal role in the treatment and care of a terminally ill individual. Their technical expertise enables them to help patients conceal scars and blemishes and thus increase self-esteem. Their work consists of more than the application of technical information and camouflage skills. The relationship that develops between the therapist and the patient as the two work together is in itself therapeutic.

It is helpful to remember that "groom-

Dr. Blacker is Professor and Chairman of the Department of Psychiatry at the University of California Davis Medical Center in Sacramento, California, and training and supervising analyst at the San Francisco Psychoanalytic Institute. He is a graduate of the University of Utah School of Medicine, the Langley Porter Neuropsychiatric Institute, and the San Francisco Psychoanalytic Institute. He is a member of the American Psychoanalytic Association, the American Psychiatric Association, and the American Psychoanalytic Society. His professional activities include examiner for the American Board of Neurology and Psychiatry and consultant for psychiatric residency training programs of the American Psychiatric Association. He is chairman of the annual Mid-Winter Program in Continuing Education for Psychiatrists, chairman of the Committee on Research and Special Training at the San Francisco Psychoanalytic Institute, and chairman of the Committee on Physician Health at the University of California, Davis, School of Medicine. His research interests include patterns of cognition observed in psychotherapy and in individuals with panic and anxiety disorders.

ing" behaviors are basic components of all animal interactions. Removing leaves, twigs, insects from one another's fur is not only hygienic, but the touching and stroking are soothing. Touching and attending to one another have important psychological and social meanings. Grooming behaviors are soothing behaviors. Mothers groom their young; peers and mates groom one another. Jane Goodall's graphic films of enraged chimpanzees being calmed as they are groomed by other members of the troop illustrate this process.

The movie "Steel Magnolias" presents a sensitive and powerful portrait of the relationships and emotional support generated among a group of women in a beauty parlor in a small southern town. In this grooming salon, women "let their hair down." While they are being groomed they talk, and these conversations facilitate the development of emotional attachments that help them face the basic issues in their lives. The interactions between a camouflage therapist and a dying patient, particularly as they develop over time, may serve a similar function.

In addition to applying one's technical skill, the primary task while working with a dying patient is to listen. Listen not only to the content of the words, but also to the sound, to the inflection, to the qualities of the voice. And listen with your eyes. These expressive communications as well as the words tell us what a person is feeling — what a person wants from us.

Fortunately, some guidelines can help us listen. They show us where a patient is emotionally in accepting the facts of a terminal illness. For example, a patient at one time may wish to talk directly about his or her illness, while on another occasion will want to deny it. We need to be attuned to the needs of the patient.

These guidelines were developed by Dr. Elisabeth Kübler-Ross. She explored the emotional experiences of dying patients by carefully inquiring into their thoughts and feelings. Her experience led her to postulate that there are five stages, or five primary issues, that a dying patient experiences or moves through.

The first is the stage of denial. Often when a person is told that he or she has a fatal disease, his reaction will be, "No. It can't be me." Usually in this stage the individual does not wish to talk about illness or death. The second is often a stage of anger. "Why does this have to happen to me?" "What have I done?" There may be feelings of bitterness, rage, and envy. In some, this anger may be much more muted, or an individual may even see approaching death as a punishment, possibly even deserved.

The third is the stage of bargaining: an attempt to bargain with the assumed powers that control our lives; an attempt to use magic. An individual may promise he will do only good if he is permitted to live. Often there is expression of a wish for a magical rescue. There may also be an awareness of the futility of such wishes.

The fourth is a stage of depression. In this stage a person detaches himself from his surroundings to relinquish responsibilities and begins to mourn the anticipated loss of the important people in his life. This stage is often characterized in its later segments by an increasing preoccupation with one's own life coming to an end. The individual thinks about the meaning of life and existence. The depression may be mild or severe.

The fifth is the stage of acceptance. At times the patient may be somewhat euphoric and very much at peace. This stage often offers the opportunity for rapprochement among family members and a sense of completeness and fulfillment.

Knowledge of these stages of dying can guide us in our listening. By understanding this sequence, we will not be surprised if at one point a patient does not wish to talk about his or her terminal illness, while at another point a patient might surprise us with the directness of his/her statements. Anger may be present at one phase, a sense of acceptance and compassion at another.

Through all of the phases, our task is to be competent, caring professionals. We should be emotionally available and supportive. Remember, the patient suffers less from carcinoma than from skin rashes, scarring, hair loss, and weight loss. They worry less about their diseases than they do about disfigurement and discomfort. It is the loss of self-esteem and these discomforts and insecurities that our technical skills can ameliorate and psychological support can sooth.

The opportunity to work with a terminally ill patient does not need to be a difficult, uncomfortable task. It can be an exciting professional opportunity to provide technical assistance to cover disfigurement. In the context of providing technical assistance the presence and support of a professional contributes importantly to the well-being of a patient.

REVIEW

You should now be familiar with:

- psychological aspects of working with physically challenged patients.
- the importance and the components of clear communication.
- how to interact with difficult patients.
- special ways of dealing with particular physical challenges.

Cosmetology Therapy with Disfigured Children

Rochelle B. Wolk, Ph.D.

This chapter will introduce the camouflage therapist to concepts that are important in achieving a successful outcome when working with disfigured children. When working with adults, the camouflage therapist must deal with the ambivalence, anger, and hope of that individual. When working with a child, the camouflage therapist must deal not only with the child's wishes and needs, but those of the parents as well. In addition, the immaturity and the dependency of the child, and the less well-developed verbal skills, may inhibit or prevent the child from being aware of, or discussing, her/his concerns. The camouflage therapist's awareness and understanding of these issues plays a vital role in creating a positive outcome to therapy, and in avoiding negative feedback to the referring physicians.

THE IMPACT OF DISFIGUREMENT — SOCIAL STEREOTYPING

A great deal of research supports the view that physical attractiveness, particularly facial attractiveness, gets positive reactions from others. It is no secret that physical attractiveness is seen as a highly desirable quality. In our society, the concept of beauty has replaced the concept of goodness as the measure of a person. Television, magazines, and billboards all promote hiding imperfections in appearance because of their negative impact on social desirability. Bull

Dr. Wolk is Assistant Clinical Professor, Division of Behavioral Pediatrics, Department of Pediatrics at the University of California, San Francisco, Medical Center.

(1979) has shown how much desirability is reduced with even a small facial scar. The impact is not limited to any one racial group. Langlois and Stephan (1977) found similar stereotypes about attractiveness among Black, Hispanic, and Caucasian children. Udry (1977) found them among adult Blacks. The relationship between "attractive physical appearance and good mental health has been well documented" (Cash, 1985).

Individuals with facial disfigurements have reported that strangers react to them in negative ways; indeed, the effects are not limited to strangers. Research findings indicate that teachers often respond less positively to disfigured individuals than to others, and give them higher grades. "Unattractive" children are punished more often than their "attractive" peers. Disfigured individuals are seen as less adept in a wide range of activities and behaviors; they are seen as less sociable, more dishonest, less able to solve their own problems, as well as less attractive; their friendship is less sought, and they are often socially isolated.

EFFECTS IN CHILDHOOD

Childhood is a time when a personality is shaped. Many intellectual and personality characteristics of children have their limits defined by the genetic inheritance. Within those wide limits, however, personality characteristics are molded through interaction with people and things in the environment. The child grows and changes very rapidly in a very few years. In that time, the experiences of childhood and adolescence shape and mold feelings and thoughts about the self and others, which will affect that child throughout the course of her or his life.

The child's first relationship is with her or his mother. MacGregor (1953), Moncada (1987), and Solnit and Stark (1977) have all reported that the loving bond between mother and child may be disrupted by the mother's negative feelings that arise when she views or interacts with a disfigured child. This is understandable, given the tremendous impact of physical attractiveness on social acceptability. Certainly not all mothers react with negative feelings and difficulty in bonding with their disfigured children. However, many children suffer the stigma of facial disfigurement from their first days of postnatal life. Hildebrand and Fitzgerald (1977, 1979) reported that "cuteness" can affect the type of care an infant gets. As Kershaw (1973) pointed out, sometimes the disfigured child "can never look for more than an outward show of parental affection."

Parents of disfigured children often try to protect them from potentially negative social interactions. These children may develop less skill than their peers in dealing with strangers and with new situations. The beginning of the school years brings new challenges, and for children with diminished skills, new fears and anxieties. Moncada (1987) reported that facially disfigured children sometimes dread having to play with other children. Even when the experiences through the preschool years have been positive, and not different from what most children learn, the early school years can be traumatic, and shape the self concept unfavorably.

School peers inevitably give some negative feedback. Children, like adults, have stereotypes associated with disfigurement. Young children are curious and rarely have a well-developed sense of social sensitivity. They poke, pry, and question insistently; they may tease, run from, or ostracize the disfigured child. These reactions can have a devastating and permanent impact upon a child's current and future social adjustment.

The distress may well continue into middle school. Peer relationships in those grades is often determined by appearance; overweight, wearing "wrong" clothes, or physical disfigurement elicit social rejection. Teachers as well as peers may be influenced by appearance. To the child having difficulty dealing with these social pressures, school can be a nightmare. The child is under constant pressure to deal with stresses of social interaction, at the same time that academic expectations are increasing. Some children express their distress in problem behaviors, such as inattention or aggression. Others withdraw; they may be reluctant to leave their homes each day, and remain excessively dependent upon parents and/or siblings.

EFFECTS IN ADOLESCENCE

Adolescence brings its unique problems. The rapid physical changes that accompany adolescence affect body image — the mental picture one has of one's appearance. Physical characteristics are of more concern to adolescents than social or intellectual skills. Lerner and Karabenick (1974) discovered that the appearance of the face was the second most important body characteristic to adolescent boys and girls. Indeed, only overall appearance was seen as more significant. School demands continue to increase, but the impact of the disfigurement does not diminish; indeed, all the body image concerns are magnified. Separation from the family becomes more difficult when rejection has been experienced everywhere else. The negative stereotypes about disfigurement may also reduce vocational options; employers may be unwilling to hire a facially disfigured individual for jobs with high exposure to the "public." Facially disfigured teens are often unwilling to attend group social functions. They may deny their longings for committed emotional relationships. Some teens, in their efforts to obtain peer group approval, become excessive risk-takers to get attention and prove their worth. Others find themselves unable to maintain a tolerable self-image, and give way to life-threatening despair.

THE USE OF COSMETIC CAMOUFLAGE

Facial disfigurement can be a severe stressor to a youngster, as well as to parents. The negative stereotypes associated with disfigurement can have damaging impact at every stage, and in every activity, of childhood. Reconstructive surgery becomes an option for many at adolescence. Some professionals report unqualifiedly excellent outcomes to surgery. However, MacGregor (1953) found that many adolescents had great difficulty accepting surgery. They felt that having surgery negated their previous efforts in adjusting to the emotional stress of the disfigurement. Some adolescents who accepted surgery were disappointed when improved appearance did not immediately bring along with it improved social status. They were not aware that surgery altered only their appearance; it could not change the behavior patterns they developed to protect themselves from the emotional pain of social interactions, and from their feelings of diminished self-worth.

Given the enormous impact of disfigurement upon the developing sense of self, it is clear that visually minimizing the disfigurement can improve self-concept and even foster a more positive parent-child relationship. Graham and Kligman

(1987) have demonstrated the positive impact on adults of cosmetic therapy. It can also be used to enhance a child's chances for a successful social and academic career. It is essential to note that an unblemished face is not a guarantee of a good relationship with one's parents and peers. It does not guarantee academic or social success, despite what Madison Avenue would have us believe. The minimizing of facial disfigurements serves to give a child a fair chance, an opportunity to use her/his skills and abilities on an equal basis with peers, free from the impact of negative stereotypes. However, a number of important variables must be considered in order to optimize the positive outcome of cosmetic therapy.

VARIABLES AFFECTING EFFECTIVENESS

Certainly, a major variable in determining the success of camouflage is the type of disfigurement. In this section, the impact of variables originating with the child and with her/his parents will be considered.

Parent Variables

The impact of the parent upon the successful outcome of camouflage therapy is enormous, since the parent may be involved in every stage of the process. Often the decision to seek such therapy is made by the parent, particularly when the child is young. Parental assistance is often required to apply cosmetics. The parents pay for the services, provide transportation to and from appointments, and, to the child, are among the most important respondents to the question "How do I look?" They often also provide feedback, positive or negative, to the referring physician, if one has recommended that they seek cosmetology services.

A variable of major importance in determining the parent's response, and one over which the camouflage therapist has no control, is the manner in which the parent has been able to cope with the child's disfigurement. There are three major ways of coping a parent might use: minimizing, exaggerating, or accepting.

Minimizing Defenses

A parent whose personality style does not permit her/him to have an imperfect child might select a minimizing strategy. This strategy might also be used by a parent who feels responsible for, or guilt about, the disfigurement, and has not resolved those feelings. Such a strategy allows the parent to unconsciously deny the prominence or impact of the facial disfigurement. When asked about the disfigurement, this parent might disparage its impact, deny its size, color, prominence, or even its existence, and tell the child that it isn't very noticeable. Incidentally, this becomes a real emotional conflict for the child, who then looks in the mirror and sees something quite different than the parent said. This type of parent might avoid exposing the child to strangers in order to forestall potentially negative or curious responses, which might then force the parent to confront the reality of the disfigurement.

Even though the child of such a parent is referred by the treating physician for cosmetic camouflage, the parent may continue to deny or minimize the need for such treatment unconsciously, even if she or he agrees to obtain such services. Such a parent might regularly fail to keep appointments or arrive late. Such a parent will "forget" what is taught, "forget" to buy necessary materials, and misplace them if purchased. Such a parent will rarely find time to assist the child in practicing proper application, and will disparage the results, even when the child is receiving positive reactions from others. Such a parent might well complain about the cost of the therapy or about the time involved, even when neither is a factor or real concern.

The problem becomes intensified when the child is pleased with, and wants to use, camouflage, while the parent must deny or minimize the need for it. In trying to respond to the child's wishes, the camouflage therapist will be forcing the parent to confront what she or he wishes to deny. If the parent's needs to deny are met, the child will not receive the best care possible.

The best way for the camouflage therapist to balance these two sets of demands is to respect the parents' unconscious needs while providing care to the child. Attention should not be focused upon the magnitude or prominence of the disfigurement; rather the camouflage therapist must focus upon the desire most parents have to make their child more comfortable personally and socially. The child's discomfort with the disfigurement, rather than the disfigurement itself, should be addressed. The parent should be praised in her or his responsiveness to the child's needs.

The camouflage therapist should be alert to signs of emotional and physical child abuse. The parent's guilt may be caused by something she or he actually did to the child, or did not try to prevent. Such an occurrence might be direct abuse or neglect. In addition, the camouflage therapist must be sensitive to the subtle emotional abuse that can arise from a parent's refusal to provide necessary relief from emotional distress. As Navarre (1987) has pointed out, psychological abuse can result from an assault on a child's well-being, or from the imposition on a child of a distorted perception of the self or the world.

The camouflage therapist has a clearly defined legal as well as moral responsibility for alertness to, and reporting of, suspected or actual child abuse. While everyone should report suspected child neglect or abuse, it is a crime for mandated health professionals not to do so in most states. In California, for example, a camouflage therapist working in a hospital setting is a mandated reporter; she or he has no options about reporting. A reasonable suspicion of abuse or neglect must be reported to a child protective agency, such as the county welfare department, county probation department, police department, or sheriff's department, by telephone, immediately or as soon as is practically possible. The telephone call must be followed up with a report, in writing, mailed to the reporting agency within thirty-six hours. A mandated reporter who fails to report may be punished by a jail term, a fine, or both. Camouflage therapists must check with their local child protective agencies for details of the laws in their states.

Maximizing Defenses

Some parents with a high need for perfection, an inability to tolerate less than that in their children, may respond to a disfigurement by magnifying its impact. They may see it as more prominent than it is. They may call attention to the imperfection at inappropriate times, or in emotionally disruptive ways. They may force the child to keep thinking about the disfigurement rather than coping with it. These parents might seek to camouflage very minor disfigurements, such as chicken pox scars or minimal blemishes. They may seek camouflage and insist that the child use cosmetics when the child is developmentally inattentive to the disfigurement, or has not developed the necessary visual-motor skills. This parent is dealing with her or his own fear of, or feelings of, inadequacy, and requires a perfect child to validate his or her being and parenting skills.

For the camouflage therapist, this parent, too, presents difficulties. Such a parent is rarely satisfied with the outcome of camouflage, because the parent is not focused upon real disfigurements, but upon her or his own emotional needs, needs that cosmetics cannot fill. This parent is often likely to give negative feedback about the benefit of cosmetic therapy to the referring physician, because such a parent is not realistic in her/his expectations of the benefits of such therapy. Often, the child of such a parent resists the cosmetic camouflage, because the child is unwilling to agree to the parent's message that the child must be perfect in order to be acceptable.

In addition, the camouflage therapist must be alert to manipulation by the parent into providing camouflage for minor blemishes, since this can be emotionally detrimental to the child. It is potentially damaging for a child to learn that her or his physical appearance does not please her or his parents, particularly when what is seen in the mirror is not notably atypical. The camouflage therapist must not join with the parent in the unwitting abuse of the child's self-esteem. The camouflage therapist must use good clinical judgment and seek input from the referring professional, as well as a mental health specialist, when confronted by a parent who is resolving her or his emotional difficulties through a child.

The camouflage therapist must explore with the parents their expectations for the cosmetic camouflage. The parent should be asked to write down these expectations for discussion and to prevent later misunderstandings. The camouflage therapist must interview the child to assess her or his wishes and perceptions. The camouflage therapist must respond verbally and in writing to each point made by the parent. If the child is too young to speak about concerns, below four years of age, the camouflage therapist should confer with a mental health professional about the appropriateness of camouflage therapy. Most young children live in a relatively restricted world and meet relatively few new people. They are least likely to receive negative feedback about their appearances. With such a young child, the major issue is the parent's inability to accept the child, not the inability of others to do so. If the parent seems uncomfortable with the limitations set by the camouflage therapist, it is wise to wait before initiating cosmetic therapy, and to refer the parent to a mental health professional to clarify the underlying issues.

Realistic Coping Defenses

A parent who has made a healthy adjustment to a child's disfigurement recognizes its impact upon the child's social and emotional development, but does not minimize or exaggerate it. The parent recognizes and acknowledges that the child looks different from peers, but does not equate difference with unacceptability. Such a parent will have consulted with the child's wishes and needs. The parent who is coping well feels comfortable discussing camouflage as a way of reducing discomfort the child has experienced due to disfigurement. Such a parent does not expect that physical perfection will lead to social popularity, nor does a healthy parent require that of the child. Rather, the healthy parent is aware that children are easily traumatized by the feedback they get from others; this parent also realizes that interaction with other children is essential for normal emotional growth and development. This parent seeks camouflage therapy as a tool to help the child experience more normal and appropriate social interactions than might otherwise occur. Such a parent acknowledges that the child will nevertheless have to earn acceptance, but should not have to experience rejection because of the negative stereotypes associated with physical disfigurement.

Child Variables

The developmental level and age of the child are crucial to the outcome of cosmetic therapy for several reasons. The fine motor and visual-motor skills necessary for independent application improve with age. Immature children may not have the neuro-development necessary to sit still during application. More important, however, is that most young children do not perceive the need for such an intervention because they have either not yet experienced stigma or have not perceived it as negative when it occurred. Since young children lack the cognitive maturity to anticipate possibilities, they presume that future social encounters will be as positive as prior ones have been.

Young children also are often resistant to change of any kind unless they have initiated it. If the child actively rejects the process of camouflage, even with a substantial degree of disfigurement, it is unwise to coerce the application, even upon parental request. Rather, the camouflage therapist should initiate the child into the use of the cosmetics and their application with doll play to introduce techniques and the concept of change gradually. If the child is not responsive and the disfigurement is substantial, referral of the parents to a mental health professional is indicated, so that the parents can learn techniques to make camouflage more acceptable to their child with her or his unique needs and history.

With a less prominent disfigurement, with less possibility of frequent and stigmatizing feedback from others, parents and camouflage therapist might consider waiting for several months and then making another attempt. If the child is responsive, it is important that the effect of camouflage be slight rather than drastic, because young children have difficulty accepting changes in their own appearances; many become distressed with costumes that include masks, because those change their facial appearance, although they are delighted with costumes that cover their bodies. A series of minimal to moderate changes will be accepted much more readily than a single, striking modification.

The camouflage therapist must develop a unique program of cosmetic application for each child. As a rule of thumb, most children under the age of ten will require assistance with the fine-motor aspect of application; they will have some difficulty in manipulating the cosmetic application tools, and may lack the esthetic balance necessary to produce a well-blended and harmonious appearance. The camouflage therapist should always involve the parent in teaching and demonstrating application, so that both the parent and child receive instruction, and each can give feedback to the other.

Periods of instruction must be tailored to the child's ability to sit still. Application tools such as pencils and crayons are preferred to brushes, because younger children are more familiar with them and have more practice in their use. All but the youngest children need to have a role in the application process; the camouflage therapist will need to find at least one step the child can perform independently. With increasing fine-motor and visual-motor skills, as well as increasing maturity, the number of steps performed by the child independently should increase. The adults should provide feedback rather than doing the application themselves. In order to enhance the child's ability to perform independently, the steps of the application should be broken down into a simple, numbered sequence. The steps should be presented in written form, like a checklist, as well as in a series of colored diagrams, so either the words or picture can be followed, if the child prefers one form of presentation. Some children and their parents might prefer a voice tape of the process, so that they can follow the verbal instructions as they work. Others will respond best to a video tape, so that they can view the process as they work. If the equipment is available, a video tape with sound is most engaging for a child between the ages of six and twelve. For the younger child, viewing herself or himself having appearance altered somewhat can be anxiety provoking, and should be avoided.

Occasionally a parent will wish to take full responsibility for the application, even though the child has the skill and maturity to so. The camouflage therapist must wean the parent away from overprotectiveness by teaching the process a step at a time, and letting the parent become accustomed, gradually, to the child performing the task.

An entirely different set of age-related variables occurs around adolescence. As the child seeks increasing independence from the parents, the child is increasingly likely to resist even the most reasonable parental suggestions. With adolescents, the most useful strategy is to provide information about the services available and establish communication so the adolescent can make the request for service her- or himself, through the parent, or through a physician or other health-care professional. Written parental consent must be obtained prior to initiating independent contact with an adolescent.

The camouflage therapist should be aware that it is often difficult for adolescents to request assistance from adults directly, or to acknowledge their emotional needs. The term "saving face" certainly is appropriate here. The camouflage therapist should be alert, and responsive to, subtle indications from adolescents that they would like to try cosmetic camouflage, but cannot acknowledge that wish directly. The camouflage therapist might suggest that the adolescent try an application "just this once," not as coercion, but as a way to let the adolescent see the outcome without having asked directly for it. An adolescent might say that she or he does not want to try application but is agreeing only because of parental insistence. This may be a "face saving" way of asking for an application without acknowledging the wish for it. The camouflage therapist must be alert to the intensity of the adolescent's refusal, and use the behavior, the readiness with which the adolescent "gets into it," as well as the words as an indicator of whether to proceed.

As noted above, adolescents sometimes resist cosmetic camouflage because they believe such measures undercut the adjustment they have already worked for; they believe using camouflage makes a statement that appearance is the most important aspect of an individual. It is important that these adolescents be supported emotionally in their desire to be accepted as they are; however, they should be given information about the ways camouflage can be useful to them. They often find it helpful to learn that camouflage enables them to make more satisfactory initial contacts, so that relationships have the opportunity to develop. They often are willing to consider using camouflage when they realize that the alternative is often cutting off potentially wonderful relationships because of unconscious, unrecognized, stereotyping.

Gender

The issue of gender and use of cosmetics is becoming less significant as men are encouraged to use more and more cosmetics in their daily grooming routines. However, gender issues are apt to emerge in adolescent males, who might well consider camouflage unmasculine. Some of the stigma can be relieved by careful application of a minimum of cosmetic products, presented with information about their usefulness in social relationships. Concerns about the camouflage being too obvious, or requiring frequent reapplication, should be addressed directly. Equipment and supplies packaged with a more "masculine" image might well be used, and might be more comfortable in larger male hands.

Life-style

The child's life-style has an important bearing upon the decision to use cosmetic camouflage as a part of the daily grooming regimen. The camouflage therapist must consider such things as the frequency of application necessary to maintain appearance, given each child's unique pattern of participation in sports and recreational activities. Need for parental assistance to apply the camouflage materials must be considered if the child spends long periods away from home, as at a summer camp, in full-day child care, or traveling between homes in the case of divorced parents. A program of cosmetic camouflage that does not address such issues is doomed to failure, because it will not be integrated into the daily life of the child and the family.

Child's Wish for Cosmetic Camouflage

Never attempt to coerce a child into using cosmetic camouflage. Never try to involve the parents in coercing the child to accept camouflage. Respect the resistance and understand that the child has reasons for the refusal. Sometimes it is the child's normal resistance to change. Sometimes it is a statement about resisting parental pressure, or a denial of the disfigurement. The child who has made a healthy adaptation to a disfigurement will be able to talk about it, and recognizes her/his difference from other children, but is not obsessed with it, either in denial or overemphasis. The child who has made a healthy adaptation may be willing to reconsider an application, after discussion of the potential benefits. If the child refuses after discussing the matter, suggest another appointment in several months, to re-evaluate feelings. Leave the youngster with a sense that she or he has a choice that will be respected; let her or him know that the option to change the decision will also be respected.

Temperament

The camouflage therapist has no control over the temperament of clients, but should be aware of major temperament styles to make sessions proceed more smoothly. Chess and Thomas (1981) identified three basic temperamental styles — easy, difficult, and slow-to-warm-up — in infants. Although these styles are modified somewhat by maturation, they can still be identified in adults. The easy child will be least resistant to change and most willing to take the risks of a novel experience. Feelings and behavior are most likely to match. Such a child usually gets good reactions from adults, values that positive feedback, and will be more compliant initially.

The slow-to-warm-up child keeps a distance initially, while assessing the situation. Such a child may be very resistant to change and require several sessions of getting to know the camouflage therapist before permitting a cosmetic application. With such a child, it is important to allow sufficient time to demonstrate what will happen, to practice on a doll or model, and to give the child a chance to become familiar with the tools and cosmetics. Since such a child will usually respond apprehensively to a new situation, such a child should not be asked about his feelings and thoughts during the initial meetings. As comfort increases, this child will express thoughts and feelings, but will remain more likely to withdraw under pressure. Go slowly with such a child, and respect the need for distance and control. If parental pressure is being applied, be certain to remain neutral, and not ally with the parent.

Children of difficult temperament are difficult for many reasons. Some are neuro-developmentally immature and re-act catastrophically to change. They are often uncomfortable with their bodies, and a disfigurement becomes one more way in which this discomfort is manifested. Many are very active physically and do not adapt well to routine. The immaturity may show in delayed or clumsy fine-motor skills, low frustration tolerance, and inconsistent attention. All of these variables would make the consistent use of cosmetic camouflage difficult. Children of difficult temperament generally improve in their self-control as they get older, so it is best to wait as long as possible before teaching a camouflage routine, unless the child is receiving a great deal of negative feedback from others about appearance.

Such a child should be taught the techniques of camouflage in brief periods, rather than fewer, longer sessions. A single step per session is sufficient. The child should be encouraged to practice often, for brief periods, on a doll or model, to learn the techniques involved. Since difficult children often have mild learning problems, the camouflage therapist should teach the child by verbally describing, demonstrating, and having the child practice. By using all three major learning modalities, hearing about, looking at, and doing, the camouflage therapist will help the child learn techniques most easily and with the least stress.

Many youngsters requiring cosmetic camouflage have had brain injuries. These youngsters also frequently present with short attention span and low frustration tolerance, but they may also show difficulties in memory, reduced motivation, a low level of personal initiative, and rapid shifts of mood. Such youngsters are often receiving services from a mental health professional; with parental consent, the camouflage therapist might consider consulting with the treating professional for guidance on approaching and teaching the youngster. The recommendations provided above for dealing with the tem-peramentally difficult youngster are usually applicable to the brain injured child, but may be insufficient, since each child presents with a unique combination of symptoms.

Given the drastic negative impact that facial disfigurement often has upon self-concept, social, and academic achievement, it is clearly valuable to provide treatment that can reduce the pain of social interaction, within the family as well as in the peer group. Cosmetic camouflage can make a dramatic change in a child's self-esteem and the way she or he learns to view family and friends. However, in dealing with children who are disfigured, the camouflage therapist must always remember to take into account the wishes and needs of the parents, as they are expressed in behavior as well as in words, and to remain alert to what is not said or is not done. The child's developmental level, adjustment to the disfigurement, temperament, and wish to undergo camouflage must also be considered. The camouflage therapist is in a unique position to help the child and the family deal with a major trauma. When the response to the disfigurement is unrealistic or excessive, when inappropriate emotional pressure is applied to a child, or when parents are not willing to respond to the child's request for treatment, referral to a mental health practitioner can facilitate emotional healing and reduce the potential for abuse. Abuse or neglect must be reported, so that a family can be helped to find better ways to deal with distress. The camouflage therapist can have the enormous satisfaction of using an art to help a child learn that she or he is a worthwhile human being, with a chance to make relationships without having to experience rejection because of society's negative stereotypes about disfigurement.

COSMETIC CAMOUFLAGE NEEDS INVENTORY

PARENT FORM
Rochelle B. Wolk, Ph.D.

Child's Name _____ Date of Birth _____

School Grade _____ Sex _____ Age_____

Parent (s) or Guardian (s) Name _____

Address _____

Telephone : Day_____ Evening _____

Child's primary physician: Name _____

Address _____

What about your child's appearance is of concern to you?

Who suggested seeking camouflage therapy? _____

In what way do you expect camouflage therapy to modify your child's appearance?

How do you think camouflage therapy should affect your child's life, on a day-to-day basis?

How did your child react when told of this appointment?

What concerns has your child verbalized about his/her appearance?

What kind of feedback does your child usually get about his/her appearance?

Why do you believe your child wants to use cosmetic camouflage?

How much time do you have in your daily schedule for applying camouflage with your child? Please specify the times of the day, as well as days of the week.

What are your child's primary recreational activities?

Does your child enjoy coloring, drawing, and writing? What have been his/her teacher comments about these skills?

Does your child have a best friend? If so, and your child requested it, would you permit that friend to join your child at a camouflage therapy session?

How much do you think camouflage materials will cost each month? Is that sum within your budget?

Are you anticipating cosmetic surgery for your child in the future? If so, what type and when?

Who referred you to this office? _____

_____ _____
                              Signature   Date

Thank you.

CLIENT FORM
(AGE 10 AND ABOVE)

Your name_____ Today's Date_____

School_____ Grade _____

Age _____ Date of Birth _____

With whom do you live? _____

Mother's Name: _____

Address: _____

Telephone (Day/Evening) _____

Father's Name: _____

Address _____

Telephone (Day/Evening) _____

What about the way you look displeases you?

When did you start to feel that way about your appearance?

Who suggested trying camouflage therapy?

How do you expect camouflage therapy to change the way you look?

How do you think changing your looks will change your life?

Who made this appointment? If your parent did, how did you react? If you did, how did your parent(s) react?

What have other people told you about how you look?

How do your parents feel about your appearance?

How do you know they feel like that?

How do other kids feel about your appearance?

How do you know they feel that way?

How do you feel about using cosmetics?

What cosmetics do you use now?

How do you like to spend your free time?

Do you enjoy making and doing things with your hands? What do your teachers say about your handwriting?

Do you have a best friend? Would you like your friend to come to a camouflage therapy session with you? Why?

_____ _____
Signature   Date

Thank you.

REVIEW

You should now be familiar with:

- ■ the impact of physical disfigurement.
- ■ how children in particular are affected by physical disfigurement.
- ■ when cosmetic camouflage can be effective with children.
- ■ the parents' role in the cosmetic camouflage process.

4 Documentation, Medical Terminology, and Record Keeping

A clinical esthetician/cosmetologist is responsible for providing professional esthetics care to patients with disfigurements within a salon, medical practice, or hospital setting. All services provided by the clinical esthetician or cosmetologist must support the patient's physician and his or her medical therapy of the patient. The clinical beauty professional works directly with the physician and other health-care personnel to provide the patient with quality care.

IMPORTANCE OF MEDICAL DOCUMENTATION

A record of all contact between a clinical esthetician or cosmetologist and a patient is very important for a number of reasons. In order for the camouflage therapist to determine what the patient's problem is and how to treat it, information must be systematically documented for review and evaluation. Medical records also provide a vital link between the camouflage therapist and other health-care providers.

The record is a focal point for all medical information. It includes direct examination of the patient, the assessment, and the plan (follow-up care). Other information in the patient's chart may include reports from the patient's physician and background information.

The patient's medical record also has important legal significance. Information that is obtained from the documentation is often requested from insurance companies. If a lawsuit involves the patient's health condition, lawyers for the attending physician may request the patient's records to present in court.

Medical records should always remain in the possession of the clinical beauty professional, not the patient. The patient may request a copy or may review his or her personal records at any time. Records can never be released to anyone without the written authorization of the patient.

Derogatory or irrelevant information about the patient, his or her family, or any member of the treatment team should never be included in the medical record. Written comments regarding negative aspects of the patient's personality should also be omitted from the patient's record.

Because of the legal significance of medical records, they must not be tampered with in any way. Whenever entering information, be extremely careful about accuracy and neatness.

At the conclusion of the patient's treatment, all documentation must be complete. Incomplete records can have devastating consequences in court if a patient initiates legal action challenging his or her care. Inaccurate documentation may confirm the patient's claim.

Nothing must ever be erased on a record. If a change needs to be made, cross out the original line and then write the correct entry next to it.

PATIENT RECORDS

The patient's records should contain the following:

- Date of the patient's appointment: month, day, and year (on each page).
- The patient's name (on each page).
- The patient's address and telephone number.
- The referral source.
- The name and title of the health-care provider.
- The signature of the camouflage therapist/clinical esthetician or cosmetologist.
- A written description of the patient's problem (from the patient's point of view).
- Physical observations of the problem site made by the camouflage therapist/clinical esthetician or cosmetologist.
- Systematic, orderly collection and analysis of data.

- The camouflage/esthetic solution (method used to resolve the patient's esthetic problem).

FILING PATIENT RECORDS

The patient's charts should be filed in alphabetical order, with the patient's last name first. The full name of the patient should be written or typed neatly on the label and adhered to the file folder tab. It is critical to file medical records properly in order to be able to find them quickly and to retrieve information accurately. When a patient or another health-care provider calls or writes with a question regarding the patient's care, the camouflage therapist must be able to respond by locating the patient's file in order to release the information to the authorized inquirer.

If any piece of the record is taken out of the patient's chart, a notation should be made and inserted into the file stating what was taken, on what date, and why it was removed. If the entire folder is removed from the files, a "marker" should be put in place of the folder indicating where the patient's chart can be located.

SHARING PATIENT INFORMATION WITH OTHERS

If the patient requests that medical information be sent to a third party, you may not refuse this request because the information is confidential. You must comply with the patient's request, but original medical records should never be released. The patient's requests should be documented in his or her file. Telephone inquiries may be answered if the patient has expressly authorized this communication and his or her authorization has been documented. The identity of the person calling for information must be verified. This can be accomplished by taking the person's telephone number and calling back.

OBTAINING THE PATIENT'S MEDICAL HISTORY

When preparing for an appointment with a new patient, it is often desirable to obtain a medical history from the physician who referred the patient to you. This is not always necessary, but in some cases you may need this information. A clinical beauty professional who is involved in a patient's care has the right and the duty to be fully informed about that patient's condition.

Ask the patient to sign a consent form authorizing the doctor to release the information. Send the doctor the form along with a letter informing him of the name of the patient you will be treating, with a request for the patient's medical history and any information that he or she may feel will be useful to you.

Below is a sample of a patient's consent form.

Patient's Consent for Release of Medical Information Form

Date _____

I herewith authorize Dr. _____ to release to my camouflage therapist/clinical esthetician/cosmetologist _____ any medical history or any other pertinent information regarding the medical consultations or treatments that I have received.

Signed_____

PATIENT RELATIONSHIP

The camouflage therapist/patient or the clinical esthetician/cosmetologist/patient relationship may be characterized as an unwritten contract. The patient should feel that he or she is being provided with the best possible service. The camouflage therapist/clinical esthetician or cosmetologist is responsible for unraveling the patient's problem, devising an esthetic solution, and clearly communicating about available options to the patient.

It is not legally allowed to discriminate on the basis of race, national origin, religion, or because of an individual's attributes that are not relevant to the type of care involved. However, the clinical esthetician/camouflage therapist is not legally required to accept patients who need services that are beyond the scope of that individual's expertise or experience. The camouflage therapist/clinical esthetician or cosmetologist, when working on a patient, should never make a medical judgment, institute a course of medical therapy, or perform an procedure that is beyond his or her qualifications.

If a patient is self-referred (as opposed to physician-referred), the nature and limits of clinical esthetics must be made clear to the patient. No statement should ever be made to the patient or anyone connected to the patient that could be interpreted as a promise or guarantee.

The camouflage therapist/clinical esthetician or cosmetologist should never criticize another health professional providing care to the patient or the type of medical treatment the patient is receiving. If the clinical esthetician/cosmetologist is concerned about any aspect of the patient's treatment those concerns should be expressed to the patient's physician directly.

Confidentiality

Information exchanged between the camouflage therapist/clinical esthetician/cosmetologist and the patient is confidential and must never be discussed with the patient's family or friends, particularly in a social setting. The patient must give permission to the camouflage therapist or clinical esthetician to discuss the patient's condition with a relative or friend of the patient.

A patient's chart should also be protected and out of access to unauthorized persons. If the patient's chart is left where someone could look at it, it is a breach of confidentiality.

S. O. A. P. - PROBLEM ASSESSMENT AND PLAN FORMULATION

For purposes of documentation, the patient's problem is individually described and evaluated, and an initial plan is formulated. All subsequent data: orders, plans, progressive notes, etc., are recorded in the body of the patient's record. New entries and the majority of this information follow a specific format (S.O.A.P. is the acronym), as indicated below:

S. (subjective) — The patient's age, nationality, gender, and the problem from the patient's point of view.

O. (objective data) — The physical observation of the potential treatment site and any other pertinent physical observations.

A. (assessment) — Analysis of data for the purpose of devising a camouflage or esthetic solution.

P. (plan) — Therapeutic plan and prescribed follow-up treatment.

Subjective

Subjective data provide a written description of the patient and his or her goals for treatment. This section begins with a portrait of the subject (the patient's age, nationality, and gender) and then identifies in the patient's own words his or her condition. It also should include any expectations the patient may have about the treatment.

Objective

Objective data is the physical findings, observations, and any other pertinent information regarding the patient's condition (area of involvement). If the patient is being treated for a disfigurement with cosmetic therapy, objective data would include a description of the color, texture, size, and location of the patient's disorder.

Assessment

A patient's goals for treatment will fall into two categories: wants and needs. It is the role of the clinical cosmetician to help the patient recognize that sometimes not all wants will be able to be met. Expectation discrepancy is the psychological term used to describe the difference between what the patient expects from treatment and what is realistically possible (what he or she will actually receive). The camouflage therapist must be careful not to overstate what can truly be accomplished by using makeup. Therefore, the first of six areas to be investigated during the interview process, and certainly the most important, will be the patient's emotional/psychological state and the results expected from treatment. This is followed by the patient's communication skills, social and leisure activities, prior makeup experience, financial status, now and in the future, skin condition — allergies or sensitivities — and any pertinent medically-related information.

Emotional/Psychological State

To determine the patient's emotional state ask him or her to describe in detail the condition to be camouflaged. Listen objectively and observe the body language, including posture, facial expressions, and stance (open or closed). Does the patient appear overly anxious, impatient, irritable, or depressed? Try to evaluate whether the patient sees himself as a victim — with little or no control — or someone who wishes to participate in his own recovery process. Does the patient appear interested and willing to correct the condition? Ask the patient what he or she expects from the treatment. While you want to be as encouraging and positive as possible, it is important to advise your patient, if you think expectations are too high, about the limitations of an esthetic service or a camouflage treatment.

Communication Skills

The second category, communication skills, will determine the patient's ability to understand and carry out simple instructions. Evaluate the patient: Does he or she have any language barriers, physical or mental disabilities that will hinder the application process? If so, the appointment time will have to be extended.

Social and Leisure Activities

The third category of investigation will be into the social and leisure activities of the patient, with special emphasis on peer group and place of employment, and finally, any hobbies or sports he or she may be involved in. Environmental factors will influence the lighting required during the application; also the need for additional sunscreen should then be assessed. The need for sunscreen depends on how much time is spent outdoors and how susceptible the patient's condition is to ultraviolet light. Questions to ask include: How much of your time is spent in the sun, the office, at home? What sports do you participate in? Are your social activities formal or casual?

Prior Makeup Experience

The fourth category to investigate is the patient's experience. Is the patient using cosmetics? If the patient is wearing makeup, it must be evaluated. What is the patient's current makeup routine? Notes should be taken on which areas of the patient's application need improvement. Patients should be questioned to assess their prior experience in applying cosmetics and with color. Ask the patient how much time he or she would be willing to devote to camouflage techniques.

Financial Status of the Patient

The fifth consideration is the patient's socio-economic level. How much can the patient reasonably afford to spend on his or her camouflage solution? Is the patient employed? Does the patient have an insurance plan that will cover camouflage sessions and the supplies he or she will continue to need to perform the camouflage therapy/esthetic procedure? Does a payment schedule need to be set up for the patient?

Medically-Related Information

The last of the six areas to be investigated is the patient's medical history. Is the patient currently taking any medications that could interfere with the application of camouflage products by temporarily altering the patient's skin tone or skin texture? Is the patient using a topical application of medication, and if so will it interfere with a satisfactory result by diluting the cover cream and reducing its opaque appearance? Most importantly, does the patient have any sensitivities or allergies to cosmetics or any of the substances that may be used in treatment?

Plan

The plan is the final phase of the appointment. It is the description of what can be done to assist the patient. It is the record of what esthetic procedure was performed, what instruction was given on the procedure to the patient, which if any, cosmetics were used, and any other esthetic recommendations that were made to the patient. It should also indicate if any other follow-up sessions were recommended and the dates of those sessions.

FACIAL OR BODY DIAGRAMS

A photograph or line drawing should be included in the patient's file as a visual reminder of the patient's condition. Only the areas of involvement need to be drawn or photographed to present a clear picture. A rubber stamp of the body and face can be made by a stamp company. A medical template can be purchased at a medical university bookstore or medical supply store, or the following diagrams can be used for documentation purpose.

1. posterior median line of trunk B
2. subcostal plane C
3. transpyloric plane C
4. supracristal plane C
5. intertubercular plane C
6. interspinal plane C
10. frontal region A
11. parietal region A B
12. occipital region A B
13. temporal region A B
15. orbital region A
16. nasal region A
17. oral region A
18. mental region A
19. infraorbital region (below orbit) A
20. buccal region, (cheek area) A
21. zygomatic region A
24. submandibular triangle A
25. carotid triangle A
26. muscular trigonum A
27. submental trigonum A
28. sternocleidomastoid region A
29. lesser supraclavicular fossa A
30. lateral neck region A
31. omoclavicular triangle A
32. neck region B
34. presternal region C
35. infraclavicular fossa C
36. clavipectoral trigonum C
37. pectoral region C
38. mammary region C
39. inframammary region C
40. axillary region C
41. axillary fossa C

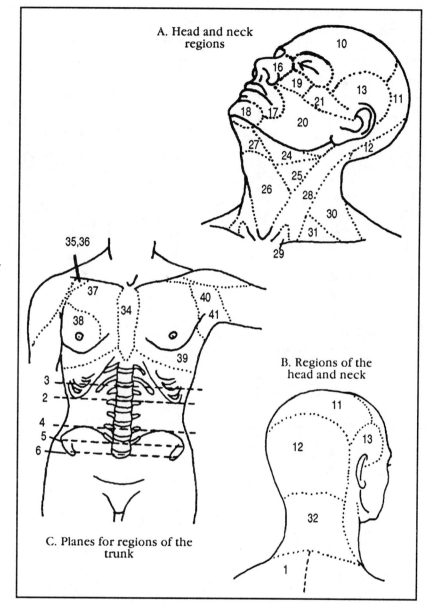

A. Head and neck regions

B. Regions of the head and neck

C. Planes for regions of the trunk

2. hypochondriad region B

3. epigastric region B

4. lateral region B

5. umbilical region B

6. inguinal region B

7. pubic region B

9. vertebral region A

10. sacral region A

11. scapular region A

12. infrascapular region A

13. lumbar region A

16. anal region C

17. urogenital region C

19. deltoid region B

21. anterior brachial region A

22. posterior brachial region A

24. anterior elbow region B

25. posterior elbow region A

26. cubital fossa B

27. lateral (radial) bicipital B

28. medial (ulnary) bicipital B

30. anterior antebrachial
region A B

31. posterior antebrachial
region A B

35. anterior carpal region A

36. posterior carpal region B

38. back of hand B

39. palm of hand A

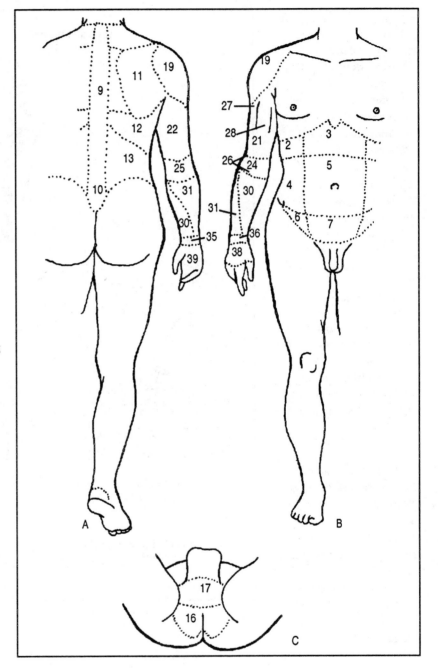

2. gluteal region A
3. gluteal groove A
5. anterior thigh region B
6. femoral trigone B
7. posterior femoral region A
9. anterior knee region B
10. posterior knee region A
13. anterior crural region B
14. posterior crural region A
15. sural region (calf) A
18. heel A
19. dorsum of foot B
20. sole of foot A

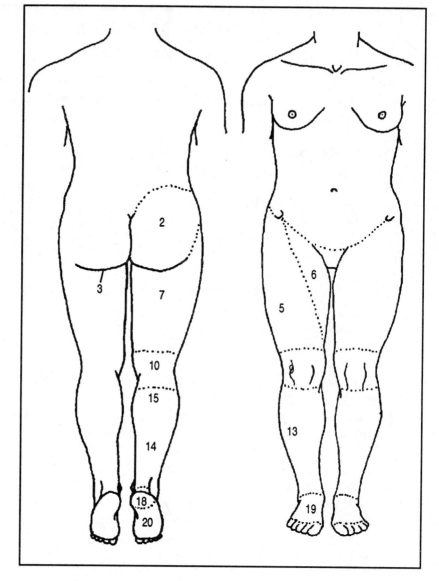

PHOTOGRAPHIC DOCUMENTATION

Sigi Torinus

The use of photography in connection with scientific and medical documentation has its roots in the second half of the nineteenth century, where it made significant contributions to medical knowledge. Aside from documenting psychological reactions and mental aberrations, the camera was used especially in investigating external conditions. Here camera images were used mainly as before-and-after records, representing the appearance of different phases of a disease or skin condition.

Within the context of cosmetic therapy, photography becomes important for documenting application results. It can have informative/demonstrative as well as therapeutic functions.

For documenting changes undergone during treatment, before-and-after shots are most suited since they provide the possibility of comparison; you can see how successful the cosmetic application has been. Comparisons work best if a certain number of parameters are fixed. The distance between the photographer and the patient should remain the same, as well as the light source, the camera lens size, the exposure time, and the type of film used. The background — preferably white — should also be the same. Different-color backgrounds can change the entire atmosphere of the picture as well as add a different hue to the skin. This also applies to the patient's clothing. It's a good idea to always take pictures in the same location in your office so your pictures are consistent. You can mark the floor with tape for your own orientation.

Many people find it very intimidating to be photographed, so it is important to have the patient feel as comfortable as possible. When photographing children, it is especially advisable to have everything ready in advance. Before your start taking pictures, the patient should have time to get used to the situation. If you have been carrying on a conversation, continue with it as before. That way the patient won't feel self-conscious or scrutinized by the photographic procedure.

Once the patient is seated, remember that you are not taking a portrait. The idea of the picture is to document application results; therefore your decisions about proper lighting will not be the same as when taking other photographs.

LIGHTING

The first decision is whether to use natural or artificial light. Natural light, also known as available or ambient light, has a vast range of effects that are dependent on the time of day you are taking the picture, the position of the sun in the sky, and the interference of atmospheric particles. Though photographs taken with existing lighting have a more natural appearance than those taken with artificial light, natural light will not guarantee the consistency you are looking for when taking before-and-

Sigi Torinus is a photographer and visual artist who resides in San Francisco, California. She holds fine arts degrees from universities in Germany and the United States and has exhibited extensively in the United States and in Europe. She has taught photography to both beginners and advanced students, has been part of a film team that worked in Jamaica, and is currently involved with large-scale theatrical productions in San Francisco.

after shots; by the time the cosmetic application is completed, the light will probably have changed significantly.

Both morning and evening light are warmer in color than midday light, which is a cooler blue. Strong direct sunlight should be avoided, since it tends to flatten tonal values and lights face and body features unevenly. It produces extremely strong contrasts between light and shade, often to a point where most films cannot reproduce both ends of the tonal range simultaneously. The result is pictures with little depth.

The advantage of using artificial light is that you can control lighting conditions. Of the large variety of lighting systems available, the two most commonly used are electronic flash and tungsten.

Electronic Flash

Electronic flash enables you to use daylight film. A drawback is that it is initially more expensive than tungsten light. While a setup with two tungsten lights might cost around $80, a small portrait strobe setup will cost at least $300. This would include two lights, stands, umbrellas, and a power pack. The pack is the heart of the flash system, into which several flash heads can be plugged. Common forms of flash heads are sign units — the flash equivalent of spotlights — which provide directional light. Here, too, direct (face-on) lighting should be avoided. It tends to flatten out the face and remove slight shadows that mark detail on the skin. The most popular form of light diffusion is the lighting umbrella. For photographing scars or disfigurements, a small grey lighting umbrella should be used, since it produces a harsher shadow and gives more light. White umbrellas soften the appearance of the skin, thus masking the detail you need. If you are using a flash that is connected to your camera, tilt the flash so that the light bounces off of a light surface such as a ceiling, a wall, or an umbrella, or wrap a piece of white cloth around your flash head for taking extreme close-ups. It is better, though, to light the patient from two different angles for more even lighting. Take care not to have the light shine directly into the camera, as this would change the exposure considerably, lending the skin a very dark tone or creating a silhouette.

The cheapest source of artificial daylight is daylight bulbs that are mounted on silver heads, the setup costing around $50. These light bulbs get very hot, so you will need thick leather gloves to handle them. Furthermore, they have a low life expectancy, which means the number of bulbs used will soon amount to a price greater than the investment in an electronic setup; for this reason it's worth considering alternatives to this method.

Tungsten Lighting

Tungsten lighting is a lot cheaper than electronic flash, but it has a few drawbacks that should be considered. With daylight bulbs, the heat buildup can become uncomfortable for the patient; it might cause the cosmetic application to run and the camera lens to pick up moisture. Thus it is important to use a well-ventilated room and to work quickly. Tungsten lights have a short life expectancy and are extremely fragile to handle. They should not be moved around too much once they are hot, since they will blow at a single jolt. The same might occur if they are switched on and off frequently. It is therefore good to have a number of spare bulbs handy. Since tungsten emits a different, much warmer, light color than that of daylight or flash, you will need a tungsten transparency film or a blue filter to correct it. There is no tungsten color negative film available, which might be a decisive factor for your choice of light source.

Overhead Light

When using electronic flash or tungsten light sources, it is important to switch off the overall lighting in your office or use color correction filters. Fluorescent lamps are especially tricky to work with and make it almost impossible to reproduce skin tones with any accuracy. Color filters for correction are not that useful since fluorescent lamps change their color slightly with age and are therefore not consistent. In addition to this, they flicker; the flicker is not visible to one's eye but will affect your exposures. This makes exposure times of at least 1/60 second necessary.

THE CAMERA

The camera most suitable for photographing cosmetic applications is the 35 mm SLR (single lens reflex) camera. Cheaper alternatives are Polaroid or instamatic cameras. These have the advantage of the convenience of operation; both have the disadvantage that they offer only a limited focal range; most often they have a wide-angle lens, so that you cannot take close-ups of skin areas, for instance. You also have less control over exposure. Since with these cameras you do not see through the lens, you do not know exactly what you will see on the picture.

Polaroids tend to be unpredictable in film color and will show little definition of skin texture. Makeup appears to stand out in Polaroid photos because Polaroid-type

film has a slight green undertone, which makes the contrasting red-based flesh tones come forward. Yet you have an instant picture and can show it to the patient immediately and talk about your application results. Sometimes this can be very important for the therapeutic process. A good way to work might be to use both a 35 mm and a Polaroid camera.

Most 35 mm cameras have built-in light meters that suggest the aperture and shutter settings. You can either use the suggested setting or change it and thus have complete control over the exposure. Many cameras come with automatic exposure controls, which ensure proper exposure, including flash settings. This can be extremely helpful if you want to concentrate more on your interaction with the patient. The same applies to auto focus cameras. Make sure you take an exposure reading of only the skin area you will eventually photograph — this is especially important when photographing patients with dark complexions. Many cameras give you the option of designating which part of the picture will determine the exposure reading. This is a very helpful feature.

A further disadvantage of the 35 mm camera is that you essentially see the picture before you take it. With the right exposure, pictures will not differ too much from the way they looked through the viewfinder. A 35 mm camera comes with a standard 50 mm lens, which covers a view angle similar to the human eye and is fine for photographing applications on the skin.

FILM

The choice of film depends on what you will want to do with the pictures later on. The best skin tone definition you will get is with reversal (slide) film, since a transparency (a slide) is actual film on which the image was recorded. If you have a print made from a negative, you will have an image that is already one step removed from the original and is therefore less accurate. If you will only be working with prints, though, a color negative film will suffice; having a negative film developed takes the least time and is cheaper than transparency film — including processing and having prints made. Another disadvantage is that to a great extent colors can still be corrected in the print development process. If, for instance, the skin appears to have a green hue, you can have a print made from the negative with instructions to the lab to filter out the green so that the skin will have a more natural color rendition. Kodak Ektar 125 or Fuji Reala are good, fine-grain, color films.

Transparencies offer a larger range of possibilities for uses later. You can have prints made, and you can project them on a large screen for discussing application results. Very good daylight transparency films are Kodachrome 25 and Kodachrome 64. Both are known for their exceptional color purity, resolution, and fine grain, which means they will work best to reproduce cosmetic applications accurately. Grain is the granule-like mottling that appears in photographs. The larger the grain, the less detail a photograph can reveal. The two films suggested are "slow" films, so they require substantial lighting. If the light available is lower you will need to shoot on Ektachrome stock, which is available up to 400 ASA. A rule that applies to both color and black-and-white film is *the slower the film, the finer the grain*. However, some high-speed black-and-white films are surprisingly grain-free, such as T MAX 400, which still gives fine-grain results if exposed at 800 ASA.

If the lighting conditions are extremely unfavorable (fluorescent light that cannot be switched off or low light), you may need to revert to a black-and-white film. Generally, though, a black-and-white film is less suited to reproducing cosmetic applications, since color plays such an important part in their utilization. Working with tungsten lighting requires using tungsten film, such as Ektachrome 160 tungsten or, if you are using a daylight film, a blue filter (Filter 80A) to correct the difference in color temperature. An amber colored filter (Filter 358) converts tungsten light to daylight.

All considerations concerning photographic documentation of cosmetic applications can only function as an initial orientation. Your decisions will depend on your working environment (lighting conditions, space available), your budget, and how you want to use the photographs. When you are purchasing equipment, let the person helping you know exactly what you are going to do with the equipment, so that you can get as much advice as possible on what to get and how to use it. You should run a few tests with friends or relatives before you photograph patients to avoid disappointments for both you and the patient. Write down all the parameters — including location, light source, film type, exposure setting, and distance between camera and patient — for each picture, so that later on you can draw on the good results and develop a system that works best for your specific situation.

Patient's Consent to Photograph Form

I hereby authorize my attending physician or a person designated by my attending physician to take photographs, videotapes, and/or motion pictures of me for purposes of diagnosis, treatment, and medical education and research.

I understand that negatives, tapes, and prints of these pictures may be viewed by others in order to promote my own health and well-being or to advance medical knowledge.

I understand that photographs made from these negatives, videotapes, or motion pictures may be published or exhibited as part of reports of advances in medical science and that, should such a publication occur, every reasonable effort will be made to disguise my identity.

Date_____ Hour_____ _____
                                                Signature of patient or
                                                patient's parent or guardian.

If signed by other than parent please indicate relationship.

_____ _____
Witness

PATIENT'S OUTLINE OF THE CAMOUFLAGE PROCEDURE

At the end of the treatment session, the patient should be given an instructional sheet illustrating how to duplicate each step of the cosmetic therapy procedure. This form should also include a record of what products were used and where to obtain them. Any applicator or additional cosmetics should also be listed. A copy of any materials or teaching aids that were given to the patient must be retained in the patient's permanent record.

MEDICAL CORRESPONDENCE

A physician's report (written documentation of the treatment given to the physician's patient) must be sent to the patient's doctor. This information will indicate to the referring physician whether or not the esthetic service proved satisfactory to his or her patient. The following forms are samples of an initial visit, interim visit, and final report form.

INITIAL VISIT REPORT

Patient_____ Date_____

Dear Doctor_____

    I had the opportunity to see your patient today in consultation. Together we developed the following goals and treatment plan:

Goals:

Treatment Plan:

    Thank you very much for this referral.

Sincerely,

INTERIM REPORT

Patient_____ Date_____

Dear Doctor_____

    This is a report to update you on the progress of your patient.
Status:

Progress:

Problems:

    Thank You again for this referral. I will keep in close touch as the treatment progresses.

Sincerely,

FINAL REPORT

Patient_____ Date_____

Dear Doctor_____

    This is the final report on your patient as we have completed our treatment plan.

Status:

Problems:

Future Plans:

    Thank you again for this referral. I greatly appreciate your support and look forward to working with you again in the future.

Sincerely,

TERMS USED FOR CHARTING

The following terms are commonly used in charting the skin, head, and neck regions:

Description	Term
normal complexion	smooth, well-hydrated, healthy color
patchy, red, puffy skin	rash, erythema
allergic rash, hives	urticaria
colorless skin	pale, pallor
bruises	ecchymosis
retention of fluid in tissue with swelling	edema, edematous
very small amount	scant, slight
medium amount	moderate, usual
large amount	profuse, excessive
forehead	frontal region

region over temple	temporal region
back of head	occipital region
back of neck	neck region, nuchal region
plane around eye	orbital region
plane just below eye	infraorbital region
nose area	nasal region
area over zygomatic arch	zygomatic region
cheek area	buccal region
area around mouth	oral region
chin area	mental region
neck	neck region, nuchal region

PROFESSIONAL SYMBOLS AND ABBREVIATIONS

Clinical estheticians or cosmetologists in the course of performing their professional duties will encounter many titles and abbreviations. The conscientious camouflage therapist/clinical esthetician/cosmetologist will want to understand the importance and meaning of each.

Medical Abbreviations This list of current abbreviations represents some of the more common abbreviations a clinical cosmetician may use. There are, however, many possible meanings, and new definitions are being added on a regular basis.

This list of abbreviations is not an endorsement of their legitimacy nor a guarantee that the intended meaning is appropriate. There are many variations of a given abbreviation. Each abbreviation may have more than one meaning; below are some of the many:

A

A	age anterior assessment	ACSW	Academy of Certified Social Workers
Abd	abdomen	AD	right ear
abnor.	abnormal	adol	adolescent
ABx	antibiotics acute	AE	above elbow (amputation)
ACC	accident		
ACS	American Cancer Society	AHN	assistant head nurse

AIDKS	acquired immune deficiency syndrome with Kaposi's sarcoma	AODA	alcohol and other drug abuse
AIDS	acquired immune deficiency syndrome	AP	attending physician
		A&P	anterior and posterior
AK	above knee (amputation)	APH	alcohol-positive history
AKA	all known allergies	AP&L	antero-posterior and lateral
AL	left ear	appr.	approximate
ALL	allergy	appt.	appointment
AM	adult male	aq	water
AMA	American Medical Association	aq dest	distilled water
		ARB	any reliable brand
AMP	amputation	ARC	AIDS related complex
AMSIT	portion of the mental status examination:	ARV	AIDS related virus
	A- appearance,	ARW	Accredited Rehabilitation Worker
	M- mood,		
	S- sensorium,	ASAP	as soon as possible
	I- intelligence,	ASS	assessment
	T- thought process	asst	assistant
AN	anorexia nervosa	ATS	anxiety tension state
ANS	answer		
Anti bx	antibiotic	AU	both ears
ANX	anxiety anxious	avg	average
		AZT	zidovudine (azidothymidine) drug therapy for AIDS patients
AOB	alcohol on breath		

B

B	both	BC/BS	Blue Cross/Blue Shield
B/C	because		

BCC	basal cell carcinoma	BM	black male
BCCa	basal cell carcinoma	BMK	birthmark
BCD	basal cell dysplasia	BP	benzoyl peroxide birthplace
BCE	basal cell epithelioma	BPD	borderline personality disorder
BCP	birth control pills	BR	brown
BCS	battered child syndrome	BRO	brother
BCU	burn care unit	BS	before sleep
BD	birth date birth defect	BSA	body surface area
BE	below elbow	BSB	body surface burned
B↑E	both upper extremities	BSC	burn scar contracture
B↓E	both lower extremities	BSN	Bachelor of Science in Nursing
BEA	below elbow amputation	BSW	Bachelor of Social Work
BIL	bilateral	BU	burn unit
BKA	below knee amputation	BUE	both upper extremities
Bkg	background	BWS	battered woman syndrome

C

C	Caucasian	CDC	Centers for Disease Control
CA	carcinoma or malignant growth	CE	community education continuing education
CAM	Caucasian adult male		
CA/N	child abuse and neglect	C&E	consultation and examination curettage and electrodesiccation
CANC	cancelled		
CC	chief complaint chronic complainer	CF	Caucasion female
CCW	child care worker		

CH	child (children) chronic	CNA	chart not available
c̄ hold	withhold	CND	cannot determine
Chemo-Rx	chemotherapy	C/O	complained of
CHG	change	COMP	complications compress
CHPX	chicken pox	CONG	congenital
chr.	chronic	cont	continuous
Circ	circulation	COTA	Certified Occupational Therapy Assistant
CL	cleft lip		
Clav	clavicle	CP	Certified Paramedic cleft palate
CL&P	cleft lip & palate		
cm	centimeter	CR	chief resident
CM	Caucasian male centimeter (cm)	CRNP	certified registered nurse practitioner
CME	continuing medical education	CU	cause unknown
CMM	cutaneous malignant melanoma		

D

D	daughter day divorced	DK	dark
		DLE	discoid lupus erythematosus
DAC	disabled adult child	DMD	Doctor of Dental Medicine
d/c, DC	discontinue		
DCFS	Department of Children and Family Services	DN	down
		DNA	does not apply
		DNC	did not come
DCYS	Department of Children and Youth Services	DNR	did not respond
		DNS	doctor did not see patient do not show
DERM	dermatology		
DI	date of injury	DO	doctor's order
DIL	drug-induced lupus	D/O	disorder
DIR	directions	DON	director of nursing

DORx	date of treatment	DS	disoriented double strength
DPA	Department of Public Assistance	Dx	diagnosis
DPB	days postburn		
DPH	Department of Public Health Doctor of Public Health		

E

E	edema eye	ERP	emergency room physician
E&A	evaluate and advise	ex	examined
EDP	emergency department physician	exam.	examination
		EXT	extraction
EE	eye and ear		

F

F	facial female finger	FH	family history
		FMD	family medical doctor
FA	forearm	FT	family therapy follow through
FACS	Fellow of the American College of Surgeons	FTKA	failed to keep appointment
F.A.C.P.	Fellow of the American College of Physicians; highest honor that can be conferred upon a physician	F/U	follow-up
		FUN	follow-up note
		FUOV	follow-up office visit
FASHP	Fellow of the American Society of Hospital Pharmacists		

G

GA	general appearance	GRN	green
GOT	goals of treatment	Gyn.	gynecology or gynecologist

H

HA	hearing aid	H/O	history of
HAT	head, arms, and trunk	H2O	water
		H2O2	hydrogen peroxide
HC	handicapped	HOPI	history of present illness
HEENT	head, eyes, ears, nose, and throat	HT	height
HI	hearing impaired	Hx	history
HL	hairline	HYG	hygiene
HN	head and neck		

I

IC	incomplete	IR	infrared
IMP	important	irreg	irregular
inj	injury		
IPOP	immediate postoperative prosthesis		

K

KS	Kaposi's sarcoma	KS/OI	Kaposi's sarcoma and opportunistic infections

L

L	left	LES	lupus erythematosis systemic
LB	left breast		
LD	learning disability learning disorder	LFA	left forearm
LE	left ear left eye lupus erythematosus	LHS	left hand side
		LI	learning impaired

LL	left leg	LOV	loss of vision
	lower lid	L.P.N.	licensed practical
	lower lip		nurse
LLL	left lower lid	LS	left side
LLLE	lower lid, left eye	L&U	lower and upper
LLOD	lower lid, right eye	LUA	left upper arm
LLIS	lower lid, left eye	L.V.N.	licensed vocational
LLRE	lower lid, right eye		nurse

M

M	male	MI	mental illness
	married	MO	mineral oil
	mother		month (mo)
MD	medical doctor		months old
MED	medical		mother
	medication	MR	medical record
	medicine	MS	medical student
	medium		
MH	mental health		

N

N	negative	norm	normal
	normal	NPH	no previous history
NA	Native American	NR	no report
	not available		no response
	nursing assistant	NRN	no return necessary
NB	nail bed	NS	not seen
ND	nothing done		not significant
NK	not known	NSI	negative self-image
NKA	no known allergies	NSR	not seen regularly

O

O	eye	OB	obese
	often	Obj	objective
	open	OC	office call
O&A	observation &	OD	doctor of optometry
	assessment		

OG	obstetrics-gynecology	OTC	over the counter (sold without prescription)
OK	all right approved	OTR	occupational therapist, registered
OP	outpatient	OU	both eyes
OPC	outpatient clinic	OV	office visit
OPP	opposite		
OR	operating room		

P

P	para peripheral plan	PLS	plastic surgery
		PLSURG	plastic surgery
PAR	paraffin	PM	afternoon evening
PAT	patient	POp	postoperative
P&B	pain and burning	post op	postoperative
PCP	patient care plan	PP	poor person
PDR	Physician's Desk Reference	prog.	prognosis program progressive
Peds.	pediatrics		
PG	pregnant	pros	prosthesis
PH	past history personal history poor health	PS	plastic surgery (surgeon)
PHAR	pharmacist	PT	patient
Pharm	pharmacy	PTS	prior to surgery
PHx	past history	PWS	port-wine stain
PI	package insert poison ivy		

R

R	right	REC	recommend record
Ⓡ	right		
RA	right arm	REF	referred refused
R&B	right and below		
RE	right ear right eye	ref>	refer to
		REP	repeat

RES	resident	RPTA	registered physical therapist assistant
RET	return		
REV	reverse review	RS	right side
		RT	right
RH	right hand	RUQ	right upper quadrant
RHS	right hand side		
RIF	right index finger	RV	return visit
RL	right leg	Rx	drug medication pharmacy prescription therapy treatment
R>L	right to left		
RLQ	right lower quadrant		
RM	radical mastectomy		
RPT	registered physical therapist		

S

S	subjective findings	SOAPIE	subjective, objective, assessment, plan, intervention, and evaluation
SCC	squamous cell carcinoma		
SD	scleroderma		
SG	skin graft	SS	sliding scale
SHEENT	skin, head, eyes, ears, nose, and throat	ST	skin test
		STG	split-thickness graft
SOAP	subjective, objective, assessment, plan	Subcu	subcutaneous

T

TB	total body	Tx	therapy
trach.	tracheal tracheostomy		

U

UA	upper arm	ULQ	upper left quadrant
UK	unknown	ULRE	upper lid, right eye
U/L	upper and lower	UNK	unknown
U&L	upper and lower	UTD	up to date

UV	ultraviolet	UVB	ultraviolet B light
UVA	ultraviolet A light	UVL	ultraviolet light

V

VG	very good	VS	very sensitive

W

w	white	wk	week
WF	white female	WWAC	walk with aid of cane

Y

Yel	yellow	YTD	year to date
YOB	year of birth		

Miscellaneous Symbols

↑	above	≥	greater than or equal to
	elevated	<	less than
	high	≤	less than or equal to
↓	decrease	∧	above
	lowered	∨	below
→	to the right	≈	approximately
←	to the left	?	questionable
‖	parallel	1°	first degree
⌐	right upper quadrant	2°	second degree
⌐	left upper quadrant	3°	third degree
⌐	left lower quadrant	♂	male
>	greater than	♀	female

REVIEW

You should now be familiar with:
- ■ why medical documentation is important.
- ■ how to file patient records.
- ■ how to obtain a complete medical history.
- ■ the importance of photographic documentation.
- ■ medical terms used for charting.

CHAPTER

5 Understanding Color

To fully understand the importance of color, try this simple exercise: Close your eyes and try to imagine a colorless world. Picture a landscape in black and white, the top of a mountain range against the backdrop of a dull, gray, and lifeless sky. At the base of the mountain is a lake surrounded by dense foliage and patches of colorless flowers. Now imagine the same landscape, only alive with vibrant colors. Picture the sun setting behind the range of dark purple mountains, only this time, the sky is ablaze with a multitude of colors: blue against yellow, red against purple, purple against orange. Visualize the once colorless lake, which now reflects the sky like a mirror, producing a kaleidoscope of colors on the water. Imagine dense greenery with patches of brightly colored flowers covering the ground and surrounding the borders of the lake.

Did you notice that as you began visualizing the mountain scene in color you were able to imagine it in more detail? No doubt you became more aware of finer points of the mountain scene, which you may have left out when you pictured it in black and white. The diversity of color assists us in recognizing objects in proportion and in relation to one another. Differences in colors, their brightness, and especially their lightness or darkness make us more conscious of the shape of objects. Diametrically opposite colors attract attention to outlines, whereas two colors with similar values make edges appear less distinct. Cool colors, that is to say blue-based colors, make more of a contrast than warmer colors (yellow-based colors) when used on or around borders.

From the beginning of time, man has been fascinated with color. The ancient Egyptians were aware of the power and influence of color, as evidenced by the colored halls in their great temples. These special rooms were designated places where color was researched. The Egyptians practiced an ancient form of color healing.

Today color studies are still being conducted by physicians and scientists; experiments are being performed to monitor the therapeutic use of color through the application of colored light transmitted through the body. The aim of this color science is to combat disease by restoring the normal balance of color energies within the body. Chromatherapy focuses on directing light at the root of a problem, the opposite of the traditional method of treatment, which is to counteract a disease by treating its symptoms.

Certain electrical devices have been designed for the purpose of producing light rays for therapeutic use. Colored light such as infrared light comforts the body, whereas red light (radiation) inhibits the growth of tumors; ultraviolet light is used to tan the skin, to destroy germs, and to speed up the healing of superficial skin disorders.

To understand how light is transformed into what we distinguish as color, we must look back to the seventeenth century, when Sir Isaac Newton, a young college instructor, accidentally made a revolutionary discovery while investigating ways to improve the telescope. His simple experiment would ultimately forever change the way we perceive color.

The first part of Newton's experiment involved passing sunlight through a glass prism, producing a spectrum of colored light. This light was a rainbow of seven different colors: red, orange, yellow, green, blue, violet, and indigo. During the second part of the experiment, he attempted to pass the colored spectrum through a second prism. He thought this would produce even more colors, but, instead, he was only able to reconstruct the original beam of sunlight. This resulted in his theory that light contained all color and that color was light. Until the time of Newton's experiment, it was believed that color was held in the object that contained it.

Newton, as it turned out, was only partially correct. Light rays, although responsible for color, are not color. Color is based on the reflection of light into the eye, which then transports information to the brain and creates the perception of color as we know it. The part of the eye called the retina is a light-sensitive extension of the brain. The brain analyzes the sensations created by light and interprets it in the mind as color.

The appearance of color is always influenced by surrounding light. The eye adjusts to the intensity of light in a manner similar to that of a camera. In a camera the quantity of light is controlled by the aperture; in the eye, however, light is controlled by the iris. If, in a camera, the amount of light is not sufficient, a different film speed can be used; if the eye needs adjustment a physiological mechanism corrects the perception of light. This is called "chromatic adaptation." Three types of receptors called cones (there are seven million of them located in the retina) are sensitive to different spectral sectors of light. Cones sensitive to longer wavelengths, for example, see red; cones that are sensitive to medium wavelengths see green; and cones that are sensitive to short wavelengths see blue.

In addition to the cones, there are cells called rods in the retina. Rods help determine the difference in brightness. They are thin photoreceptors that respond to low levels of illumination and are like tiny antennae. There are approximately 15,000 rods in one square millimeter of retina. These cells receive light rays, allowing optical impressions to occur. These impressions are carried to the brain by nerves, bringing about the sensory perception of color.

Nature creates colors by reflecting certain wavelengths and filtering out others. This process is accomplished by molecules (photopigments) that selectively absorb and reflect particular parts of the light spectrum. The color of an object results from two factors: the way in which the object absorbs and reflects light and the type of light that makes the object visible. When light illuminates an object, some of the light rays are absorbed, while others are reflected. The reflected light rays are what gives the object its color quality. For instance, let us look at the color of a lemon. A lemon absorbs all the colors of the spectrum except yellow; therefore it is the color yellow that it reflects. White objects reflect almost all the colors in light; black objects reflect none of them.

The second factor that gives objects color is the light illuminating them. The color of objects can be influenced by light that has been altered by passing through a window treatment such as a colored curtain, a shade, or stained glass. Evening light or moonlight gives objects a bluish cast, firelight or candlelight (incandescent) gives off a yellowish cast, and fluorescent light gives off a green tint. Because it contains the full spectrum of hues, the light from the noonday sun is considered the purest and vastly colored light.

The light spectrum is a dispersion of light wavelengths that form a progressive series of colors, from red-orange at one end to orange, yellow, green, blue, and violet at the other end. The most familiar light spectrum is the rainbow. On each end of the light spectrum is light wavelengths that are too long or short to be visible. Wavelengths longer than red-orange are known as infrared and produce heat; wavelengths that are shorter than the color violet are known as ultraviolet. The prefix "infra" refers to the warmest end of the spectrum, and the prefix "ultra" refers to the coolest end of the spectrum. Both "infra" and "ultra" are beyond the color spectrum and therefore cannot be perceived by the human eye as having color; however, some of these light rays are visible to other life forms, such as insects, certain birds, and some mammals.

The color distinctions made by the human eye are categorized as primary colors, fundamental primary colors, and pigment primary colors. Red, yellow, blue, green, black, and white are known as the fundamental primaries; because visual reproduction of black light creates shadows while white light allows objects to appear closer, both black and white are considered primaries because their qualities define objects. Red, yellow, and blue are referred to as the pigment primaries. In theory all colors can be produced by mixing any or all of these three hues together.

The normal eye sees three sets of color pairs: light and dark, red and green, and yellow and blue. An individual who sees all three of these color sets is called a trichromat, and a person who is only able to see just two of these color systems is called a dichromat. A monochromat is a person who can only distinguish light from dark. This limited ability to react to light is referred to as color blindness and is found more often in men than in women. It has been estimated that as many as 7 percent of men are affected by either color blindness or some other form of color weakness, while less than 1 percent of women are affected. In many instances partial color distinction is hereditary. Persons who have only the color receptors for yellow and blue are considered red-blind; persons who have problems perceiving all colors (causing them to confuse colors such as red, blue-green, and gray) are considered green-blind.

While man has always been surrounded by color in nature, it really was not until the nineteenth century that we were able to produce the number of dyes and pigments available to us today. Before then, richly colored fabrics or materials were only available to the most affluent. Now, with the use of coal-tar derivatives and metallic oxides, any object can be stained, painted, or colored either wholly or in part. As a result of color technology color is everywhere, and today we are subjected to literally thousands of color messages daily.

Color has become an integral part of all of our lives because of its psychological effect. When vibrations of light enter the eye certain impulses are conveyed to the brain. The brain then transmits these impulses, and we are affected, regardless of our mental attitude at the time of the exposure. We are constantly struggling to orient ourselves to color whether we are aware of it or not. The effect of light on the brain, in fact, is so powerful that it can even affect our perception of time. The influence of green or blue lights can cause us to underestimate time, whereas red or orange lights can make time seem as if it is passing slower, as anyone who has ever waited for a red traffic light to change can attest.

Color is a powerful instructional tool. One of the many ways color is used in our society is to communicate instructions to motorists. To a driver, a red traffic light means stop, a green traffic light means go, and a yellow traffic signal means slow down and proceed with caution. A sidewalk curb painted green indicates that a car must not be parked in that space for more than 10 minutes or the owner of the automobile will be cited. Color is also used to define space by placing an emphasis on a specific area. For example, a blue curb indicates that the painted area is reserved for the handicapped only, and a yellow curb specifies that only certain vehicles with special permits can park at all. Parking garages also use colored signs to indicate the appropriate direction in which to drive, where to exit by way of the stairs or elevator, and where we left our car.

Before we are even aware of it, color acts on our subconscious. The feelings that are generated by our response to color produce a wide variety of reactions. We cannot prevent being affected by color since light is constantly being reflected back to us by our surroundings. The presence of this continuous stimulus can result in harmony or confusion, can create excitement, or can cause depression. For example, most of us can identify with the feeling of joy when the sun comes out after a series of gloomy, overcast days. It brightens up the sky, turning it a light blue color, and all that extra light makes the colors in nature appear more vivid. The air itself somehow seems to be crispier and cleaner, and we tend to feel refreshed and renewed. A bright sunny day will enliven the spirit and quicken the muscles and organs of the body, while a dark, gloomy, overcast day will most likely tend to depress the spirit and make us feel less alert and even somewhat sluggish.

We also strongly associate temperature with color. Pale colors are considered lighter and cooler, while warmer, richer, darker, colors carry more weight and create a feeling of heat. Imagine checking into a hotel suite in Anchorage, Alaska, during the freezing winter months and finding that the color scheme used to decorate your room is made up of only cool colors, icy blues and the palest shades of green. The walls of the room, including the window treatments, all the furnishings, as well as the upholstery and the bedspread are all in these cool colors. This color scheme would actually make the temperature in the room seem colder than it really is, and you probably would not feel very warm or cozy. Now imagine the same hotel suite decorated in vibrant, warm colors such as yellow, yellow-orange, and orange. Just envisioning a room decorated in those sunny, warm colors can make you feel warm in comparison. Warm colors, whether used to decorate a room or worn as clothing make people feel more comfortable.

Man's acknowledgment of color's powerful effect on the subconscious has encouraged many small businesses and large corporations to engage the services of advertising companies. These advertising companies have conducted extensive marketing research to determine which colors have the greatest possible effect on today's consumer. The results of these studies confirm what had always been suspected; certain colors are loaded with hidden meanings. Blue, white, and green for example, are colors that are associated most often with cleanliness; therefore most packages that contain products for disinfection and hygiene are designed with these colors. Pale yellow, certain yellowish greens, pale green, tan, brown, vermilion, and orange are used to color food because these colors tend to stimulate the appetite.

The human eye is most naturally attracted by striking, bold colors. This is why bright colors are used most frequently to grab the consumer's attention. Because of today's competitive market color has become the number one sales tool worldwide, drawing the eyes of the consumer to a multitude of different products.

Our ideas and associations with color result from social conditioning. Research has revealed that persons who belong to the same culture react in much the same way when exposed to certain colors. For example, warmer colors tested as more attractive to persons of Spanish, French, Italian, Portuguese, and Mexican cultures, while cooler colors were preferred by the English, Irish, Norwegian, and Americans. Colors such as yellow, red, orange, and green were proven to produce the strongest effect on persons of all nationalities and were voted the most popular. Researchers concluded from their experiments that color in general has the capability of expressing a very powerful pictorial language that can be used to amplify subliminal messages.

In our culture, bright, vibrant colors are symbolic of good health, vitality, and constant activity. Cheerful, vivid colors are frequently worn by models and actors in magazine advertisements and television commercials to promote athletic equipment, sporting goods, vitamins, and other health aids. High intensity, brightly colored uniforms are worn by professional athletes as well as weekend sports enthusiasts. Warm hues, as a general rule, tend to raise our spirits and stimulate us to be more active. Psychologists have reported that young children who were tested in brightly painted rooms achieved higher I.Q. scores than those tested in drab, colorless, dark rooms. The benefits, then, of having child-care centers, preschools, and elementary educational facilities decorated in bright yellow, orange, green, and blue color schemes would seem to be obvious.

Extroverts (individuals with outgoing personality traits) tend to lean toward warmer, attention-getting colors, while introverts, who are shy, shun flamboyant colors and favor cool colors that are more in keeping with their personality type. Beige, tan, ivory, and off-white make us feel more subdued and quiet than colors such as red, orange, and yellow, which make us feel assertive and more active. Dark colors tend to represent authority and appear conservative, like the policeman's navy blue uniform or the long, black robe traditionally worn by a judge during trial. Conservative colors such as traditional beige, camel, brown, taupe, gray, charcoal, black, and navy-blue are predominantly worn by career men and women employed by cautious corporations with strict dress codes who frown on their executives wearing loud or garish colors during business hours.

Soft colors, light blues and soothing green tones, are considered restful colors by many health-care professionals, which is why so many hospitals and physician's offices are decorated in these hues. These colors promote rest and relaxation, and, as a result, many professionals involved in health care believe their presence can speed up the healing process and aid in a quicker recovery.

In religion color also plays a significant role. Christianity, for example, recognizes the following five canonical hues: white, the symbol of light — innocence, purity, joy, and glory; red, symbol of fire and blood — charity and generous sacrifice; green, symbol of nature — hope of eternal life; purple, gloomy cast of the mortified — affliction and melancholy; black, symbol of death — and sorrow. Even astrology uses color to define the twelve signs of the zodiac: Aries, red; Taurus, green; Gemini, brown; Cancer, silver; Leo, gold; Virgo, variegated colors; Libra, clear green; Scorpio, vermilion; Sagittarius, sky blue; Capricorn, black; Aquarius, gray; Pisces, sea blue. Other popular color associations are red — piety and sincerity; gold — honor and loyalty; green — with youth and hope; white or silver — with faith and purity; purple — with royalty and rank; and black — grief and endurance. From these few examples it is clear that color has an enormous impact on our thinking, and so on our lives.

THE COLOR WHEEL

Colorists reproduced the spectral band of colors in the form of a circle to make it more convenient to work with color. Every camouflage therapist should have a color wheel on hand to refer to during camouflage therapy. The color wheel is to the clinical cosmetician what the stethoscope is to the doctor, scissors are to the tailor, and the drill is to the dentist.

The color wheel has two distinct divisions, a warm side that centers around the color orange and a cool side that centers around the color blue. The hues are summarized as follows: starting at the top of the color wheel is the color yellow, and proceeding clockwise, yellow-green, green, green-blue, blue, blue-violet, violet at the base of the wheel, red-violet, red, red-orange, orange, yellow–orange, and again back to yellow.

COLOR SCHEMES

Color schemes allow both you and the patient an opportunity to use a sense of order when working with color as a camouflage tool. Most typical color schemes fall into one of two separate categories, related or contrasting.

Related Color Schemes

A related color scheme is a combination of several colors near each other on the color wheel, used together. Harmony can be easily created with color when one or more closely related hues are skillfully combined.

A monochromatic color scheme evolves when variations of just one color are used. The hue is lightened by tinting with white or darkened by shading with gray or black. Because only one color is used, unity and harmony are almost always guaranteed. To avoid monotony, combine this color scheme with diversified values and intensities, and incorporate interesting textures and patterns.

Analogous color schemes have a little more variety than monochromatic because they are based on three or more hues containing a common color. Using the color wheel, you select any color segment of the wheel that is less than halfway around it. For example: if blue were to be used as the common color, the neighboring, closely related colors would be blue-green, blue-violet, and violet, because they all contain some degree of blue. See Figure 5-1.

Contrasting Color Schemes

A contrasting color scheme is based on creating drama and interest by combining colors that are far apart or opposite each other on the color wheel. See Figure 5-2. The camouflage therapist and the patient can use this type of color scheme to divert attention away from the patient's disfigurement by establishing another point of interest with color.

A complementary color scheme is created when any two colors directly opposite each other on the color wheel are

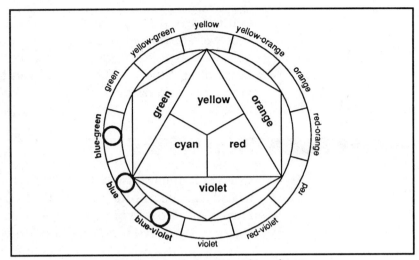

Figure 5-1. Analogous color scheme

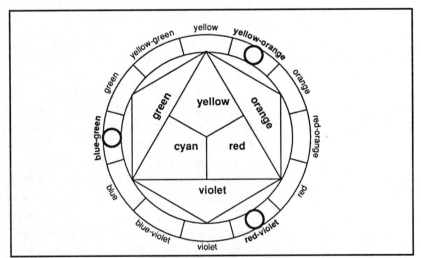

Figure 5-2. Contrasting color scheme

used together, Figure 5-3. Possible color combinations could be red and green, orange and blue, or yellow and violet.

Double-complementary color schemes are built on two sets of complements, two colors next to each other on the color wheel incorporated with the two colors positioned opposite on the color wheel. See Figure 5-4. Blue and blue-green combined with their complements orange and red-orange is an example of a double complementary color scheme.

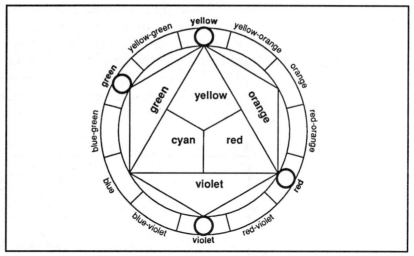

Figure 5-3. Complementary color scheme

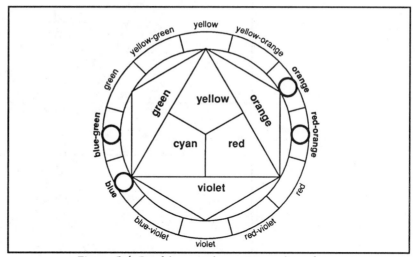

Figure 5-4. Double complementary color scheme

Split-complementary color schemes evolve from combining a color with two colors opposite each side of that color's complement color. See Figure 5-5. For example, the complement of yellow is violet; to create a split complementary color scheme using yellow you would look to each side of violet and select those colors. The result would be a color scheme that combined yellow with red-violet and blue-violet.

Triad color schemes are established by combining three colors that are equally distant each other on the color wheel.

See Figure 5-6. A good example of a triad color scheme would be the combination of yellow, red, and blue.

Tetrad color schemes are developed when any four colors are combined that are equally spaced from each other on the color wheel. See Figure 5-7. An excellent example of a tetrad color scheme would be yellow-orange combined with green, blue-violet, and red.

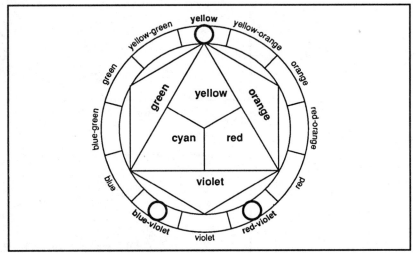

Figure 5-5. Split complementary color scheme

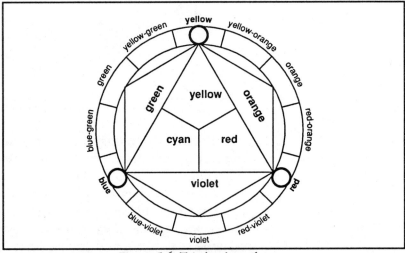

Figure 5-6. Triad color scheme

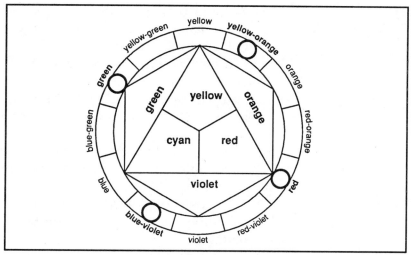

Figure 5-7. Tetrad color scheme

MIXING COSMETIC PIGMENTS

Many outside influences must be taken into account when mixing cosmetic pigments. Consideration must be given to the lighting the patient will be seen in, the characteristics of the surrounding skin tone (ruddiness, freckled, or thin skin outside of the area being treated), and the texture. (A smooth skin texture will reflect light differently than a textured area, making it difficult to camouflage a scar with just one color). For these reasons the major considerations when mixing colors are a camouflage therapist with good eyesight, having the ideal light source present, and addressing difficulties that might arise from color matching areas that are textually different.

Adequate Eyesight Since our state of health can affect our perception of color, disorders such as headaches, colds, or fever can cause us to see colors differently than they actually appear. The results of countless scientific experiments have proven that loud noises, strong odors, and tastes can also affect our ability to perceive colors properly. Eyestrain or fatigue must be carefully guarded against by the camouflage therapist because it is easy to unconsciously abuse the eyes while performing such precise color work. The eyes should be rested between color matches by looking at a piece of black cloth (preferably felt or velvet) or by closing the eyes momentarily in between color matches. Tension or mental strain can also impair color vision. All sense of urgency and fearfulness over obtaining the perfect color match should be discarded while engaging in exacting color blending work.

In order to ensure success when combining cover cream colors you should first familiarize yourself with the pigments you will be working with. Each cosmetic manufacturer will have a different range of colors mixed in different vehicle binders. The base to which pigment has been added will affect the appearance of that pigment; therefore, vision, understanding, and practice are important requisites in mastering the art of color mixing.

You will need to have a clear understanding of the particular colors you will be mixing together to obtain the color match desired. To evaluate what colors were used to make up the flesh tones in your cover creams, have a colorist depigment your makeup palettes and cover cream shades for you. This process breaks down the pigments that make up the more popular skin tone colors. The colorist will match the pigments with oil paints. (Usually two or three different pigments will be used to make up one of the cover cream shades.) You will notice that most of your cover cream colors can be matched by blending different variations of artist's paint in colors such as gold and yellow ochre, raw sienna, Naples yellow, mars brown, Davy's gray, and white.

A more complete understanding of pigment in cover creams can be reached by evaluating these color mixtures and by basic analysis and deduction of what is just the right amount of each pigment required to result in the same color as the cover cream. You will become more experienced mixing colors as you practice combining different color combinations.

Lighting

Consideration must be given to the light source that the patient will be viewed in during the time he or she will be wearing cover creams. When mixing cosmetic colors to match the patient's skin tone, remember that incandescent lighting, or any lighting with warm tones, will intensify red, yellow, and orange hues and neutralize violet and blue. Fluorescent or any lighting with green or blue tones will intensify violet, blue, or green and will neutralize warmer hues such as red, yellow, or orange. Be sure to have a suitable lighting system that will accommodate color blending for all lighting situations.

Texture One of the most difficult problems you will encounter in color matching is caused by differences in skin texture on different areas of the patient's body. Certain areas will appear quite different from others because of their refractive indexes (the bending of a ray of light when it passes from one medium to another) and the skin's color absorption qualities. Atrophic (inverted) scars or hypertrophic (raised) scars will be more difficult to conceal because the edges at the base of the scar are on a flat plane and reflect light differently than the raised or indented scarred area. The color of rough or irregular skin texture will also appear quite different because of the way these textured skin surfaces absorb light. When working on this type of scarring always tell the patient beforehand that you anticipate these problems and that you will need to conduct some preliminary experiments with several cover cream color combinations before you will be able to obtain the best results.

COLOR TERMS

Specific terminology is associated with the study of color just as medicine has its own language. Complete knowledge of color depends on understanding the correct definitions of commonly used terms. To clearly comprehend color, you must become familiar with the language of color. The following definitions will help you to expand your color vocabulary.

Achromatic — devoid of color, colorless.

Achromatic adaptation — the visual adjustment to altered light qualities.

Acuity — the capacity to discriminate fine details of objects.

Advancing colors — colors that give the illusion of coming forward. Warm colors with a predominating red-orange pigment are advancing colors.

After-image colors — a visual effect occurring after light has been removed.

Analogous colors — colors closely related to one another because they all share the same primary color.

Color — the way the brain interprets the wavelength distribution of light entering the eye. This general sensation perceived by the eye and the mind includes all hues, tints, tones, and shades.

Color blindness — a disorder of the retinal cones in the eye, which results in the inability to discriminate between certain colors, an inherited trait. The most common form of color blindness is dichromatism, sensitivity to only two distinct colors. The ability to distinguish all three colors is needed to match all the colors in the spectrum.

Color constancy — the tendency to perceive a familiar object under different light conditions.

Coloring strength — the strength of a pigment in coloring a light or white base.

Compatibility — pigments are considered compatible when they are chemically capable of blending well with one another and existing in a base without producing a harmful reaction.

Complementary colors — any two colors that have nothing in common and are opposite each other on the color wheel. A mixture of any two primary colors is the complement color of the remaining primary color. When two complements are mixed together in equal amounts they will produce neutral gray.

Cool colors — colors in which blue predominates. These are considered cool because of their association with ice, water, sky, etc.

Cones — photoreceptor cells in the retina that provide sensitivity to detail.

Cornea — the cornea is the transparent part of the coat of the eyeball. It covers the iris and the pupil and is a part of the eye's focusing system.

Cosmetic colors — colors that are given names by cosmetic companies to define makeup shades for foundations, eye shadows, lipsticks, and blushers.

Dark and light adaptation — the eye's ability to adjust to changing light conditions. This adjustment is made possible by changes in the size of the pupil.

Dark colors — colors low in value, usually pertaining to hues that are shaded with black or gray.

**Plate 1.
Herpes
Simplex.**

*Courtesy
of
Timothy
Berger,
M.D.*

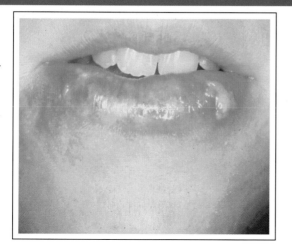

**Plate 4.
Acne.**

*Courtesy
of
Timothy
Berger,
M.D.*

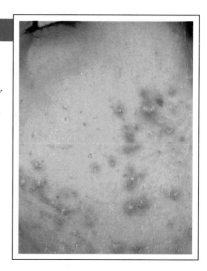

**Plate 2.
Impetigo.**

*Courtesy
of
Timothy
Berger,
M.D.*

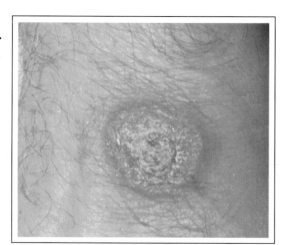

**Plate 5.
Comedo-
nal Acne.**

*Courtesy
of
Timothy
Berger,
M.D.*

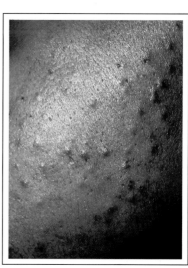

**Plate 3.
Psoriasis.**

*Courtesy
of
Timothy
Berger,
M.D.*

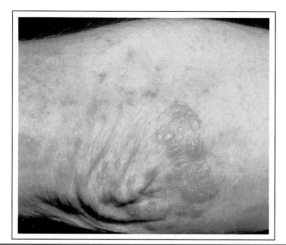

**Plate 6.
Acne
Rosacea.**

*Courtesy
of
Timothy
Berger,
M.D.*

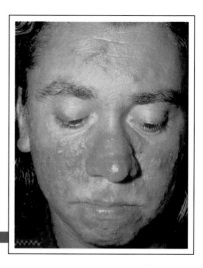

Plate 7. Discoid Lupus with hair loss.

Courtesy of Timothy Berger, M.D.

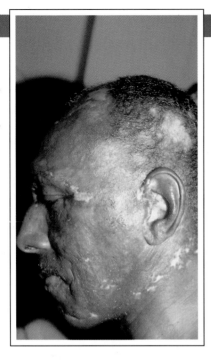

Plate 10. Hypopig-mentation.

Courtesy of Timothy Berger, M.D.

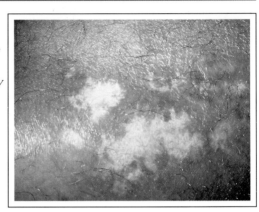

Plate 8. Basal Cell Carcino-ma.

Courtesy of Timothy Berger, M.D.

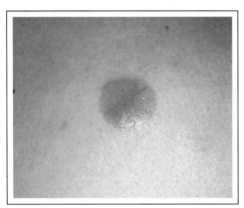

Plate 11. Hyperpig-mentation.

Courtesy of Timothy Berger, M.D.

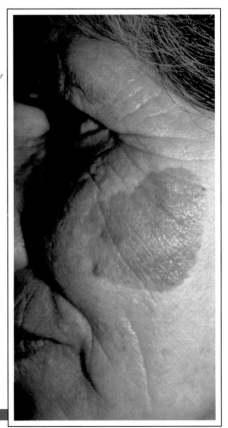

Plate 9. Squamous Cell Carcino-ma.

Courtesy of Timothy Berger, M.D.

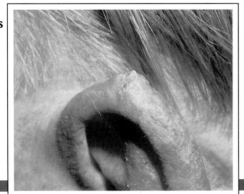

Plate 12.
Dark
Circles.

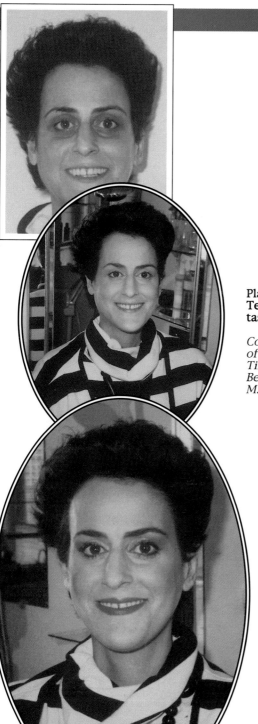

Plate 13.
Dark
circles,
normal-
ized cos-
metic
applica-
tion.

Plate 14.
Dark
circles,
enhance-
ment
makeup.

Plate 15.
Melasma.

*Courtesy
of
Timothy
Berger,
M.D.*

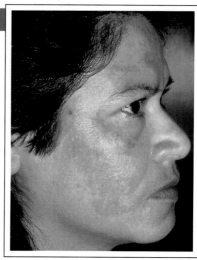

Plate 16.
Telangec-
tasia.

*Courtesy
of
Timothy
Berger,
M.D.*

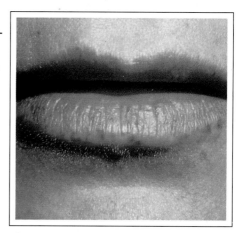

Plate 17.
Acne
Rosacea.

*Courtesy
of
Timothy
Berger,
M.D.*

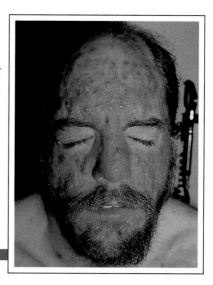

**Plate 18.
Portwine
stain —
before.**

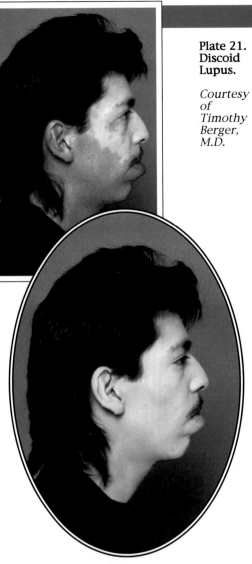

**Plate 21.
Discoid
Lupus.**

*Courtesy
of
Timothy
Berger,
M.D.*

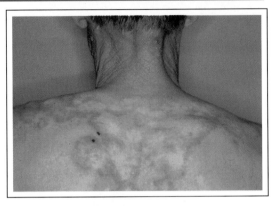

**Plate 19.
Portwine
stain --
after.**

**Plate 22.
Contact
Derma-
titis --
Poison
Oak.**

*Courtesy
of
Timothy
Berger,
M.D.*

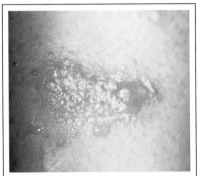

**Plate 23.
Seborrhea.**

*Courtesy
of
Timothy
Berger,
M.D.*

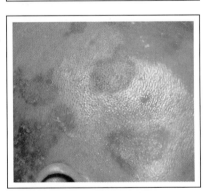

**Plate 20.
Acne
scarring.**

*Courtesy
of
Timothy
Berger,
M.D.*

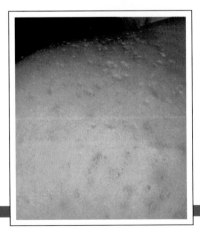

**Plate 24.
Photoder-
matitis.**

*Courtesy
of
Timothy
Berger,
M.D.*

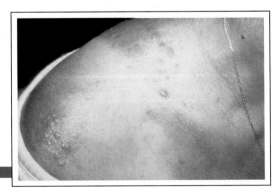

Deep colors — colors that are strong in pigment with no apparent presence of black.

Diffused light — scattered or dispersed light that is extended over a considerable area or space.

Dominant color — a superior color that dominates.

Double split-complementary — all four points of the color wheel are embraced to create this harmony. Two complements are chosen, and the colors on both sides of each of those complements are used to create a color scheme. For example, one of the complements chosen is yellow and the other is violet. The two neighboring colors to yellow are orange and yellow green; when these are combined with the two neighboring colors to violet (purple and blue violet), they create what is called a double split-complementary.

Dull colors — dull colors are those colors that have been grayed and muted, such as dusty blue or dusty pink.

Earth tones — colors formulated by the influence of nature, relating to the brown color family.

Focal point — the center of interest.

Full color — a color that is pure.

Glare — a harsh, dazzling light or reflection.

Hue — a label used to distinguish one color from another; a synonym for color.

Intensity — the impact a color makes, its force, strength, and saturation.

Iris — the eye tissue behind the cornea that contracts, regulating the amount of light entering the eye.

Irradiation — the optical illusion created when a bright object appears against a dark background and the object appears larger than it actually is.

Lifting tone — changing the general character or quality of a color by lighting it with another color other than white.

Light — a small band in the electromagnetic spectrum, with wavelengths ranging from approximately 400 to 700 millimicrons, containing all of the visible colors. The electromagnetic spectrum includes radio and x-ray as well.

Medium value — a color that is between a light and a dark color.

Monochromatic — the use of one color in different shades.

Munsell color system — a system that arranges or assigns colors by numbers and letters.

Neutral — a dull or grayed color of medium value that is neither warm nor cool.

Nuance — a small degree of difference in a color.

Opacity — the quality or state of being opaque.

Opaque — colors that are opaque are said to be incapable of being penetrated or affected by light. Certain reds and yellows have unusual opacity.

Optical illusion — a visual perception in which there is an unusual discrepancy between the real object and the perceived object.

Pale — having a light value of color and lacking in intensity.

Palette — a board made of wood, porcelain, or metal, on which pigments are arranged and mixed.

Pigment — coloring matter made of animal, vegetable, or mineral, used to impart visible color. The term comes from the Latin word "pigmentum," meaning "paint."

Photopigments — molecules that favor different wavelengths of light by absorbing or reflecting them.

Photoreceptors — cells located at the back of the retina that contain light-sensitive pigments. When light is absorbed by these pigments they undergo a reaction that triggers nerve impulses, resulting directly in vision.

Primary colors — primary colors are the colors considered most important. To an interior designer, an artist, painter, chemist, and printer, they are crimson red, yellow, and blue, and are the colors from which all other colors are made.

Pupil — the hole in the center of the iris that controls the amount of light passing to the interior of the eye. The size of the opening is governed by the iris.

Receding colors — colors that appear distant, that seem to move back or away from the observer. Cool colors in which blue predominates are receding colors.

Refractive index — the degree of speed of light in air compared to the speed of light in another substance. It is a measurement that varies with each light ray. For example, red has the least refractive index, while violet has the greatest. Dark object surfaces absorb light, and light object surfaces reflect light. Transparent surfaces bend or reflect light. All are examples of refractive index.

Retina — the innermost layer of the eye, and the location of light-sensitive rods and cones.

Rods — straight, slender photoreceptors that respond to low levels of light that reflect back black and white responses.

Saturation — a way of referring to the intensity or purity of a color. One measure of a color's richness is the amount of white or gray found in the mixture.

Secondary colors — any two primary colors combined will create a secondary color. For example, yellow and red will produce orange, and blue and yellow will produce green. Orange and green are secondary colors.

Sensation — the visual perception of color caused by the stimuli of light on the mind through the eye.

Shade — darkness or dimness of illumination that darkens the value of a color. Dark colors are referred to as shades. This term is also used to denote color.

Sheen — the quality or condition of shining by reflected light. A subdued luster.

Simultaneous contrast — the visual effect caused by colors being influenced by other colors situated near or next to them.

Spectral colors — the rainbow of colors produced when a ray of sunlight is passed through a prism.

Spectrum — a series of colors formed (a rainbow) when white light is dispersed into its components. Each component is a different wavelength of light, producing a different optical effect. The result is a progressive series of hues beginning with red-orange at one end, progressing through orange, yellow, green, blue, and ending with violet.

Split-complementary — a split-complementary is a color scheme created by combining a key color with the two colors that are next to its complement. For example, if the key color is yellow, its complement is violet. On one side of violet is red-violet, and on the other side is blue-violet; therefore the split-complementary would be the three colors yellow, red-violet, and blue violet.

Surface color — the outside color of a material object.

Texture — the feel and appearance of a surface; also the effect of certain methods of pigment application.

Tint — a pale or light value of a color that has been altered by the addition of white. Colors of light values are referred to as tints.

Tone — an intermediate hue. A degree of color on the value scale.

Transparent — clear enough to permit light to pass through. Some pigments have this transparent quality.

Triadic colors — colors such as red, yellow, and blue that form a equilateral triangle on the color wheel. Triadic colors are the most effective if only one color is allowed to dominate.

Undertone — a low, subdued tone that bleeds through other colors on top of it, altering their effect.

Value — the lightness or darkness of a color, its tendency to reflect or absorb light.

Vehicle — the medium that holds a pigment and makes it adhere to a surface.

Vivid — the brightness or the intensity of a color.

Warm colors — red-orange hues. They are referred to as warm colors not only because of their association with heat (such as the sun and fire) but also because they actually radiate heat, which can be demonstrated by a very sensitive thermometer.

Wavelength — the measurable distance between vibrations of light that produce visible color sensations on the retina. Red-orange has the longest wavelength, and violet the shortest. The wavelengths that are longer than red-orange are called infrared, and the wavelengths shorter than violet are called ultraviolet.

REVIEW

You should now be familiar with:

- the theory of color.
   a. dispersion of light wavelengths.
   b. how we perceive color.
- the psychological effects of color.
- systematic organization of color.
- mixing cosmetic pigment.
- color terminology.

6 Materials

In this chapter, materials and equipment that will be needed by the clinical esthetician/cosmetologist to provide a patient with a camouflage treatment will be reviewed. Physical requirements, such as the setup of the treatment room, its furnishings, as well as the appropriate lighting systems, will be discussed.

The clinical esthetician/cosmetologist will need to be familiar with the wide variety of cover creams on the market. This understanding is necessary in order to be able to perform camouflage therapy. A list of the various camouflage solutions and their manufacturers is also provided for each reference.

MATERIALS CHECKLIST

The camouflage therapist will need to equip him- or herself properly with the materials needed to perform cosmetic procedures. He or she will also need to know where to obtain them. The following table will provide that information.

Sterilization Materials to Sanitize Implements

MATERIAL:	AVAILABLE AT:
Ethyl alcohol (70%)	Drugstore
Quaternary ammonium compounds (QUATS)	Beauty supply
Autoclave system	Medical supply
Ultraviolet light	Beauty/Medical supply

Skin Care Supplies

MATERIAL:	AVAILABLE AT:
Cleanser - (oil in water) (water in oil)	Distributor, Department store, Pharmacy

Sunscreens, SPF 15 or higher (UVA and UVB protection)	Pharmacy, Department store, Distributor
Astringent and toner	Beauty supply, Distributor, Department store, Pharmacy
Moisturizer (Aging, dry, oily skin)	Beauty supply, Distributor Department Store, Pharmacy

Cosmetics and Makeup Implements

MATERIAL:	AVAILABLE AT:
Synthetic and sable brushes Dusting powder brush, Flat-tipped contouring brush, Blush brush, Artist's flat paintbrush, Flat angle eye-shadow brush, Oval tapered eye-shadow brush, Sponge eye-shadow applicators, Two-sided eyebrow brush and comb, Firm eyebrow brush, Lip-lining brush, Brush cleaner	Theatrical makeup store, Beauty supply
Wedge disposable sponges	Beauty supply, Department store, Pharmacy
Powder blusher	Beauty supply, Distributor, Department store, Pharmacy
Cream rouge	Same as above
Lipsticks	Same as above
Lip-lining pencils	Same as above
Powder shadows, matte only	Same as above
Eyebrow pencils (in blonde, taupe, gray, light brown, dark brown, and black)	Same as above
False eyelashes (individual and strip upper and lower)	Theatrical makeup or hair replacement center
Artificial eyebrows (in blonde, auburn, brown, gray, and black)	Same as above

Crepe hair (for eyebrows, mustaches, and beards)	Same as above
Mustaches (blonde, brown, auburn, gray, black)	Theatrical makeup or hair replacement center
Eyelash and brow dye (black and brown)	Beauty supply
Eyedrops	Pharmacy
Petroleum jelly	Pharmacy
Liquid mascara waterproof (black and brown)	Beauty supply, Distributor, Department store
Cake mascara (black and brown)	Beauty Supply, Distributor, Department store

Disposable Items

MATERIAL:	AVAILABLE AT:
Small plastic spatulas	Beauty supply
Cotton swabs Roll of cotton	Pharmacy
Latex exam gloves	Medical supply

MAKEUP KIT

The camouflage therapist will need a storage kit for his or her camouflage materials. The most efficient portable container for all your supplies is a large tackle or tool box with separate compartments. The sectional trays will allow the clinical esthetician/cosmetologist to transport his or her camouflage materials without spilling or breaking them. Make sure that the kit you choose is large enough to hold all your makeup tools, with additional space for extra items.

If the camouflage therapist is not planning to move his or her materials outside his or her treatment area, it is not necessary to house makeup or supplies in a portable container.

ROOM EQUIPMENT

While camouflage therapy can be done anywhere, the procedures described in this textbook are the result of a practice performed in several medical institutions over the past five years and are based on that standard. The room and the procedures reflect the highest standards in patient treatment.

Patients who seek out cosmetic therapy are suffering from a condition that has caused them emotional discomfort and embarrassment. They may have experienced humiliation and rejection as they searched through department stores and drugstores to find a cosmetic solution for their specific problems. These individuals have come to the camouflage therapist either by a referral from a physician or on their own. Whether it is a temporary or permanent condition, the immediate need is the same: The patient needs to feel that he or she is no longer being stared at and that he or she has finally found a place that offers a real solution for the problem. Therefore, one of the most important considerations in performing camouflage is to create a private environment where the patient will feel comfortable enough to concentrate on the instructions given. This can be done by setting aside a private area in a hospital, doctor's office, or salon. Ideally, this is a separate room that accommodates all of the equipment and supplies required without the esthetician having to leave the patient alone in the room.

Physical requirements, such as the setup of the treatment room, its furnishings, as well as appropriate photographic and lighting systems, are discussed below.

THE ROOM

Figure 6–1 shows an example of a room set up within a clinic or physician's office: The room should be a separate area where privacy can be maintained for the patient.

The treatment area should include the following items:

1. *Makeup station with mirror:* A makeup station is a work space similar to that used in the theater for the application of stage makeup. The counter provides a flat surface to work from with storage drawers and cabinets underneath to hold supplies. Attached to the counter is a wall-mounted mirror with three lighting panels — one on top and one on each side. A standard

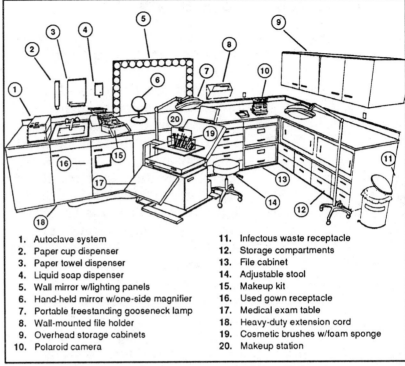

1. Autoclave system
2. Paper cup dispenser
3. Paper towel dispenser
4. Liquid soap dispenser
5. Wall mirror w/lighting panels
6. Hand-held mirror w/one-side magnifier
7. Portable freestanding gooseneck lamp
8. Wall-mounted file holder
9. Overhead storage cabinets
10. Polaroid camera
11. Infectous waste receptacle
12. Storage compartments
13. File cabinet
14. Adjustable stool
15. Makeup kit
16. Used gown receptacle
17. Medical exam table
18. Heavy-duty extension cord
19. Cosmetic brushes w/foam sponge
20. Makeup station

Figure 6-1. Room set up within a clinic

panel can hold up to six non-heating bulbs. Several types of bulbs can be used to produce different lighting effects. A warm, fluorescent lighting system will imitate natural daylight, while fluorescent bulbs recreate an office environment. (See lighting in the color chapter.) No more than 17–40 watt bulbs should be used around the mirror. A dimmer can also be used to soften or intensify the lighting used during the application of camouflage makeup.

2. *Two portable goose-neck lamps:* Goose-neck lamps are used in conjunction with the stationary lighting system to further highlight a patient's face and neck area, and in cases when the stationary lighting is not satisfactory, such as parts of the body. Portable lamps are essential in cases where the clinical esthetician/ cosmetologist will not have access to a stationary system. Optimally, a goose-neck lamp would be placed on each side of the patient, providing maximum lighting.

3. *A small, portable, lighted makeup mirror with daylight, office, and evening lighting panels designed into the unit:* This unit can be used in place of the stationary mirror and lighting system and can be transported easily when performing camouflage therapy in several locations. It is important to remember that lighting is a crucial factor in the success of camouflage work, since makeup tones will change depending on the patient's environment. Take the time to experiment with different lighting systems and make sure you can recreate various environments, including daylight, office, home, and evening.

4. *A double-faced hand mirror, with one side a magnifier:* The hand-held mirror is used by the patient to view the application of the camouflage techniques used during the treatment.

5. *File cabinets:* One file cabinet should be large enough to keep an inventory of all the products and supplies needed to perform camouflage therapy. A second cabinet will provide enough space to file all the required documentation on a patient in an efficient and organized manner.

6. *Utility table:* It will be helpful to have a portable table to keep extra materials close at hand during the appointment.

7. *Extension cord:* An extension cord for the goose-neck lamps and for the portable makeup mirror will be needed.

8. *Waste disposal:* Two separate waste disposal units will be needed; one for hazardous waste (which the hospital or doctor's office should already have), and a regular waste receptacle for tissue and disposable materials.

EQUIPMENT AND INSTRUMENTS

For easy reference, a table is provided below of all the instruments and equipment needed to set up a camouflage treatment area and where these supplies can be purchased.

MATERIALS NEEDED

PRODUCT	WHERE TO OBTAIN
Medical exam table or facial lounge chair	Beauty or medical supply company
Makeup station and wall-mounted mirror with lighting panels, using 17–40 watt warm fluorescent bulbs on top and sides only	Lighting and fixture supply company
Two portable free-standing goose-neck lamps with warm fluorescent bulbs	Hospital supply company
Two file cabinets for makeup storage and patient files	Office supply store
Hand-held mirror with one-side magnifier	Drugstore, Beauty supply
Extension cord	Hardware store
High-backed director's chair	Furniture store, Beauty supply
Trash receptacle (for hazardous waste)	Hardware store

CAMOUFLAGE COVER CREAMS

Cover creams vary in thickness, texture, and color depending upon the manufacturer. Certain cosmetic manufacturers offer more of a color selection of cover creams than others. Some cosmetic manufacturers offer tints, shades, and color correctors that can be used to alter the cover cream shades that they provide. Different product lines will vary in consistency; some will be heavier, while others will provide lighter coverage. Regardless of the cover cream products you choose, they must be hypo-allergenic, waterproof, opaque, and formulated to adhere to non-absorbent, slick, scar tissue. No one product line can address all the cosmetic needs of each and every patient; therefore, more than one cover cream line of products is recommended. Experiment with the various brands until you are familiar with their strengths and weaknesses. The following information will serve as a resource guide for the clinical esthetician/cosmetologist to obtain the necessary cover creams, both to use in treatment and to give or sell to the patient as a start-up supply.

The camouflage therapist should telephone or write several of the manufacturers for information and a free catalogue or a brochure. Because many new products are in the developmental stage, this list is by no means complete, and should be updated periodically.

- *Ben Nye Company Inc.*
  Mr. Dana Nye, President
  5935 Bowcroft St.
  Los Angeles, CA 90016
  (213) 839-1984
  Coverette base cream foundation is available from Ben Nye Company in four shades; ultra fair, fair, medium, and tan. Two color correctors, Mellow Yellow (a flesh-colored cover cream with strong undertones of yellow to neutralize redness) and Mellow Orange, which conceals bruising and tattoos. Several setting powders are also available: Colorless translucent, fair with pigment; and coco-tan for darker skin tones. Ben Nye also makes an excellent brush cleaner available in bulk size (16 oz.).

- *Cabot's Clear Perfection Corrective Cosmetics*
  1989 West Cabot Cosmetics Association
  Central Islip, NY 11722
  Cabot's cover cream skin system is called "Clear Perfection." It offers eight cover creams with a range of colors from very fair to very dark. Each jar contains 450 units of Vitamin E. They also carry a full line of skin-care products.

- *Corrective Concepts by Pattee Products*
  Pattee Patrik Henderson, Director
  European Crossroads — Bordeaux Building
  2829 West Northwest Highway
  Dallas, TX 75220
  (214) 352-9880
  Corrective Concepts offers a complete line of skin-care products for post-burn patients.

- *Cosmetic Specialty Labs*
  210 Southwest Texas Ave.
  P.O. Box 187
  Lawton, OK 73502
  (800) 654-4507

The Cosmetic Specialty Labs call their cover cream line the best, long-wearing foundation. It comes in ten shades that range in color from Ivory to their darkest shade, called Rachel. The cover cream system includes two types of setting powders, tinted powder (available in four shades), and colorless translucent powder. Coversticks also are available in light, medium, and dark shades. The skin-care line includes a special cleanser for the removal of cover creams, toners, astringents, and moisturizers.

- *Dermablend Corrective Cosmetics*
  N. Craig Roberts, M.D., President
  P.O. Box 3008
  Lakewood, NJ
  (800) 631-2158
  Dermablend cosmetic camouflage system consists of nine different cover cream shades for the face and six for the legs and body. All cosmetics are 100 percent fragrance free. The face creams are packaged in jars; the leg and body makeup is available in tubes. Dermablend also offers "Quick Fix" concealer (stick cover creams) in three shades: light, medium, and dark. Dermablend's setting powder can be ordered in a shaker (loose) dispenser or in a compact (compressed). Both forms are colorless. Maximum Moisturizer sunscreen with a SPF of 15 is also available, as well as a special cover cream cleanser with aloe vera for the removal of the makeup.

- *Dermacolor*
  Christine Heathman, Distributor
  Advanced Aesthetics
  5167 Clayton Rd. Suite D
  Concord, CA 94521
  (800) 676-9667
  Dermacolor offers the widest range of cover cream shades available. Their complete cosmetic line also includes seven tinted setting powders and a colorless translucent. Lipsticks and eye shadows with higher concentrations of pigment can be extremely beneficial in concealing pigmentary problems around the eyes and on the lips. Dermacolor also manufactures its own cleansing removal lotion and moisturizer.

- *Derm Essence, Inc.*
  4901 Marina Blvd.
  Suite 811
  San Diego, CA 92117

(619) 270-1662
(800) 275-3376
Derm Essence distributes a skin-care cosmetic line called Resources that was formulated by a dermatologist. These products are mineral-oil free, will not promote blemishes, are fragrance-free, and are hypo-allergenic. The line includes a gentle facial cleanser, astringent or toner, light day moisturizer, night cream, with high potency amino acids and anti-oxidants, exfoliant scrub, and a sun protector cream that does not contain PABA but blocks U.V.A. and U.V.B. rays for all skin types.

- *Hide and Sleek*
  R..H. Cosmetics
  Richard Soloman, Owner
  80–39th St.
  Brooklyn, NY 11232
  (800) 537-5537
  R.H. Cosmetics formulated a line called *Hide and Sleek*. These cover creams address skin irregularities of every age group, from adolescents with acne to senior citizens. Their cover cream products differ from other lines in that they are waterproof, but do not contain oil. They are completely opaque and contain a PABA-free sunscreen. The line has four shades: fair, beige, tan, and dark. Cover sticks are available in light, medium, and dark. A colorless, translucent powder is also part of their line. Included are four color corrector wands, mint to neutralize red, white as line fill, lavender for neutralizing age spots, and beige for concealing minor imperfections. Beige, alabaster, and mint under-eye concealers can also be used for camouflaging.

- *Fashion Fair Cosmetics*
  820 South Michigan Ave.
  Chicago, IL 60605
  (312) 322-9444
  Fashion Fair manufactures a complexion corrective cream called Cover Tone that conceals a wide range of skin imperfections and flaws, including scars and burn marks, blotches, blemishes, dark undereye circles, age spots, birthmarks, broken capillaries, varicose veins, tatoos, and post-surgery discolorations. Cover Tone is waterproof, compatible with all skin types, non-greasy, and fragrance free. It comes in a range of ten shades from ivory to ebony

brown, to match most skin types. Cover Tone can be blended with different shades to obtain an exact match.

- *Joe Blasco Cosmetics*
  Joe Blasco, President
  1708 Hillhurst Ave.
  Hollywood, CA 90027
  (213) 222-5537
  Joe Blasco manufactures a line of cover creams called Dermaceal. They are available in ten different shades. Because the cream contains 70 percent pigment concentration, it contains less oil and waxes than other cover cream products. The line also includes ten different shades of setting powder. Ultra Formula base offers even more of a selection, with a variety of different shades to choose from in 50 to 55 percent pigment concentration. Six color correctors are also available (three for red undertones and three for blue undertones) to neutralize skin discoloration. Pink, orange, yellow, and dark skin color correctors can be used to counteract undereye and facial shadows. A body makeup is also included in the line, which is designed especially for use on the hands and neck. It is called Hanz-N-Neck. Joe Blasco also makes a brush cleaner available in large economy size or convenient refill sizes if you want to economize.

- *Feather River Company*
  133 Copeland
  Petaluma, CA 94952
  (707) 778-7627
  (800) 762-8873
  Feather River Company is a distributor for several cosmetic and skin-care companies. They have printed a small pamphlet of common ingredients found in most cosmetics and skin products. This glossary will conveniently fit into your portable makeup kit and can be used as a reference guide.

- *Keromask Cover Cream*
  Innoxa Ltd.
  202 Terminus Road
  Eastbourne, Sussex BN21 3DF, England
  0323 639671
  Keromask is produced in eight shades (three cover creams and five foundations for the surrounding areas) along with three pre-mixed shades and a translucent setting powder.

- *IL Makiage Cosmetics*
  Ilana Harkavi, President East Coast
  Ellen Caron, President West Coast
  323 Geary Street, 6th Floor
  San Francisco, CA 94102
  (415) 399-8744
  (800) 722-1011 (New York)
  (800) 685-4673 (San Francisco)
  Twenty years in the business, IL-MAKIAGE is the manufacturer of a comprehensive line of professional cosmetics. Their cover system includes Creme Makiage and Dual Finish, available in five shades each. Both creme and dual finish powder base have matching pigments, are smudge resistant, and have a high meld point for arid and humid climates. The Makiage cosmetic line also contains two color correction systems: TV Touch and Even Tones, with a total of twelve colors. All products contain dimethicone, a pharmaceutical grade carrier that is nonocclusive and maintains a matte finish. Transparent colors are available in thirteen shades ranging from white to natural pigments.

- *Lydia O'Leary/Covermark*
  1 Anderson Ave.
  Moonachie, NJ 07074
  (800) 524-1120
  (201) 460-7713
  Covermark offers fourteen different cover creams in a variety of skin shades, with two setting powders. Face Magic is a line of foundations that contain sunscreens and can be used to mask minor skin problems. Lydia O'Leary's Leg Magic (available in seven different cover cream shades) is a line of camouflage creams designed specifically for the body. Lydia O'Leary/Covermark also manufactures cover creams in pencil applicators (cover-sticks). By writing or calling the company, you will receive a color chart, a full price list, and a brochure on their full line of cosmetic products.

- *Natural Cover Cosmetics*
  Linda Sidel, President
  L.S. Cosmetics
  P.O. Box 32203
  Baltimore, MD 21208
  (301) 664-3010

Natural Cover produces twelve shades of cover creams, eight skin tone shades, and four tints. The line also includes three different shades of coversticks, three shades of powder, and an oil-base cleanser for the removal of cover creams.

- *Spencer Forrest Laboratories, Inc.*
8306 Wilshire Blvd. Penthouse
Beverly Hills, CA 90211
(213) 201-0444
Spencer Forrest Laboratories manufactures a cover cream masking lotion for alopecia patients called COUVRE (pronounced Coovray). Alopecia Masking Lotion is available in the following colors: black, dark brown, medium brown, light brown/blonde, and grey. This product reduces the visibility of fresh scars and grafts on the scalp and provides an alternative for spot baldness other than artificial hair replacement or transplants.

- *Veil*
Annette Hansen, Distributor
Atelier Esthetique
350 Fifth Ave, Suite 3406
New York, NY 10118
(800) 626-1242
Veil differs from other camouflage cosmetics because it is lighter in texture and contains a sunscreen. It is available in nineteen natural skin shades. The line also offers both a white and a black opaque cover cream for tinting and shading, along with green, rose, and yellow cover creams that can be used for mixing, restoring natural skin coloring, or correcting color. A colorless, translucent setting powder is also available.

REVIEW

You should now be familiar with:

- ◼ materials needed to perform cosmetic procedures.
- ◼ how to equip the ideal environment for camouflage therapy.
- ◼ some sources for supplies.

7 Corrective Makeup

Corrective makeup techniques are valuable aids to patients with disfigurements, birthmarks, or any signs of physical trauma that can occur from surgery.

Each patient will have different physical characteristics that will require special cosmetic considerations. This chapter will address how to select the appropriate foundation base for the patient, how to correct and balance facial features using highlighting and contouring techniques, and how to select the right cosmetic shades for each patient.

MAKEUP FOUNDATIONS

The purpose of a foundation base is to provide fresh, even color to give the complexion a brighter, clearer appearance. Cream foundations are better for dry skin, and liquid foundations are better for oily skin. A foundation base can be applied with a slightly damp sponge to give a lighter finish or with a dry sponge to add more color.

There are three predominant skin shades: pink-red undertones, cream-neutral undertones, and olive-golden undertones. If you are in doubt about the patient's coloring, ask him or her to stand before a bright, sunlit window and hold a white sheet of paper next to his or her cheek and look into a hand mirror. The patient should be able to see a reflection of his or her skin undertone on the paper. If his or her coloring does not fall into the pink or olive catagory he or she probably has a creamy undertone.

When selecting makeup foundation, choose a shade in that color family. Be sure that it complements the deepest tones of the patient's skin color. Apply the foundation to the patient's jawline, matching the color to the color of the neck. Make sure that the shade is not so dark that it leaves a line of demarcation or that it isn't so light that the patient's skin will look chalky. Remember, because the foundation in the container is concentrated, it will always appear much darker than when it is applied on the skin. If the patient's complexion is sallow, suggest a pinkish shade or add a small amount of mauve color corrector to the makeup base. If, however, the patient's skin is ruddy, suggest an ivory shade to tone it down or apply a green color corrector to the skin before applying the foundation.

Regardless of the type of foundation base you select, be sure that you inspect the patient's face carefully after applying it, to ensure that you have created a smooth, even finish. The foundation should appear natural and well-blended, without any obvious streaks of color.

Sometimes too much suntanning produces yellow or brownish discoloration around the mouth area or across the bridge of the nose or along the upper lip. The application of a lighter, more opaque foundation in any one of the areas affected will conceal discoloration, producing more even coverage.

BONE STRUCTURE

To create or alter facial features you will need to be familiar with the bone structure of the face. The easiest way to do this is to examine a human skull, concentrating on the facial bones (irregular and angular), which form the framework of the face. See Figure 7-1. One of the most thorough ways in which to learn about the structure of the human form is to take a class in sculpture or anatomy. The *Pocket Atlas of Human Anatomy*, published by Georg Thiem Verlag, Stuttgart and New York, can also be an invaluable aid in providing such clarification.

HIGHLIGHTING AND CONTOURING

The shape of the face can be altered by highlighting and contouring facial features. Creating dimensions with light and dark is the basic principle behind highlighting and contouring. Light brings objects forward, making them appear closer, and dark makes objects recede, making them appear further away.

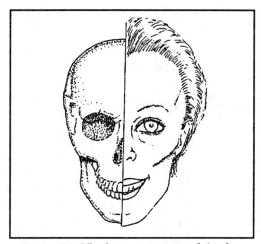

Figure 7-1. The bone structure of the face

Highlighting

Highlighting is a way to add fullness to depressed contours. It can be used to minimize deep facial lines, partially block out shadows, and accentuate bone structure. Highlighting is achieved by using a color a shade to a shade-and-a-half lighter than the actual skin color. Highlighting should always have shadow on one side to soften it. For example, if a line in the face is highlighted, it should also be shadowed along the perimeter that surrounds it. The camouflage therapist needs to recognize that it is impossible to conceal any shadow completely.

Highlighters are available in liquid, cream, powder, or pencil. Highlight can be applied either before or after powder. It is generally applied to the bone beneath the eyebrows or above the cheekbones. It can also be used in the crease of the nasolabil fold (the lines between the corners of the nose and the corners of the mouth) or any lines in the face. An eye-liner brush or an artist's flat brush is an effective way to apply it.

Contouring

Contouring creates definition through shading. It is more effective when used with highlighting. Shadows should always be created with highlighting on at least one side. Contouring is used to minimize swelling by making the area appear as if it is receding. It is achieved by using a color a shade to a shade-and-a-half darker than the actual skin color. The face can be contoured with liquid, cream, powder, or pencil.

Blending   Subtle and dramatic changes can be made by both highlighting and contouring, but blending is important to create a natural appearance. When contouring or highlighting becomes obvious, the purpose has been defeated.

FACE SHAPES

There are seven different face shapes: heart, triangular, square, diamond, round, oblong, and oval (which is considered the only perfect shape). To make the the perfect oval shape from any of the other face shapes, superimpose an imaginary oval over the face. See Figure 7-2. Any area that falls outside of this imaginary oval should be shaded to make it recede, while those areas that do not meet the border of the oval will need to be highlighted to appear as if they do. For example: A round face can be de-emphasized by using a small amount of contour around the sides of the forehead, in the cheek hollows, and on both sides of the jaw.

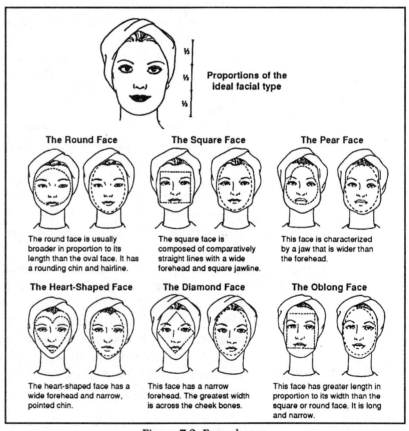

Proportions of the ideal facial type

The Round Face

The round face is usually broader in proportion to its length than the oval face. It has a rounding chin and hairline.

The Square Face

The square face is composed of comparatively straight lines with a wide forehead and square jawline.

The Pear Face

This face is characterized by a jaw that is wider than the forehead.

The Heart-Shaped Face

The heart-shaped face has a wide forehead and narrow, pointed chin.

The Diamond Face

This face has a narrow forehead. The greatest width is across the cheek bones.

The Oblong Face

This face has greater length in proportion to its width than the square or round face. It is long and narrow.

Figure 7-2. Face shapes

CORRECTIVE MAKEUP TECHNIQUES

Other facial imperfections can be corrected by using the following principles:

Wide Forehead

Narrow the appearance of a wide forehead by applying contour (foundation a shade to a shade-and-a-half darker than the skin tone), powder, blusher or cream rouge to the sides of the forehead and blending it in toward the hairline.

Double Chin

Use contour to shade the area just under the jawline using a lighter application at the outside and deepening it as you move toward the center.

The Nose

Long nose — shade around the nasal bone and highlight the bridge between the eyebrows to draw attention upwards.

Wide nose — shade both sides of the nose and highlight down the center.

Bulbous nose — shade down both sides of the nose and stop at the nostrils. Use a highlighter down the center of the nose to make it appear longer.

Crooked nose — shade the area on the nose that has the bump and highlight the area that does not need to be corrected.

ADDING ADDITIONAL COLOR

Blush color does two things: It gives the face additional color and adds dimension to the face by shaping it.

Cream Rouge and Powder Blushes

After applying foundation, contouring and highlighting is necessary to restore the patient's natural color tone to give the skin a healthy appearance. This can be accomplished with the use of powdered blusher, a water-base gel, or a cream rouge. Powdered blushers or gels are more appropriate for oilier skin types, and cream rouge is preferable for mature patients or those with dry skin.

Selecting the Appropriate Shade of Powdered Blusher or Rouge

The shade of blusher or rouge you choose will depend on the patient's coloring. The paler the patient's skin, the lighter the shade should be. Select bronze, terracotta, coral, or peach shades for patients with cream or olive skin tones and rose, pink, or mauve shades for patients with pink undertones.

How to Apply Gels or Rouge

Creams or gels can be applied to the cheek area with the fingertips and blended out toward the hairline with a wedge makeup sponge.

How to Apply a Powdered Blusher

A powdered blusher can be applied with a brush or disposable cotton ball by using long, even strokes and extending the color from the cheekbones into the hairline. To remove powdered blush from the container, scrape off what you need with a small makeup spatula. Scratch the surface of the cake, turn it over, and transfer the loose powder to the palm of your hand.

CORRECTIVE TECHNIQUES FOR THE EYE AREA

The following contouring and highlighting techniques with eye shadows or eye creams can be used to balance and reproportion the appearance of the eyes.

Eye Cosmetics

To select the appropriate eye-shadow shade for the patient use the eye color as a guide.

For patients who find that cream eye shadow forms a crease on their eyelid, select a powdered eye shadow. Compressed, or powdered, eye shadows are made of talc with oil and emulsifiers. They are packaged in individual cakes or matching color combinations in compact cases. A shadow that spreads easily will be silky to the touch, as opposed to one that feels chalky and will not be as smooth and easy to apply.

For mature patients or patients with dry skin, select a cream eye shadow. Cream shadows are made with a thick oil (castor, vegetable, or mineral) and wax and provide a nice alternative for older patients, whose eyelid-skin tends to be dry and can look crepe-y with a powdered shadow. It is not recommended to use frosted shadows on older patients since they reflect light and will make the skin appear drier. Instead, use eye shadows with a matte finish (without shine) in the following colors: beige, peach, brown, medium brown, dark gray, dark green, navy blue, and mauve.

To apply eye shadow, work with disposable cotton swab makeup applicators, or artist's flat brushes. Lighter, more neutral, eye shadow or cream shades such as beige, peach, and mauve tones can be used for highlighting and to imitate flesh tones. Darker colors such as brown, gray, green, and navy-blue can be used to contour, outline, and define the eye area.

Brushes   A good selection of brushes for contouring and shading the eye area is essential for corrective makeup and camouflage work. The following eye-shadow brushes are recommended. See Figure 7-3.

Artist's flat brush — These brushes are available in a variety of sizes and can be used for contouring the eye area, filling in scars, and lining the lips. They can be made from sable or from synthetic materials. The bristles must be fine, tapered, and springy.

Flat angle eye-shadow brush — These brushes can be used for contouring and defining the eye area.

Oval tapered eye-shadow brush — These brushes can be used to blend eye shadow and to add additional color to the eye area when needed.

Sponge tip eye-shadow applicators — These can be used to soften the appearance of eye shadow by moistening the sponge tip first before dipping it into

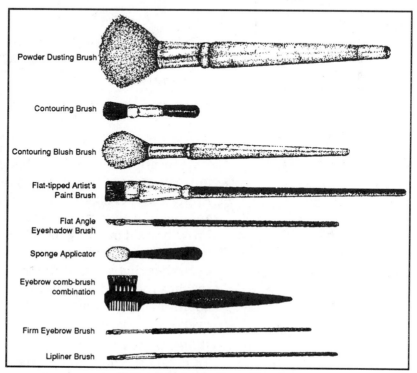

Figure 7-3. A selection of brushes

the eye shadow. This technique works well for mature patients or patients with dry skin. It prevents the skin from appearing crepe-y after the powdered eye shadow has been applied. It is also excellent for blending eye-shadow shades.

Contouring and Highlighting with Eye Shadows

The lighter, more neutral eye shadows such as beige, soft peach shades, and light mauve tones can be used for highlighting and to imitate flesh tones. See Figure 7-4. Darker colors such as brown, green, gray, teal, and navy-blue can be used to contour, outline, and define the eye area, depending on the patient's eye color.

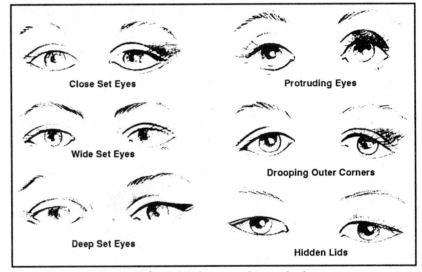

Figure 7-4. Highlighting with eye shadows

1. *Close-set eyes*
   Start by applying a lighter shade of eye shadow to the inner corners of the eyes and on half of the eyelids. Apply a darker shade to the outer corners of the eyes and blend it upward toward the outer edge of the brow bone. Line only the outer half the eyelids by using a liner pencil to draw a line right next to the eyelashes that starts at the iris and thickens as it reaches the outer corner of the eyes. Use an additional coat of mascara on the outer part of the eyelashes.

2. *Wide-set eyes*
   To create the illusion that the eyes are closer

together, apply a darker shade of eye shadow on the inner corners of the eyes and blend toward the nose. Use a lighter shade on the outer half of the eyelids and blend it outward toward the outer edges of the eyes. Apply a second coat of mascara on the inner eyelashes.

3. *Deep-set eyes*

Bring the eyes forward by using a light eye-shadow color on the entire eyelid. Apply a darker color to the outer edges of the eyes. With an eye-liner pencil draw a line on the upper eyelids closest to the eyelashes, completely outlining both eyes. Allow it to graduate into a wider line as it approaches the outer corners of the eyes.

4. *Protruding eyes*

To minimize the appearance of protruding eyes, apply a flat matte shadow in a medium shade over the entire eyelid, blending it upward toward the brow bone. Now apply a darker eye-shadow color, starting above the iris and covering the rest of the eyelids. Using a liner pencil, line both the upper and lower eyes from corner to corner.

5. *Almond eyes*

This eye shape is considered normal. Simply shadow the upper eye area along the brow bone with a light shadow. Use a medium or dark shadow on the entire eyelid, and line both the upper and lower eyes if desired.

6. *Small eyes*

To make the eyes appear larger, use a lighter shade of eye shadow under the eyebrows and on the eyelids. Along the the brow bone above the crease of the eye use a darker shade and blend the outer edges outward toward the temples. Use an eye-liner pencil to line only the outer half of the eyelids to the corners of the eyes, both on the upper eyelid and underneath the lower lashes.

7. *Droopy eyes*

To correct this eye shape, a medium or a dark eye shadow should be placed toward the outer corners of the eyes, extending upward to create the illusion of lifting the eye. A paler or light eye shadow should be applied directly under the eyebrow.

8. *Oriental eyes*
   Create the illusion of an eyelid by using an angular eye-shadow brush to apply a medium shadow shade in an arched shape that extends from one corner of the eyelid to the other. Above it, under the eyebrow, apply a light or pale eye-shadow color; below the arched line apply a second application of that pale or light color again. Line the entire upper eye with a very thin line made closest to the lashes with an eyeliner pencil. Underline the outer corner of the eyes with a soft color, extending it just a little past the outward edge of the eye.

9. *Under-eye puffiness (pouches)*
   To correct puffiness and conceal pouches under the eyes, use a foundation base half a tone darker than the face makeup and blend out the edges.

10. *Under-eye circles*
    Use a foundation base half a tone lighter than the face makeup. Do not apply purple, blue, rose, pink, or mauve eye shadows.

Eyelashes   *Eyelash Curler*

Some patients will have eyelashes that tend to grow downward or that are very straight. If an eyelash curler is not used, mascara will draw attention to this problem. Be sure that you sanitize the lash curler before you give it to the patient to use. This can be done by wiping the rubber strip with a cotton pad saturated in alcohol. Have the patient slip the thumb and finger into the handle grips and separate to open. Instruct the patient first to fit the eyelashes between the curling bows, then squeeze the grips together and hold for 30 seconds for each eye. Advise the patient never to use the lash curler after applying mascara, because it will break off the eyelashes.

Mascara

Once the lashes have been curled, mascara can be applied. See Figure 7-5. Liquid mascara is made from animal fats with color added. It comes in two types, water-soluble and waterproof. It is available in many colors, but for corrective makeup only black or brown should be used. To prevent the mascara from becoming contaminated, the container should be replaced every two to three months. You will also need to use disposable wands, since re-dipping them into a container will breed bacteria.

To avoid clumping of the lashes, mascara should be applied in the following manner:

1. Dip the disposable wand into the applicator container.

2. Use the sides of the container to scrape off any excess.

3. Start with the upper lashes. Have the patient look directly ahead and focus on a specific object to help him or her concentrate — this will prevent blinking.

4. Place the wand parallel to the lashes and lightly stroke on the mascara. Start at the roots and apply outward to the tips of the lashes. Use a lighter application first.

5. Let dry. After you have finished the upper lashes, repeat the same procedure on the lower lashes while the patient looks up and focuses on the ceiling. Move the wand back and forth in a downward motion, gently against the lower lashes until they absorb color and start to thicken.

6. Apply a second coat to both the upper and lower lashes with another disposable wand.

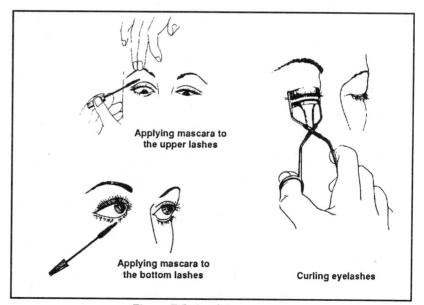

Applying mascara to the upper lashes

Applying mascara to the bottom lashes

Curling eyelashes

Figure 7-5. Applying mascara

Eyelash and Eyebrow Dye

Eyelash dyeing can be beneficial for patients with vitiligo, or for patients who are recovering from alopecia areata and need pigment restored to their eyelashes and eyebrows, or to replace color to the eyebrows or to the eyelashes of a male patient or child. In these instances, mascara may appear too obvious and would not be an appropriate method of camouflage. Eyelash dyes are available in black and brown. Brown dye only should be used on blondes and redheads.

Eyelash dyes contain mild para-phenylenediamine dyes or metallic dyes. Darkening of the eyelashes and eyebrows should be limited to once every month or the dye may be very irritating and result in an allergic reaction. This process should never be performed by a patient because the dye could easily get into the eye, possibly resulting in injury. Therefore this procedure should always be performed by a qualified skin-care specialist. See Figure 7-6.

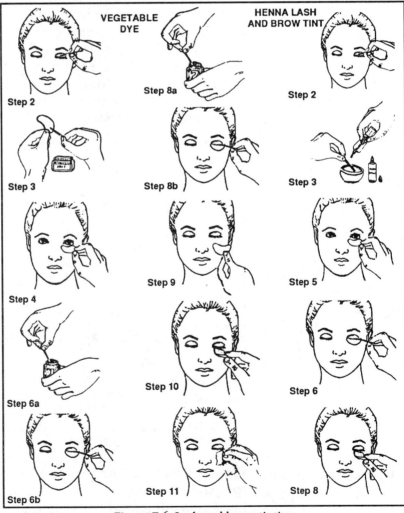

Figure 7-6. Lash and brow tinting

Although many brands of eyelash and eyebrow dyes are on the market, application procedures for only two types are discussed below, vegetable and henna:

Vegetable Dye

1. Ask the patient to sit in a semi-reclined position. This will help keep the dye out of the eyes during the application.

2. Cleanse the eye area with a non-greasy eye-makeup remover. Remove both liquid and cake mascara with a cotton swab dipped in eye-makeup remover. Gently brush back and forth across the lashes. Soaking a tissue in makeup remover, then folding it to sandwich the lash is an alternative method. Delicately rub the thumb and forefinger back and forth to dislodge mascara from the lashes.

3. Apply petroleum jelly directly to the paper shields and above the upper eyelashes to avoid getting the dye on the skin.

4. Place the protective shields or moistened cotton strips under the lower lashes. The patient's eyes should be open and should be looking up.

5. Adjust the shields or the cotton strips so that they cover any skin, and make sure the lashes are sitting neatly on top. The patient's eyes should now be closed.

6. Dip an application stick into the #1 solution. Application sticks are made by tightly wrapping the cotton around one end of the small, flat toothpick. It will look similar to a commercial cotton swab, except that the cotton should sit flat against the stick. Touch the tip of the stick on a folded tissue to remove any excess solution.

7. Gently apply solution over the lashes from the top of the lash down. Try to get as close to the lid as possible to cover the entire lash. Apply several applications, but do not use the same cotton swab again in the solution; use a new one each time you re-dip. Wait until it dries, usually 2–4 minutes.

8. Apply the #2 solution in the same manner. Wait until it dries.

9. Remove paper shields and wipe off petroleum jelly with a clean cotton swab. Have the patient close the eyes again.

10. Moisten the eyelashes with a cotton square dipped in warm water until they rinse clean.

11. Blot with tissue to dry. Remove any stains by soaking a cotton swab in the stain remover and blotting. Gently rub back and forth on the stained area and rinse.

Henna Lash and Brow Tint*

1. See step #1 above.

2. See step #2 above.

3. Squeeze 1–2 centimeters of cream out of the tube and mix with 2–3 drops of mild peroxide (10 volume or 3 percent).

4. Wait 3–5 minutes for solution to darken.

5. Apply damp cotton-wool under both eyes to prevent the dye from staining the skin under the lower lashes and have the patient close the eyes.

6. Apply dye with a lip brush or applicator stick made from tightly wrapping cotton around one end of a flat toothpick.

7. Let the dye saturate the eyelashes for 3–5 minutes.

8. Remove the dye from under the eyes with a wet cotton-wool pad; cleanse the eyes and remove any traces of dye on the skin.

* Without exception, always follow manufacturer's directions for application of eyelash and eyebrow dye.

Dyeing the Eyebrows

Coloring the brows is a procedure that should always be performed separately. It requires a great deal of concentration and a steady hand. Repeat the procedure for lash tinting. Be careful not to get either solution on the skin. Gently glide the swab over the brows, immediately removing any dye that may have missed the hair and touched the skin. A light application should be applied first, and if more color is required, follow up with a second coat. Brown dye is almost always preferable to black, since black produces a much harsher result.

False Eyelashes

False eyelashes are considered a prosthesis in the practice of camouflage therapy. They are used to replace missing lashes or to conceal a scar along the eyelid or on the lower rim of the eye. There are different types of lashes, varying in size from full strip eyelashes to small clusters, or even individual lashes. They can be purchased at a theatrical makeup store, department store, or a hair replacement center.

Applying False Eyelashes

Before applying false eyelashes you will want to curl the remaining eyelashes to make them uniform. To curl with an eyelash curler, begin by slipping the thumb and forefinger into handle grips. Separate to open. Hold it up to the lashes and insert the lashes until the metal portion of the curler rests against the eyelid and is slightly touching the lashes. Gently squeeze your fingers together. If pinching occurs, move curler further away from the skin. Hold firmly and wait 30 seconds. Spread fingers apart slowly and release clamp. Remove curler and repeat on the other eye. See Figure 7-7.

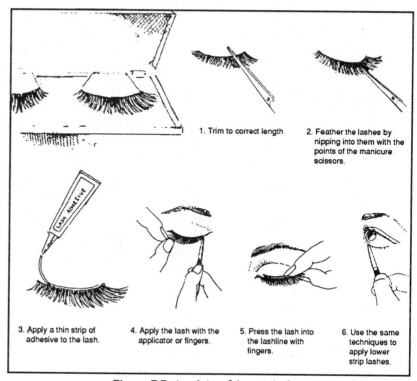

1. Trim to correct length
2. Feather the lashes by nipping into them with the points of the manicure scissors.
3. Apply a thin strip of adhesive to the lash.
4. Apply the lash with the applicator or fingers.
5. Press the lash into the lashline with fingers.
6. Use the same techniques to apply lower strip lashes.

Figure 7-7. Applying false eyelashes

Use the following method to apply false eyelashes:

1. Before application of false eyelashes, line the eyes with an eye pencil or eyeliner to conceal the lashstrip. Curl the remaining eyelashes on the upper lid to prevent a line of separation.

2. Remove the lash from the kit. It should have some adhesive still on it. It will temporarily attach to the eyelid long enough for you to measure and fit it to the eye.

3. Use either manicure or mustache scissors to trim ends that may be too full. Begin by trimming the widest edge of the lash at the outer corner and work inward. See Figure 7-7.

4. Once the eyelashes have been trimmed properly, bend and flex the lash so it will fall in line with the natural curvature of the eye. Grasp the lash with a pair of tweezers.

5. With one end of an orange stick (wooden stick used in manicures), apply surgical adhesive to the eyelash by thinly spreading it across the rim. Wait a few seconds for the adhesive to partially set. Surgical adhesive is made from latex and is routinely used to adhere false eyelashes and to apply artificial hair. It is packaged in small tubes and can be purchased at a theatrical supply store, medical supply store, or a hair replacement center.

6. Ask the patient to look down.

7. Hold the lash gently with fingers on one end and tweezers on the other end. Attach as close to the natural lashes as possible. The base of the strip should rest on the lined portion of the eyelid, about one-quarter of an inch from the inner and outer corners of the eye.

8. Remove tweezers.

9. Press the blunt end of the orange stick on the lash strip to adhere it to the skin on the eyelid.

10. Gently stretch the eyelid with fingertips to determine if there are any gaps where adhesive still needs to be applied. You can fill in the gaps by placing surgical adhesive on the tip of a flat toothpick and sliding it onto the rim of the lash, and then pressing to secure it.

Note: If the application is on a female patient, apply mascara to the lashes lightly for a completely natural look. To apply cake mascara, wet the brush and stroke it across the moistened mascara cake. Lightly brush over lashes. Repeat this procedure until the result is satisfactory. To apply liquid mascara use a disposable wand as an applicator and apply only one light coat.

Method of Application for Individual Eyelashes.

Individual eyelash clusters can also be applied by cutting two or three lashes and adhering them to the base where needed. Application of individual lashes differs from that of strip lashes or eyelash clusters. See Figures 7-8 and 7-9. The following procedure is recommended:

1. Grasp the individual lash with a pair of tweezers.
2. Apply surgical adhesive to base.

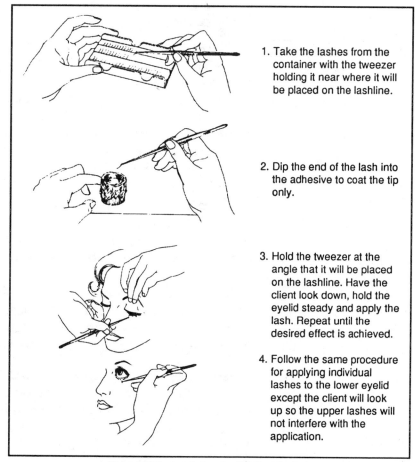

1. Take the lashes from the container with the tweezer holding it near where it will be placed on the lashline.

2. Dip the end of the lash into the adhesive to coat the tip only.

3. Hold the tweezer at the angle that it will be placed on the lashline. Have the client look down, hold the eyelid steady and apply the lash. Repeat until the desired effect is achieved.

4. Follow the same procedure for applying individual lashes to the lower eyelid except the client will look up so the upper lashes will not interfere with the application.

Figure 7-8. Applying individual lashes

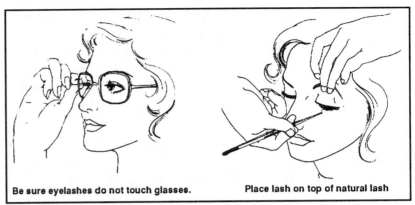

Be sure eyelashes do not touch glasses.   Place lash on top of natural lash

Figure 7-9. Applying individual lashes

3. Apply to the eyelid at the same angle as the natural lash. Start at the outer corner and work inward.

4. The lash should be trimmed so it graduates to a shorter length as you work toward the inner corner of the eye.

Corrective Techniques for Eyebrows

Eyebrows should be well shaped and balanced and in proportion with the rest of the facial features. It is important that the eyebrow follows the natural curve of the eye, the eyelid, and the line of the nose. The curve of the brow should begin at the bridge of the nose. Imagine a line straight up from the inside corner of the eye to this point. This is where the eyebrow should begin. A pencil can be used to locate where the eyebrow should be properly positioned. Hold the pencil at a diagonal angle from the side of the patient's nostril to the outside corner of the eye. The length of the eyebrow should be the distance from the pencil to the inside of the eye. If the brow is shorter than this it can be extended by penciling in the ideal length. If the brow is too long, the excess hairs can be removed by tweezing.

Gray and black, gray and brown, blonde, or a taupe pencil can be used to stroke in tiny lines. These lines should be drawn in lightly in the same direction as the natural brow hairs. A horizontal line should never be drawn.

Filling in or Correcting Eyebrows

You can fill in or correct the shape of eyebrows by using an eyebrow pencil. An eyebrow pencil is a wooden pencil filled with grease lead, yet it is harder than an eye-lining pencil. See Figure 7-10. You will need pencils in the following colors: blonde, taupe, medium brown, dark brown, gray, and black.

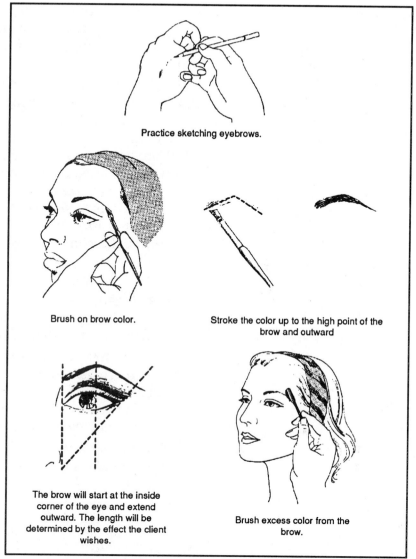

Practice sketching eyebrows.

Brush on brow color.

Stroke the color up to the high point of the brow and outward

The brow will start at the inside corner of the eye and extend outward. The length will be determined by the effect the client wishes.

Brush excess color from the brow.

Figure 7-10. Correcting eyebrow shape

You will use the pencils that match the natural hair and eyebrow color of the patient you will be working on. Pencils should be sharpened to a fine point before application.

To correct or fill in eyebrows, use any of the following procedures:

1. Using a child's toothbrush, mustache comb, or eyebrow brush and comb, stroke the brow hairs in an upward motion. This will define the direction of hair growth. A eyebrow pencil or a firm eyebrow brush can be used to re-define the eyebrows. The brush is

an alternative to the eyebrow pencil and can be used to brush on eye-shadow powder in a color that matches the natural eyebrow, giving it a softer, more natural look.

Using very short, slanted strokes, duplicate the appearance of the preexisting brow hairs. Be careful not to be too heavy handed. A gray pencil or the application of eye-shadow powder can be used to buffer the harsh look dark brown and black pencils can give. The gray pencil should be used first (lightly) and then followed up with gentle strokes using the dark brown or black pencil, depending on which color is appropriate. Eyebrows should only be darkened slightly and should frame the eyes, not stand out.

2. Eye shadow can also be used to fill in very thin eyebrows by applying the eye shadow to the brow with an angular brush in a color that matches the natural brow or the patient's hair color.

3. Long-wearing mascara does an excellent job of re-creating eyebrows, and is waterproof as well. To avoid an application that is too dark or obvious, the color of the mascara should be coordinated with the patient's hair and eyebrow color and applied by the following method:

   a. Dip the disposable wand into the applicator container.

   b. Use the sides of the container to scrape off any excess.

   c. Apply to the eyebrow by placing the wand parallel to the brow bone, and lightly stroke on the mascara. Start above the inner eye where the eyebrow begins or should be and apply outward to the end of the brow, using very light strokes.

To Correct Thin Eyebrows
Lightly draw the ideal shape by adding width both above and below the natural eyebrow. First fill in the brow with either pencil or eye-shadow powder using light, short, diagonal strokes, starting at the bottom of the brow and working upward.

To Correct Thick Eyebrows

Brush the eyebrow hairs up to determine if the brows are too thick. Remove excess brow hairs by tweezing them. Remove only the hairs that will not brush into formation. If the eyebrow needs more definition, arch it with a pencil and remove any random hairs below. If the hairs are too long they can be combed straight down until the natural arch becomes visible. Small manicuring scissors can be used to trim these hairs.

To Correct Droopy Eyebrows

Remove random hairs under the center of the brow to form a natural, curved arch. Remove any extra hairs that go beyond the diagonal line from the nose to the outside corner of the eye.

Re-creating Eyebrows

The eyes and the eyebrows are the most expressive part of the face.

For many patients the loss of part or all of their eyebrows can be devastating. Post-burn patients, patients with alopecia, and patients who are suffering from hair loss due to chemotherapy treatments may need to replace their eyebrows. The following techniques are recommend to camouflage missing eyebrows. See Figure 7-11.

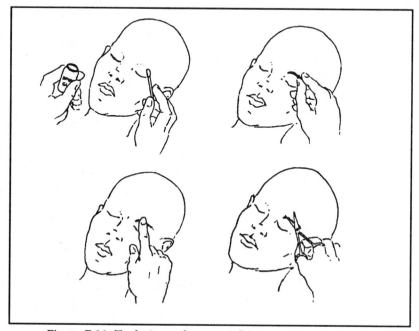

Figure 7-11. Techniques for camouflaging missing eyebrows

Eyebrows

Real or synthetic hair can be individually knotted onto a thin lace net, cut, and shaped into a strip of hair that resembles an eyebrow. Ventilated artificial eyebrows are more practical for patients who will need to apply them on a daily basis. They are available in the following shades: blonde, auburn, brown, gray, and black. They can be obtained at a hair replacement center or a theatrical makeup store. They are attached to the brow bone with medical adhesive or spirit gum. To remove them, a cotton swab soaked in medical adhesive remover can be slid underneath the brow to loosen the adhesive. Adhesive remover is made from alcohol or acetone and will easily remove both surgical adhesive and spirit gum. For patients with sensitive skin, the "extra mild" spirit gum remover is recommended. Advise the patient to close the eyes and bend over a basin when using the liquid remover. This will direct the remover away from the eyes.

Crepe Hair

Crepe hair can also be used to replace eyebrows, or to create mustaches, beards, and sideburns. It is an alternative to the pre-made hairpieces that can be purchased in a wig or theatrical makeup store. It is made from wool and comes in braided strands in a variety of natural colors that can be blended together to create a more natural shade. See Figure 7-12. To mix shades, use several colors, starting with the darkest color, and blend in the lighter colors on top.

1. In many cases you will need to straighten the hair before applying it since the packaging causes it to become kinky. For thick beard stubble or sideburns, the crepe wool can be used directly from the braid as is.

2. To straighten the hair for mustaches and eyebrows, cut the string that holds the braid together and unravel it gently.

3. Place a couple of strands between your fingers and roll them. Another way you can straighten the strands is with steam. Place the strands under a damp cloth and iron them with moderate heat, being careful not to burn the hair.

4. Comb the hair from the end of the braid with a wide-tooth comb.

5. Pull small pieces of the wool crepe out to reconstruct eyebrows or mustaches.

6. Use spirit gum or medical adhesive to apply the crepe hair to the skin. Spirit gum is an alternative to surgical adhesive. It is used in the theater to attach hair pieces and prosthetics.

   If you have used corrective cover cream first the adhesive will be brushed on over it. The camouflage application must be well powdered so the oil in the foundation will not interfere with the ability of the spirit gum to stick. Powder your fingers as well; it will make it easier to place the crepe hair on.

7. Apply in the direction of the hair growth, if hair is still detectable.

8. Allow the spirit gum a couple of seconds to become tacky.

9. Gently brush your finger back and forth to eliminate any hairs that are not firmly attached.

10. If the hairs need any additional vertical trimming, use a pair of small mustache or manicure scissors to shape and remove unnatural looking strands.

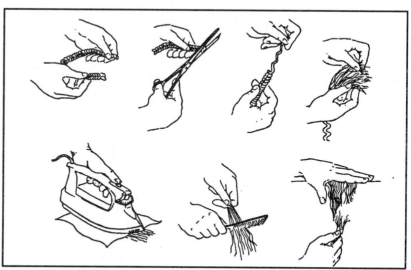

Figure 7-12. Crepe hair techniques

CORRECTIVE TECHNIQUES FOR THE LIPS

Lip Liner   A lip pencil or a lip brush can be used to outline the lips and correct their shape. Use a pencil or a lipstick color that either matches the patient's lipstick or is a shade darker, from the same color family. The lip liner should be blended into the lip color until it is undetectable.

Lip-liner pencils are made of soft grease lead and are used to define or re-shape the lips. The mouth shape can be re-defined in a number of ways with a lip pencil, but it must be re-shaped as naturally as possible, so that it does not look obvious. To restore the natural border around the lips (vermilion border), use a shade of lip pencil that closely resembles the color of the patient's lips. The lip liner should be blended into the lip color until it becomes undetectable. See Figure 7-13. A light brown, reddish brown, or taupe eyebrow pencil should be used to outline a boy's or a man's lip because it will be less noticeable and appear more natural.

Uneven Lips

When the upper and lower lips are unevenly balanced, concentrate on lining each lip separately until they are perfectly proportioned. This can be accomplished by lining the outside border of the lip that is too small to build it up and lining the inside of the lip that is too large to minimize it, until both lips appear evenly balanced.

Drooping Corners

To correct a mouth that has a droopy appearance, use a lip-liner pencil to draw in an artificial lip border that does not turn down at the corners of the mouth, and then fill it in until it looks natural.

Thin Upper Lip

If the patient's upper lip is too thin, use a lip-lining pencil to draw in an artificial lip border, which you can later fill in with lipstick, to make the lip look fuller than it actually is, until it appears equally proportioned with the lower lip.

Thin Lower Lip

Outline the lower lip with a lip-lining pencil until it is slightly fuller. Keep this artificial border as close as possible to the natural lip line to prevent it from looking too obvious.

Thin Lips

Enlarge the appearance of both the upper and lower lips by outlining and filling in color to make the lips seem fuller.

Rounded or Pointed Upper Lip

When the upper lip is either too rounded or too pointed, it will need to be softened to balance with the lower lip. Mini-

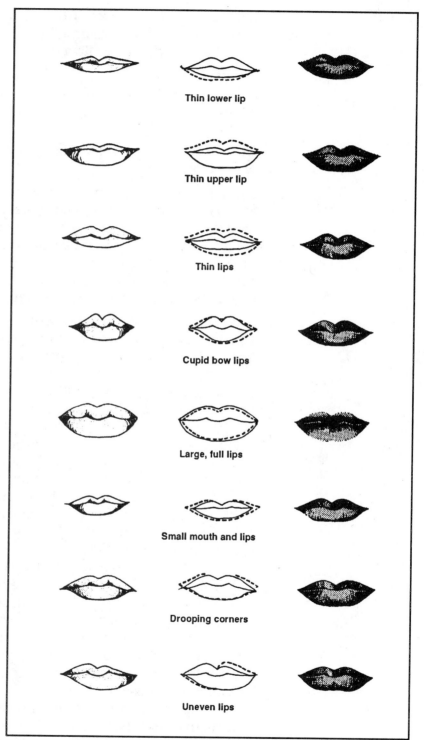

Figure 7-13. Corrective techniques for the lips

mize the extreme peaks of the upper lip by extending the border out to the corners of the mouth with a lip-lining pencil to give the upper lip a softer curvature.

Large, Full Lips
Apply soft, subtle colors that do not attract attention to the lip area.

Small Mouth and Lips
Outline and build out the sides of both upper and lower lips with color.

Lipstick

Lipsticks have an oil-wax base to which dyes and pigments are added to create color. It is the emollient (oil) added to the wax base that gives the lipstick its creamy consistency. Emollients are added to condition and keep the lips moist, as well as to prevent the lipstick from drying out. Your selection of lip colors should correspond with the shades of powder blushers and creme rouges you have in your makeup inventory.

Selecting the Correct Lip Color
Lipstick shapes the mouth and emphasizes the lips. Because lipstick is the most obvious cosmetic, careful consideration is needed to insure that the appropriate shade is selected for the patient. Fair-skinned and fair-haired patients with golden undertones to their skin will look more attractive in softer shades, such as peach and soft corals. Fair-haired and fair-skinned patients with pink undertones will look best in soft lavender, rose, or mauve shades. Patient's with darker, more vivid complexions will look better in brighter shades (although dusty shades are also becoming to patients with dramatic coloring). Patients with dark hair and pink undertones to their complexion will look best in vivid, high-intensity shades such as true reds and clear pink tones, and patients with dark hair and golden undertones will look best in warm, richer shades, such as terracotta and russet lip colors.

Always match the lip color you select to the powder blusher or cream rouge; if they are not an exact match, they must at least be from the same color family to create visual harmony and produce a natural look. If you are using the lips as the focal point to draw attention away from an area you are trying to conceal, choose a color with a brighter intensity. Most patients appear to be self-conscious about the lip area and do not like to have it exaggerated. Therefore, it is best to consult with the patient about lining the lips and the selection of lip color prior to application. Do not use frosted lipsticks, since they tend to produce a more glamorized appearance. Do not use clear gloss or petroleum jelly in place of a lipstick unless your intention is to make the lips appear larger.

It may be necessary to apply lip color on men or on small children when there is a loss of pigmentation to the lips. The selection of lip color should then be based on the remaining pigment and should appear as natural as possible (use an amber or auburn makeup pencil to fill in lips). Unless you are replacing pigment, it is best not to color the lips at all.

Applying Lip Color

1. To apply lipstick, use an orange stick, flat toothpick, or plastic spatula to remove the lipstick from the container.

2. Use the spatula as a palette from which to work off.

3. Line the lips with a lip pencil or a lip brush.

4. Dip a lip brush, or a flat red-sable brush, into the lipstick and then proceed to fill them in. To avoid heavy application, use a tissue to gently blot off excess. See Figure 7-14.

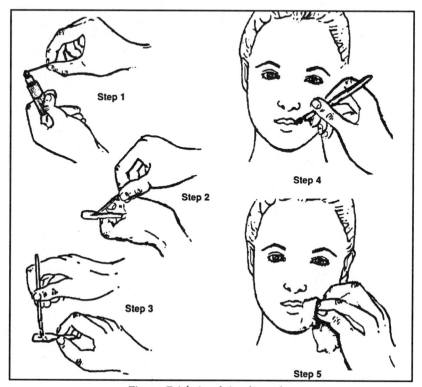

Figure 7-14. Applying lip color

REVIEW

You should now be familiar with:

- ■ how to select the appropriate foundation base for the patient.
- ■ techniques for highlighting and contouring.
- ■ corrective makeup techniques.

CHAPTER

8 Cosmetic Therapy

Cosmetic therapy is the masking of physical irregularities with cover creams by normalizing or by distracting the viewer's attention away from the lesion. This may be achieved by a number of different techniques, including full concealment with a non-transparent cover cream and subtle textural and pigment blending. Selection of the materials will not only involve the camouflage therapist's judgment of what will best cover the patient's disfigurement, but will also depend on what the patient can and will apply and how it will fit in with his or her daily activities. For example, if the patient works in a humid environment, the re-application of setting powder may be required, or if the patient has very little time to apply the cover creams, a simple application (less time-consuming) method is indicated.

WHAT TYPE OF PATIENT IS A CANDIDATE FOR CAMOUFLAGE THERAPY?

The patient who is most likely to benefit from the camouflage therapy procedure is a person who is dissatisfied with his or her appearance and is seeking a cosmetic solution to correct it. This is because camouflage requires effort on the part of the patient to perform the procedures, and he or she must incur the cost of the sessions and the supplies.

Cover creams can be used on a temporary basis to mask skin trauma from surgical procedures, in particular bruising, swelling, and redness from cosmetic surgery (face-lift, eyelid lift, etc.). Camouflage may also be used during the recuperation period from dermabrasion and chemo-abrasion (chemical peels).

It can also be used for temporary or permanent scarring resulting from skin disorders, such as herpes zoster, shingles, lupus, rosacea, acne scarring, and congenital lesions (birth-marks).

Camouflage therapy will help patients with permanent physical irregularities, such as scarring from cancer removal, lacerations (cuts), and burns.

Pigmentary problems can also be modified with the use of camouflage preparations. These include conditions such as melasma (dark pigmentation of the skin), vitiligo (a skin condition resulting in white patches), hypopigmentation (diminished pigmentation), or any pigmentary disorder.

CORRECTIVE COVER PRODUCTS AND SETTING POWDERS

Camouflage preparations have a thick, paste-like consistency and are more opaque than traditional makeup foundations. One or several of these cover creams are matched to the patient's skin and applied with a light tapping motion, instead of the traditional rubbing method. A light, translucent powder or a slightly tinted setting powder stabilizes and waterproofs the application.

APPLYING COVER CREAMS

Cover cream products vary in covering capabilities, color selection, and cost. Therefore, the greater the inventory of camouflage creams the camouflage therapist has to choose from the better chance of matching the right product to the patient's needs. The camouflage therapist should be equipped with at least three palettes from different cosmetic manufacturers to offer patients a full range of cover cream shades and a wide selection of cosmetic brands to choose from.

It is important for the camouflage therapist to buy the best camouflage products possible. Inferior grades of cover creams can cause constant difficulties. Cover creams should have a fairly thick ointment base with good concealing properties, water-in-oil solutions mixed with a combination of waxes to achieve a thick consistency. Products that contain Kaolin, magnesium carbonate, or talc absorb oil on the surface of skin, which prevents natural oils from mixing with cover creams and diluting their application. Titanium dioxide, when pigmented with iron oxides, provides good color.

Each type of cover cream will react differently once applied, depending on the amount of acid in the patient's skin and the way in which the skin's chemistry interacts with the ointment base. Because of this, the color of the cover cream will differ noticeably from the original color as it appeared in the container. Most manufacturers try to produce a wide enough cover cream selection to match each patient's skin color, but unfortunately the appropriate cosmetic color usually falls somewhere between two shades. Very rarely can an exact color match be found using just one cover cream. The variety of skin colors makes it nearly impossible to match a patient's skin coloring with one particular cover cream color. The camouflage therapist should, however, try to avoid selecting more than two cover cream shades when color blending. The patient will ultimately be performing the camouflage process alone, and using three or more colors will be too confusing; also working with three different shades will require too much time to achieve the exact color match.

CLEANSING THE SKIN

The first step in the camouflage process is to prepare the skin by cleansing, toning, and moisturizing it. See Figure 8-1. Any residue left on the surface can cause discoloration and will affect coverage. Before you can apply cover creams, you will need to cleanse the skin. This can be accomplished by using the appropriate cleanser on a damp cotton square to gently wipe away any film or preexisting makeup. Before the appointment, prepare enough moistened cotton pads by cutting cotton off a roll into 3 x 3 inch squares. Immerse them in water, then squeeze out the excess and store in a plastic, travel-size soap container or a plastic zip-lock bag. This will provide adequate storage for the moistened cotton squares, and the bag and container will fit neatly into your portable makeup kit.

The cleansing solution you select should correspond with the patient's skin type; for example, if the patient has oily or combination skin, a facial cleanser for oily skin is indicated. Below are skin-care recommendations for dry and oily skin.

Oily or Acne-Prone Skin

Patients who are acne prone or who occasionally experience flare-ups should avoid cleansers, moisturizers, and sunscreens that contain large amounts of oil. Facial cleansers are formulated for oily skin that are very effective for removing makeup preparations. Cleansing should always be followed up with

Procedures for Cleansing the Face

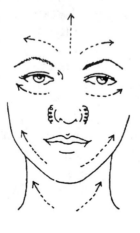

Such products as eye oils and special cleansers can interfere with makeup application. Oil control and antiseptic products may be used when needed.

During the time you are cleansing the patient's face, you can question him or her about his or her daily skin-care routine, which products they are currently using, and make suggestions about proper skin-care and makeup procedures.

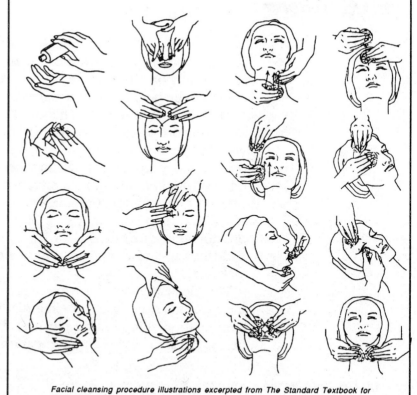

Facial cleansing procedure illustrations excerpted from The Standard Textbook for Professional Estheticians by Joel Gerson

Figure 8-1. Procedures for cleansing the skin

the use of an astringent to eliminate any remaining surface residue. An oil-free moisturizer that contains a sunscreen should be applied to the patient's skin before applying camouflage makeup.

Long-term contact with waterproof camouflage creams can lead to breakouts and will only worsen the patient's problem skin condition. Cosmetic therapy on facial areas (to cover acne scarring), must be limited to the use of non-greasy color correctors worn underneath water-based makeup foundations, such as theatrical pancake makeup or a variety of oil-free foundations. Heavier concealers that contain oil should only be used where needed and never on areas of the skin where blemishes form. Transparent powder applied over the makeup will help absorb excess skin oil and provide additional coverage.

Sensitive, Dry, or Dehydrated Skin

Dry or chapped skin tends to be sensitive and is often allergic to certain cosmetic ingredients. Question all patients about any possible allergies they may have before applying anything to their skin. Always list the ingredients in your products for the patient to review. Avoid using skin-care or cosmetic preparations that contain substances known to produce allergic reactions. For additional information on cosmetic ingredients, you should be able to find several books on the subject in your local library or neighborhood bookstore.

Patients with dry, chapped, or sensitive skin will need a cleansing solution formulated for their specific skin type. Cleansing creams are less abrasive and less irritating. The oils they contain break down the waxes and oil in cover-cream preparations without stripping natural surface oils and drying out the skin. Cleansing should be followed up with a gentle toner to remove any oil residue left behind. After the patient's skin is cleansed and toned, a moisturizer — preferably one with a sunscreen — should be applied. The SPF (sun protection factor) should be no less than 15. There are many sunscreens and sunblocks available on the market. In the evening, a light moisture lotion can be worn under cover cream as a substitute for the sunscreen. Moisturizers and sunscreens should be applied sparingly. Allow ten to twenty minutes for the cream or lotion to be completely absorbed into the skin before a cover cream is applied. To speed absorption time the excess cream can be blotted off with a tissue after a few minutes.

The skin's surface and its appearance is affected by its inner moisture and oil content. If the skin is dry and scaly, thick, opaque foundations will only accentuate fine lines, wrinkles, and flakiness. Cover creams with a higher percentage of oil will produce a better cosmetic result because they will help erase some of the surface dryness. If the camouflage cream contains its own sunscreen and is of a whipped consistency it may not be necessary to apply a thick moisturizer underneath; in this case, the addition of an emollient cream may break down some of the oils in the product and inhibit coverage. To avoid this, the esthetician should read the product manufacturer's recommendations for applying the cover cream.

MATCHING COVER CREAMS TO THE SKIN

To successfully match a cover cream to the patient's skin you must first be able to identify the underlying colors that make up his or her skin tone. Hemoglobin produces redness in the skin, keratin produces a yellowish cast, and melanin brings forth a brown pigment. The thinner the skin the more likely you are to see a red undertone and ruddiness; the thicker the skin, the more likely you will see a lot of brown pigment in it. After you have experimented with different cover cream colors, you will begin to associate certain shades with particular nationalities. For example, patients from countries north of the equator will need cover creams in light colors, such as ivory, natural, medium, and beige; patients from countries south of the equator will wear darker shades, such as suntan, tan, brown, chestnut, amber, copper, and dark brown. The secret to color matching is being aware of undertones in the skin and being able to duplicate the varying degrees of color. Each time you correctly match up a cover cream with a person's skin you will become more familiar with the various depths of color in the skin. The more you practice, the easier this process will become for you. The following information will guide you step by step through the color matching process. See Figure 8-2.

1. Protect the patient's clothing during the camouflage makeup session by draping the patient. Paper gowns can be used instead of cloth and are disposable, which will eliminate unnecessary laundry costs.

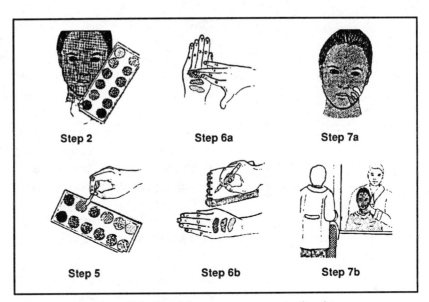

Step 2   Step 6a   Step 7a

Step 5   Step 6b   Step 7b

Figure 8-2. Matching cover creams to the skin

2. Begin by raising the cover cream palette to the area of skin that you want to cover.

3. Look slowly as you scan each cover cream; as you do, ask yourself, does this color have the same amount of brown, yellow, or red tones as the skin surrounding the lesioned area?

4. If not, move on to the next color. Sometimes you will see some resemblance, but the color may lack some yellow or pink undertones in a patient's skin. If this occurs, try to find another color that will fill that void to blend into it. Before doing so, ask yourself what proportion will be needed of the second color to correctly match the tone.

5. Take a small amount from the container (with a spatula) and place it on the back of your hand. Rub it onto the skin in a circular motion until the cover cream is malleable and spreads easily. Your body heat and the oil from your skin will soften the concealer cream, which will make it easier to apply.

6. Mix and place on the back of your hand three different color combinations of no more than two blended colors each. Be sure to record your formulas on a scratch pad.

7. Place a small sample of each of the three separate cover cream combinations on the skin. Stand back and look at the application from a distance (if on the face, apply to the jaw area, stand behind the patient's shoulder and look at the patient's face in a well-lit mirror).

8. Squint your eyes. Again, ask yourself: Does the color match the skin in value or is it too light or too dark? When you squint, the color combination that matches the skin most closely should meet the edges of the surrounding skin with no sharp distinctions. It should blend in so well that it is barely visible. Then you know you have achieved the correct color match.

9. If the cover cream color combination you have selected is too dark, add a little bit more of the lighter color of the two until it matches the patient's skin tone, or add a pinhead of white cover cream to lighten it up. If, on the other hand, it is too light, add a little more of the darker shade of the two until you have matched the color of the patient's skin tone as closely as possible.

10. Once you have selected the correct color match, you can proceed to cover the area you wish to conceal. The application of camouflage cosmetics involves the following four steps:

   a. Selection of the correct cover cream or creams to match the patient's skin color as closely as possible.

   b. The application method is a gentle dabbing motion (with the third finger or with a synthetic cosmetic sponge), to pat in the cover cream or creams on the area to be camouflaged. Sponges can be used when you have a larger area to cover to expedite the process, or for blending out the edges of the makeup.

   c. Eliminate distinct edges where the opaque makeup has been applied by blending the cover creams into the surrounding skin and feathering out the sharp edges with delicate strokes either by hand, with a sponge, or a cotton swab.

   d. Waterproof the makeup application by applying a loose powder with a dry cotton square or a disposable powder puff. To stabilize your cover cream application, liberally apply a colorless, translucent powder.

11. Set the application by waiting a few minutes for the powder to be absorbed. The setting time for the powder will depend on the patient's skin type (dry or oily). Patients who have more surface oil will require the powder to remain on their skin a little longer (approximately 8–10 minutes) to absorb some of their natural oils along with the oils in the cover creams. Patients with dry or aging skin will achieve a better result by having the cover creams on their skin longer (8–10 minutes) before setting the application with powder, because the oil in the product helps to lubricate the surface of the skin. Brush off excess powder with a powder brush or cotton ball, using a gentle, downward, sweeping motion (this will make facial hairs lie flat) from the center outward. Patients with extremely dry (flaky and cracking) skin will not require setting powder to stabilize the cover creams. Using a setting powder will only accentuate fine lines and wrinkles and make the application more detectable.

12. Re-application may be necessary if you have not achieved complete coverage. Repeat the original camouflage steps, re-setting the second application with powder. If the corrected result looks cakey and artificial, sprinkle a tissue with water by misting it and gently blot the tissue over the area. Be sure not to rub it or you may accidentally remove some of the makeup. In an hour or so, after the cover creams have had time to settle on the skin, the makeup application will appear more natural.

If you choose to select a powder with a tint, remember that it will alter the cover cream mixture you have just blended.

DUPLICATING NATURAL IMPERFECTIONS ON THE SKIN — COSMETIC THERAPY FOR CHILDREN

A child may have a congenital lesion such as a small birthmark with slight discoloration. Sometimes, he or she will outgrow it or it may eventually fade. Or the problem may be just the opposite: the patient may be suffering from a condition such as vitiligo (lack of pigmentation). In either case, cosmetic camouflage therapy can temporarily disguise the disfigurement. In some cases the clinical esthetician/cosmetologist will be asked to conceal a scar that will later be operated on. This could result from a burn or a laceration. Many surgeons prefer to wait to do scar revision since the skin on a child will stretch and expand as the child grows.

Childhood diseases produce a variety of scars, some temporary and others permanent. These scars include those resulting from chicken pox, german measles, or mumps. Although a child heals more quickly than an adult, the scar may take longer to fade, especially if the child has a dark complexion.

Sometimes camouflaging even minor irregularities on the faces of small children can be difficult. The developmental level and the chronological age of the child are contributing factors that will affect the outcome of camouflage therapy. In order to perform the application process successfully, the child will need the fine motor and visual-motor skills required to perform cosmetic procedures (children under the age of nine will need the assistance of a family member or guardian). Therefore, the camouflage therapist must develop a unique program of cosmetic application for each child or child/parent team.

Children should be instructed to only lightly cover the lesion, burn scar, laceration, or birthmark, allowing it to bleed through. Over time the child can gradually increase the application to make it more opaque. The goal, of course, is for complete concealment. By using this method less attention will be drawn to the area, rather than removing an obvious scar or birthmark all at once. This is particularly important for a child since other children can be quite cruel and the makeup could seem more of an embarrassment than a positive solution.

Regardless of the camouflage method used, the technical process should be kept simple. Only cosmetic applicators a child would be familiar with should be used in treatment, such as a pencil instead of a brush, a finger instead of a sponge. Instructions should be carefully documented on a diagram in a way that the patient will readily comprehend. The diagram can later be used as a practice tool to guide the child through the application process.

Camouflaging Acne Scars

Some adolescent patients will seek a cosmetic solution for pitted acne scars. Although the camouflage therapist will be able to conceal discoloration and pigmentary problems, acne scar formations are difficult to disguise. Corrective cover creams cannot change the texture of the skin. In fact, if an oil-based, opaque foundation is used, the patient's problematic skin condition may be further complicated because of the added oil. Patients need to be told that the only treatments that can correct this condition are dermabrasion and chemoabrasion. These procedures are routinely performed by a dermatologist or a plastic surgeon. In this instance the use of a water-based foundation or a pancake makeup over a green color corrector will obliterate the redness and will not interfere with the acne treatment prescribed by the patient's physician.

Camouflaging Hypopigmentation

Small children or men with hypopigmentation or vitiligo can use either a bronzing gel (to temporarily stain their skin) or a tinted powder to discreetly camouflage this lack of pigment. A bronzing gel will not provide coverage but will add color to the skin and can be extremely beneficial compared to a thick, opaque cover cream because it will look more natural.

If cover creams are used and if more opaque coverage is required, the camouflage therapist may have to duplicate the cover cream application slightly on the other (unaffected) side of the patient's face to achieve a completely natural result. This will balance the two sides and prevent the camouflaged area from appearing made-up.

Recreating Skin Imperfections

Camouflaging imperfections on the skin by combining two cover creams and successfully blending them to match the patient's skin without detection is only one aspect of the camouflage makeup process. Concealing problem areas on children or men requires a more complex set of makeup procedures to discreetly correct problem areas. These camouflage methods involve recognizing the subtle imperfections surrounding the treated area that constitute the natural appearance of the skin (freckles, veins, and capillaries) and reproducing their appearance with makeup.

Closely scrutinize the area surrounding the disfigurement and select the proper camouflage method to duplicate the imperfections you see over the cover cream application. Skin imperfections can easily be identified by looking for hemoglobin (such as thin skin and capillaries) that produces redness and ruddiness, or keratin, a chemical substance that gives skin a sallow (yellow undertone) look in places by producing an uneven blotchy appearance, or melanin (patches of brown pigment, freckles, brown spots, or tanned areas). By observing the pink, yellow, or brown undertones in the patient's skin you will be able to help the patient achieve a more natural result by imitating common flaws on the surface surrounding the irregularity.

IMITATING BEARD STUBBLE, FRECKLES, ROSY CHEEKS

Camouflage makeup can be applied in various ways by using different types of sponges (stipple sponges, sea sponges, and foam wedge sponges). Stipple sponges and sea sponges are smaller than average sponges and have large pores so that the makeup looks dappled rather than creating a complete coverage look. These are used to fake imperfections such as freckles or rosy cheeks, and to imitate beard growth. See Figure 8-3.

1. To stipple in color to imitate freckles, broken veins in the skin, or an unshaven look or beard shadow, press the stipple (a cosmetic sponge with large pores) sponge into the cover cream. A separate container to dip into should be set aside for sanitary reasons. Stippling must be done lightly since you do not want to completely fill the holes in the sponge. Use a rose cover cream for imitating broken capillaries, a brown

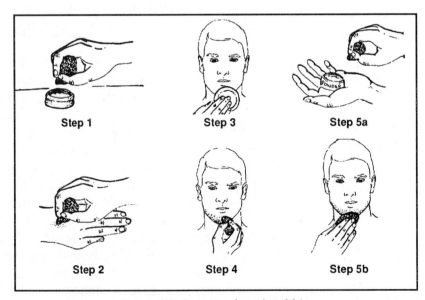

Figure 8-3. Imitating beard stubble

and yellow mixture for freckles, or, depending on the beard color, brown, dark brown, gray, or black to imitate a beard.

2. Press the sponge down on the back of your hand first to test the application. This will help you determine the amount of pressure that will be required to match the surrounding skin's surface.
3. Powder the area you wish to cover.
4. Apply by gently patting sponge onto the skin area.
5. Re-apply powder with stipple sponge.

This same procedure can also be used to hide the sharp line of demarcation that is often visible at the edge of a camouflage makeup application.

COLOR CORRECTORS

The type of cosmetic treatment you select will depend on what you are attempting to conceal. Most surgical or dermatologic surgery procedures result in temporary trauma to the skin, which results in swelling and discoloration. Color correctors can be worn underneath foundations to neutralize these skin color changes. Green color correctors will counterbalance redness or ruddiness, and mauve or lavender color correctors will offset sallow or yellow undertones in the skin.

Neutralizing Redness

The redness that often accompanies surgical procedures can be neutralized by applying a green color corrector to the affected area, setting it with powder, and applying either a light application of cover cream that matches the natural skin tone or the patient's regular makeup foundation over the powdered color corrector.

Tattoos

The most effective way to conceal a tattoo is to apply a color corrector to the area first, set with powder, allow the powder to be absorbed (depending upon the patient's skin type, oily or dry, 3–10 minutes), covering the area with a cover cream that matches the patient's skin, and then resetting with a dusting powder. To obliterate red tattoos apply a green color corrector. To erase a blue tattoo use an orange color corrector.

Neutralizing Bruising

Skin discoloration can occur from a leakage of blood after an injury or surgery. At first the blood under the skin appears blue or black; then the breakdown of hemoglobin turns the bruise yellow. A mauve or a lavender color corrector applied directly over the yellow discoloration and set with powder should help to eliminate the obvious yellow discoloration from the bruising. After applying the color corrector, use a clean sponge to apply a light application of cover cream or foundation. This should be all that is necessary to completely conceal this problem. Be very gentle when working on patients after surgery; when the skin is in the process of healing tenderness may result. A sponge or a light finger application will prevent the patient from feeling any unnecessary discomfort during the makeup application process.

Concealing Eyelid Incision Lines

If too heavy a concealer is used on the incision lines on the eyelids it will end up in the crease of the eyelid. To prevent this from occurring apply a lavender or mauve color corrector first by brushing directly over the incision line with a thin brush such as a lip or an artist's flat brush, setting with powder, and covering the entire eye area with a light, non-greasy foundation base.

COSMETIC THERAPY FOR PARTIAL BALDNESS

Cover creams can also be applied to the scalp to eliminate the contrast between the patient's hair and the scalp after a transplant or scalp reduction. By selecting a cover cream that closely matches the patient's hair color and by applying it directly to the patient's head, areas with a low density of hair growth appear fuller. This procedure can also be very effective for patients who are recovering from alopecia.

CREAM ROUGE AND POWDER BLUSHERS

Often you will find it necessary to camouflage the entire facial area, which will automatically obliterate the natural color of the skin. To restore color tone and to give the skin a healthy appearance, a cream rouge or powder blusher can be applied.

PATIENT INSTRUCTION

Only after you have completed the procedure and your patient is satisfied with the cosmetic result are you to progress with the instruction phase of the appointment. Start by guiding the patient through the removal process. The best way to teach the patient how to cleanse and remove the cover creams is by asking him or her to remove your application. This will ensure that the patient will be able to properly cleanse his or her skin alone. Because camouflage makeup is an oil-based formula, regular soap and water will not dislodge the cover creams. A water-in-oil solution removal cream is the most efficient cleanser. To avoid the possibility of irritation to the patient, select a product that is hypo-allergenic (without fragrance).

Cover Cream Removal Method

1. Have the patient apply a liberal amount of cleansing cream directly over the cover cream, massaging it in circular motion to loosen up the waxes and the oil in the product. See Figure 8-4.

2. Instruct the patient to wipe off the makeup application with moistened cotton squares until the cover creams have been completely removed.

3. The cleansing cream will leave a filmy residue on the skin. This can be removed with a toner (without alcohol) for sensitive skin and an astringent (with alcohol) for oily skin. If necessary, demonstrate to the patient the method with which to apply toner or astringent to the skin with a cotton square.

4. Follow up with a light moisturizer that contains a sunscreen.

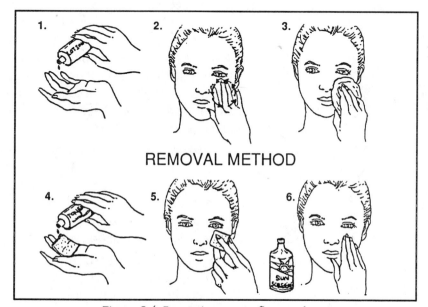

REMOVAL METHOD

Figure 8-4. Removing camouflage makeup

Guiding the Patient through the Application Process

A patient's previous experience with applying cosmetics and prior knowledge of color will influence the length of time required for the appointment and the level of complexity to be used in teaching certain makeup techniques. It is important to determine the patient's prior experience with makeup and overall comprehension of color, including both theoretical and practical applications. A patient may have more knowledge of color than he or she realizes, either through an art course or through hobbies, such as landscaping, photography, or interior design. You can determine the patient's color awareness by asking him or her about any formal color studies or personal experimentation with color. Ask questions relevant to the patient's cosmetic experience, such as does the patient have a current makeup routine? If so, how complex and time-consuming is it? The answers to these questions will give you an idea of the patient's technical experience and how much of that experience can be incorporated into the camouflage lesson.

Face and Body Diagram

The face and body diagram is an instructional tool that is offered to the patient at the beginning of the appointment. You should suggest that he or she take notes throughout the session. In addition, this document is often filled out by the camouflage therapist to illustrate some of the more technical aspects of the cosmetic process. At the end of the camouflage therapy session, the patient is given a copy of this form as a record of his or her treatment. This diagram can later be used by the patient as a visual practice tool in which to repeat the procedure. See Appendix B.

After watching you perform the initial application process, the patient should attempt the makeup process. See Figure 8-5. The following steps will help you to review the camouflage procedure with your patient and will assist you in guiding him or her through the necessary steps to complete a successful camouflage application. Remind the patient that this is a learning situation and that he or she can't expect perfection.

1. Lesson number one is organization — this is an important step. Start the lesson off right by instructing the patient to line up all his or her tools and preparations in the order in which he or she will be using them. This process will help the patient to remember the sequence of the application process.

2. Suggest that the patient document the procedure on the facial or body diagram you will provide him or her (see the documentation chapter). Recommend that the

patient take notes as you review the application process together, one step at a time.

3. Ask the patient to put small amounts of the selected cover creams on the back of his or her hand, blending them together by making small circles until they match his or her skin color as closely as possible.

4. Instruct the patient to apply the camouflage creams thinly and evenly to the surface of his or her skin using the third or fourth finger or a sponge, using a light dab-pat motion, and blending out the edges of the cover creams until they disappear.

5. Direct the patient to set the application with a powder puff or a cotton square by liberally applying setting powder over the cover creams.

6. Advise the patient to wait for 3–10 minutes (depending on his or her skin type) before lightly dusting off all traces of the setting powder with a fluffy powder brush.

7. At the end of the session ask the patient to inspect the application to make sure all the edges of the cover creams are well blended in, and to determine if any remaining traces of powder need to be brushed out of facial (beards, mustaches, or eyebrows) or body hair.

8. Be sure to have an inventory of clear plastic containers (1/4 oz.) with lids to give samples of custom blended cover creams and setting powder to your patients if

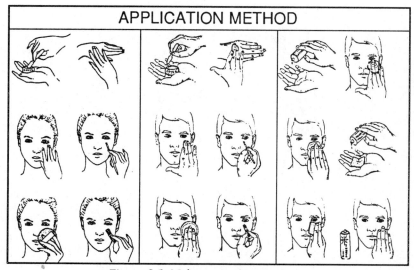

Figure 8-5. Makeup application lesson

necessary. These containers can be obtained from a packing supply company. Also, offer patients lunch-size paper bags for their cosmetics.

REVIEW

You should now be familiar with:

- how to decide if a patient is a candidate for camouflage therapy.
- the correct method to use when cleansing the skin.
- how to apply cover cream.
- techniques for duplicating skin imperfections.
- how to instruct patients in the technical aspects of camouflage makeup

CHAPTER

9 Micropigmentation

Jessica L. Elkins, R.N., BSN

Micropigmentation is an alternative that you can suggest to patients who have lost their eyelashes or eyebrows. Micropigmentation, or permanent cosmetic therapy, is the technical art of applying color to the dermis or second layer of skin with a specially designed instrument. The most ancient and widely employed form of micropigmentation is tattooing. Archaeological evidence indicates that tattooing was practiced among peoples living during the late Stone Age. Cleopatra was said to have had permanent, or tattooed, eyeliner.

In the 1990s both women and men are opting for permanent cosmetics.

The micropigmentation procedure is extremely operator dependent. The operator must be medically trained in performing anesthetic injections around the eye and lip area and well-versed in pre-operative and post-operative care. Anesthetic injections within the upper and lower eyelids and around the lip area must be performed skillfully to minimize discomfort to the patient. Educating and advising patients on what to expect during a micropigmentation procedure is essential. At this stage, a special rapport develops between the person performing the micropigmentation procedure and the patient. The patient should have complete trust in the operator's skill and knowledge of micropigmentation. A well-informed patient is aware of all possible complications that may occur during and after a micropigmentation procedure.

Jessica Elkins is a registered nurse with ten years experience in plastic and reconstructive surgery.

Medical professionals performing the micropigmentation procedure around the eyelids, brow, and lip area must be skillful and knowledgeable in makeup application techniques. For instance, the contour and shape of a patient's eye determines the thickness of color pigment applied to the lower and upper eye. In addition to being a makeup artist, medical professionals must precisely identify the appropriate pigment colors that compliment the hair, skin, and eye color of their clients.

CANDIDATES FOR MICROPIGMENTATION

Vitiligo patients are good candidates for micropigmentation procedures. Vitiligo is a skin disorder marked by stark white skin patches. The lesions are always depigmented, generally appearing over bony prominences, around the eyes and mouth, within body folds, and at sites of trauma. Although the cause of vitiligo is unknown, inheritance seems to be a definite etiological factor.

Alopecia universalis patients would benefit from micropigmentation. Alopecia universalis is a skin disorder in which hair loss occurs over the entire body. Eyebrow and eyelash alopecia is definitely a significant cosmetic defect. The etiology of alopecia is usually presence of other diseases such as granulomas, lupus erythematosus, scleroderma, and skin tumors. (See the dermatology chapter for more details on these conditions.)

Burn patients are good candidates for micropigmentation procedures. Burn patients usually have a long and painful period of rehabilitation. Many times burn patients are permanently disfigured. Loss of facial hair can be overcome with micropigmentation.

Blind patients who are unable to apply eyeliner or lipliner could permanently enhance their features with micropigmentation. In the United States blindness is legally defined as optimal visual acuity of 20/200 or less in the better eye after best correction, or a visual field not exceeding 20 degrees in the better eye. Women with poor vision who are not legally blind can also benefit from pigmentation procedures. (See chapter on visual disabilities.)

Limited mobility patients are good candidates for micropigmentation. For example, patients who have limited use of arms or hands would be suitable for micropigmentation procedures.

Arthritis patients are excellent candidates for micropigmentation procedures. Rheumatoid arthritis is a chronic, systemic, inflammatory disease primarily attacking joints, muscles, tendons, ligaments, and blood vessels. Joints usually begin to stiffen and eventually become tender and painful, making a daily activity such as makeup application very difficult.

Women with *oily skin* are also candidates for micropigmentation procedures. Conventional makeup tends to smear or fade on women with oily skin.

Allergy sufferers would greatly benefit from micropigmentation. Many times women with allergies have itching, weeping eyes, making it virtually impossible to wear conventional makeup.

Contact lens wearers are good candidates for micropigmentation. Removing and replacing contact lenses tends to smear conventional makeup as well as to irritate the eye.

Mastectomy patients are good candidates for micropigmentation. Women who have had mastectomies due to breast cancer often opt for areola reconstruction. Micropigmentation techniques can simulate the nipple-areola area.

Athletic women who want to look good during and after exercising are very good candidates for micropigmentation. Sweating tends to smear conventional makeup.

POOR CANDIDATES FOR MICROPIGMENTATION

Children are not good candidates for micropigmentation. Children's bodies, as well as their heads, are continually growing and would distort the permanent pigment. Micropigmentation procedures should not be performed on patients younger than eighteen years old.

Women with unrealistic expectations of micropigmentation procedures prove to be poor candidates. Women who believe the procedure will change their personalities or quality of life should be strongly discouraged from undergoing the micropigmentation procedure.

MOST COMMONLY USED MICROPIGMENTATION PROCEDURES

Currently, the most common micropigmentation procedures performed include lash liner, eyebrow enhancement, lip liner, nipple-areola simulation, and scar camouflage.

Lash Liner Micropigmentation is performed to cosmetically enhance the eyelid margin. Lash liner gives the appearance of fuller and thicker eyelashes. Pigment is placed along the lash line in small dots, creating a soft, subtle halo around the eyes. Heavy or light lash liner can be applied, depending on the patient's needs. Heavy lash liner is not recommended because of the permanence of this procedure. The color of the eyelashes, eyebrows, hair roots, and iris is examined in choosing the correct pigment choice.

Eyebrows Micropigmentation is performed to cosmetically re-create or fill in the brow area. Pigment is placed in the brow area with a brush-stroke technique that simulates the cilia (brow hair). Colors are blended to match the patient's hair color and skin tone.

Lip Liner Micropigmentation is performed to effectively outline as well as fill in the vermilion area. Thin lips can easily be made to look fuller. Overfull lips can be made to look smaller. Lips that have been subject to some type of traumatic injury may achieve a look of normalcy. Pigment choice is usually darker than the natural color of the vermilion border.

Nipple-Areola Micropigmentation is performed and is cosmetically effective to recreate the natural color of the areola area following breast reconstruction. The nipple is also re-created using a variety of pigmenting techniques. The pigment is mixed and should be slightly darker than that of the opposite breast.

Scars Micropigmentation is performed to camouflage scarred or depigmented areas of the skin. Flesh colored pigments are blended to closely match the natural skin tones.

PRE-OPERATIVE EVALUATION

During a patient's initial consultation, a pre-operative evaluation is performed. The patient is encouraged to ask questions and to establish realistic expectations of the various procedures. A medical history is taken. Patients are asked if they have a history of allergies, especially allergies to paints, crayons, or makeup. Since all of these contain iron, it may suggest a potential sensitivity to ferrous oxide pigments, commonly used in most color pigments. If a patient has a history of allergies, a skin test should be performed. A small amount of pigment should be applied behind the ear. The patient is rechecked two days and ten days after the skin test. If there is no reaction, the micropigmentation procedure can be performed. A variety of pigments are available for each procedure. A color analysis system is used to precisely identify the appropriate colors that uniquely complement the patient's hair, skin, and eye colors. At this point, the patient reads the consent form, which outlines all the potential risks and complications resulting from the procedure.

POTENTIAL RISKS AND COMPLICATIONS

Abrasion of the Cornea

Abrasion of the cornea can be prevented by the use of a lid plate. Cornea abrasion is the result of needle penetration into the cornea.

Eyelash Loss

Eyelash loss is most likely due to the mechanical trauma of the eyelash bulb.

Pigment Fading

Pigment fading is most likely due to pigment implanted too superficially. The pigment will slough off as the epidermis desquamates.

Unexpected Scarring

Dermal maceration may occur if the micropigmentation procedure is done too vigorously.

Inconsistent Color

Inconsistent coloring could result from improper technique.

Hematoma

Hematoma could occur from injection of xylocaine directly into a blood vessel.

Infection

Infection could occur if the patient was not compliant with post- op care or if the procedure was done with dirty needles.

Spreading of the Pigment

Spreading or fanning of pigment within the orbicularis muscle could occur from increased duration and depth of needle penetration within the skin.

If a patient is having a micropigmentation procedure for permanent lash liner, the patient must arrange transportation to and from the office. Also, the patient must remove contact lenses before the procedure. The pigment would permanently stain the contact lenses. To help patients relax, recommend that they wear loose-fitting, comfortable clothing.

LASH LINER PROCEDURE

The most requested micropigmentation procedure is for permanent lash liner application. The following is a description of the steps taken in this procedure, which is performed by a specially trained operator.

1. Several drops of a topical anesthetic are instilled into both eyes.

2. Local anesthetic is injected into the lower eyelids.

3. Steroid antibiotic ointment is applied to the eyelashes to protect them. A small amount of ointment is applied to a Jaeger eyelid plate, which is used to support the lower eyelid during the procedure.

4. The eyelid margin and eyelashes are used as landmarks for pigment placement. A three-pronged needle is usually used for permanent lash liner applications. A single needle is used when a patient requests a very light lash liner. First, the central and medial landmarks are identified and a small dot of pigment is implanted at these locations. Additional dots are added between the landmark dots beginning medially and ending centrally. Next another dot is placed at the lateral end of the proposed lash liner. The dots are applied, working from the lateral end toward the medial landmark. The dots are applied sequentially, barely overlapping. Throughout the procedure the eyelid plate should be removed and the eyelid examined. The same procedure is repeated on the opposite lower eyelid.

5. After the lower eyelids are completed, the upper eyelids are anesthetized. Most women request heavier pigment in the upper eyelids, particularly in the lateral end of the upper eyelid. The upper eyelid pigment line is produced with a single row of pigment dots within the superior row of eyelashes. To achieve a heavier liner, two or more rows may be applied.

6. After the micropigmentation procedure is complete the eyelids are cleaned of excess pigment with an eye

rinse and antibiotic ointment is applied to the pigmented areas. The patient is provided with artificial tears, which should be used throughout the day of the procedure to prevent any keratitis from the eyelid akinesia.

POST-OPERATIVE INSTRUCTIONS

Following are the standard post-operative instructions given to patients following a micropigmentation procedure.

1. Immediately following the procedure, ice packs will be placed on your eyes. Upon returning home, apply ice packs intermittently to your eyes for twenty-four hours to reduce swelling.

2. Gently apply the prescribed ointment to the eyelashes and eyelid margins twice a day for four days after the procedure. While a cotton swab may help you distribute the ointment, do not rub the skin vigorously. The purpose of the ointment is to prevent infection and to keep the wound free from crusting.

3. Do not attempt to scratch or pick away any crust along the eyelid. Early removal of pigment crusts may result in areas with insufficient eyeliner.

4. You may carefully cleanse around the eyelids in the morning with a cotton ball soaked in water. Gently dab the eyelids following cleaning with a moist cotton ball. Do not disturb the eyelashes.

5. Some blood-tinged tears are normal for the first day after the procedure.

6. Avoid swimming and sunbathing for one week after the procedure.

7. Do not wear eye makeup for three days. Use a new tube of mascara when resuming makeup application.

8. Call the office if you have any problems.

This information is not intended to be a "do-it-yourself" manual, but is meant to inform the camouflage therapist of the various procedures available through micropigmentation. Micropigmentation procedures should never be attempted without adequate training and certification.

REVIEW

You should now be familiar with:

- ■ what micropigmentation is and when it is used.
- ■ what are the most commonly used micropigmentation procedures.
- ■ the micropigmentation procedure and what to expect afterwards.

10 Adaptive Grooming Techniques for the Visually Impaired

Of all the physical afflictions mankind suffers, no people are as pitied as those who are struck by blindness. Most people stereotype individuals who are sightless, primarily because they do not understand their disability. Because of their uneasiness, many well-intentioned people avoid contact with those who are blind, and as a result they are ignorant about the capabilities of the blind. Because a person is blind, he or she does not necessarily think or feel any different than a person who can see. We all live in the same world, and we all experience many of the same problems. But because we live in a world arranged for those with sight, many people view blindness as a fate worse than death.

We live in a visually oriented culture, so eyesight is considered, of all the senses, the most important. Loss of vision is a devastating experience. As of this year, more than 80,000,000 Americans have been diagnosed with diseases in one or both eyes that will cause partial or complete vision impairment. More than 14,000,000 Americans have impaired vision that cannot be corrected by eyeglasses, 1,500,000 need assistance with daily living activities, and 800,000 are considered legally blind.

A patient who has lost sight is probably experiencing a loss that will not improve. Because of blindness, a patient may lose the ability to work at his or her current job, lose independence, and lose much self esteem. Eventually he or she must learn to cope with the loss because ultimately there really is no other choice. Grief is a process that no two people experience the same way. Reorganization is a positive step toward acceptance. In order for people who have lost their sight to feel good about themselves again, they must learn to acknowledge both their strengths and their limitations.

How people work through the loss of their eyesight and the intensity and duration of their grief will depend on two main factors: how a person copes with the stress of functioning without his or her sight and how quickly he or she adapts to the adjustments that must be made in his or her lifestyle. The support the patient receives from family, friends, and health-care professionals is also a major factor in influencing how well the patient will eventually cope with his or her visual impairment.

This chapter will discuss various causes of visual impairment and blindness, and will offer the clinical cosmetologist adaptive techniques that he or she can teach blind patients to help them develop coping strategies to make the most of what they have.

Blindness refers to the total or partial inability to see. It involves a severe loss of vision that cannot be corrected with ordinary eye glasses. More commonly, the definition of vision impairment is associated with a loss of sight of an extent that it notably hinders everyday activities.

Loss of vision, which may develop slowly or suddenly, depending on the cause, impairs central (front) vision, peripheral (side) vision, or both. When an ophthalmologist (a medical doctor or osteopath who is educated, trained, and licensed to provide total care of the eyes, including the diagnosis and treatment of the many different types of eye diseases) tests eyesight, he or she reports the results in numbers that compare the patient's eye with a normal eye: in 20/40 vision, for example, the person sees at 20 feet what a person with normal vision can see at 40 feet. See Figure 10-1. 20/20 indicates normal vision; 20/200 constitutes legal blindness. In

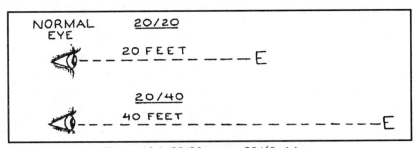

Figure 10-1. 20/20 versus 20/40 vision.

the United States blindness is defined as corrected visual acuity (perception) of 20/200 or less in the better eye, or a visual field of no more than 20 degrees in the better eye.

Loss of central vision prevents an individual from reading and being able to distinguish fine details. Loss of peripheral vision may be unnoticed by the affected person until it is well advanced, causing awkwardness of movement. See Figure 10-2.

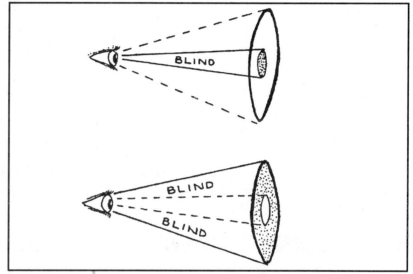

Figure 10-2. Loss of central and peripheral vision

Normal vision depends on the uninterrupted passage of light from the front of the eye to the retina. It involves two main components, the eye and the brain. As light rays reach the eye, most of the focusing is done by the cornea. The eye also is equipped with a fine focusing facility (called accommodation) that operates by altering the curvature of the eye's crystalline lens. These two systems together generate enough optical power to create an image on the retina. See Figure 10-3. Vision begins in the retina, a membrane at the back of the eye that contains light-sensitive rod and cone cells. Much of the rest of the eye is concerned with focusing the right quantities of light onto the retina. A large amount of information is sent from the retina through the optic nerve to the brain for analysis. If a person's vision is out of focus, it can be corrected by other lenses, such as eye glasses or contact lenses.

Anything that obstructs the passage of light rays from the retina can cause blindness. Blindness is one of the most feared of all human afflictions. Unfortunately it is widespread,

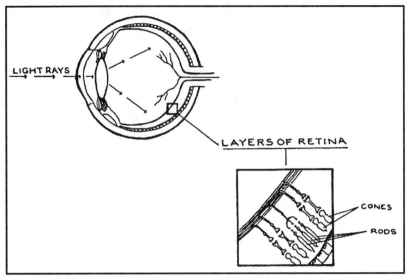

Figure 10-3. Normal vision

affecting all segments of our population. Most of us do not realize that blindness is most frequently the result of eye disease.

COMMON CAUSES OF BLINDNESS

The most common causes of blindness in the United States are glaucoma, cataracts, retinal detachment, degenerative retinal disorders, diabetic retinopathy, and accidents. Industrial accidents involving objects thrown up from high-speed machinery that penetrate the eye can cause serious injuries or blindness. Blunt trauma such as a blow can lead to bleeding behind the lens or into the front chamber of the eye; fluid outflow draining the eye can also threaten vision. Less than 4 percent of blindness results from eye injuries. Visual complications can also be due to AIDS, the largest cause being cytomegalovirus (CMV); the second largest cause is infection to the nervous system, such as that resulting from toxoplasmosis. Only a small percentage of people with AIDS will develop vision complications, however. (See the chapter on AIDS.) The following diseases are the most common causes of blindness.

Glaucoma   Glaucoma is an eye disease in which pressure from the fluid in the eye is increased enough to cause damage. The damage comes from compression and obstruction of the small internal blood vessels and/or the fibers of the optic nerve. See Figure 10-4. The result is partial or complete loss of vision.

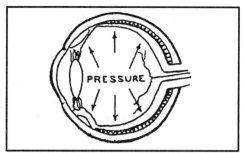

Figure 10-4. Glaucoma

Why this loss of vision occurs is something that is not completely understood.

Open-angle glaucoma is the most common form of glaucoma. This disease is caused by the unbalanced outflow and production of fluid in the front compartment of the eye over a period of years. It usually occurs after the age of 40, but can occur at any age; it is most commonly diagnosed in the elderly. Glaucoma can also be congenital. Generally there are no symptoms (it is painless), because the gradual loss of peripheral vision is not apparent until blindness is advanced. The accumulation of fluid results in a slow rise in pressure. Chronic open-angle glaucoma appears to be caused by genetic factors. Closed-angle glaucoma is a sudden rise in pressure in which pain and redness is present.

Cataracts

When the transparency of the lens of the eye is lost, the result is a cataract. See Figure 10-5. Cataracts cause loss of visual acuity (clarity) and make it difficult for the person afflicted to define images. When detail is lost, objects become blurry and fuzzy and the patient is bothered by glare. Several factors cause cataracts: aging, injury to the eye, birth defects, the rubella virus, galactosemia (sugar galactose accumulates in the body, causing the condition), prolonged

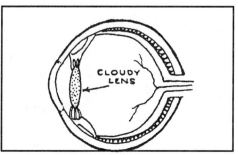

Figure 10-5. Cataracts

intake of corticosteroid drugs, and diabetes mellitus. Exposure to any form of ultraviolet light (sunlight), radiation, or X-rays can cause their development. Most people over the age of 65 have cataracts, and the majority of persons over 75 years old have minor visual disturbances. In fact, it is so common that it is considered normal. As we age the center of the lens gradually hardens, and there is an increased chance of liquid seeping through to the lens capsule. This leads to protein changes, and in the advanced stages causes the eye to appear white because of the protein fibers within the lens.

Cataracts are painless. Persons who suffer from cataracts frequently become nearsighted because, as the density of the lens increases, the light-refracting power becomes greater, often allowing persons who were once far-sighted to read without wearing glasses. Cataracts may cause some form of change in color perception by decreasing the value of blues and accentuating red, orange, and yellow colors.

Cataracts usually develop in both eyes, but one eye is sometimes more affected. Once a person has cataracts, surgery is indicated. There is no way to reverse the change with current medication. When vision is seriously affected, cataract extraction is necessary. This operation is routinely performed in a surgery center. The opacified lens is replaced with a tiny plastic implant that is fixed permanently within the eye. Not everyone can benefit from this procedure; young people may be advised against an implant because the lifespan of the implant has not as yet been determined, and a patient with a history of eye disease may be considered an unsuitable candidate for this type of surgery. As an alternative, patients are fitted for contact lenses that they can wear postoperatively. Intra-ocular lenses are used more and more in younger individuals. Other ocular disease may not preclude implant surgery. Implants can also be used later in life as a secondary procedure.

Retinal Detachment

Retinal detachment occurs when there is a separation of the light-sensitive inner surface of the back of the eye from the outer layers. See Figure 10-6. It occurs when vitreous fluid (a gel-like substance that fills the main cavity of the eye between crystalline lens and the retina) accumulates between the photo receptor layer and the underlying pigment layer, resulting in separation. It is usually proceeded by a tear or break in the retina. This condition can occur spontaneously in persons who are nearsighted because they have thin retinas, persons

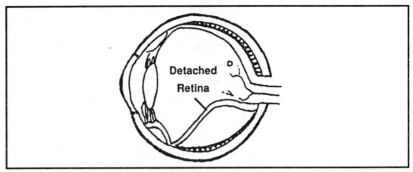

Figure 10-6. Retinal detachment

who have suffered a major injury to the eye, and in people who have had cataract surgery.

The symptoms are visual and are not painful. The first indication of this disease may be the appearance of bright flashes of light or spots. These flashes or spots are caused by over-stimulation of light-sensitive cells when the tear occurs. Sometimes these symptoms never manifest and the person affected is not aware until vision is obscured. If the retina of the central portion becomes detached it may not be fully restored. Retinal detachment is treated by laser or cryopexy (involving the application of extreme cold to fix the retina in place by causing inflammatory adhesiveness of the underlying tissues). A scleral buckle may also be indicated to push the retina back into place.

Degenerative Retinal Disorders

Macular degeneration may occur in older people, while macular dystrophy may occur in younger individuals.

There are two kinds of degenerative retinal disorders: "dry" atrophic in which there is no treatment, and "wet" atrophic in which new blood vessels leak fluid and hemorrhage, causing scarring of the tissue. See Figure 10-7. Treatment may halt

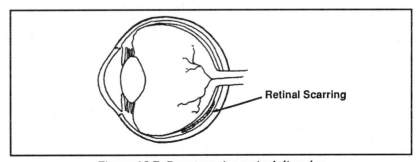

Figure 10-7. Degenerative retinal disorder

the progression of the disease but will not restore the lost vision. Early diagnosis and treatment is very important. Side vision is unaffected.

Degenerative retinal disease is a slowly progressing disorder that occurs in the central part of the retina, creating a loss of vision. It is most common in the elderly and usually affects both eyes. It is painless. Fluid leakage occurs when there is a breakdown of the layer between the retina and the blood vessels behind the retina. This causes a destruction of retinal nerve tissue by the new blood vessels growing from this layer, creating scar tissue. The effect is a circular area of blindness that enlarges until it obliterates two or three words at normal reading distance. Some cases are untreatable; however, early diagnosis sometimes makes it possible to seal-off the leakage with laser surgery. Optical or low vision aids frequently help.

Diabetic Retinopathy Diabetes mellitus may result in retinopathy (a disease or disorder of the retina); a hemorrhage of the retinal capillaries (sometimes brought about by persistent hypertension or high blood pressure) results in an aneurysm (a sac formed in a weak area of an artery or vein) of the capillaries that later hemorrhages into the retina. See Figure 10-8. New blood vessels are then formed on the surface of the retina, and these fragile vessels bleed readily. The major cause of permanent loss of vision occurs when the blood vessels hemorrhage into the vitreous gel (the gel-like substance that fills the cavity between the lens and the retina), and fibrous tissue can grow onto the gel causing proliferative retinopathy.

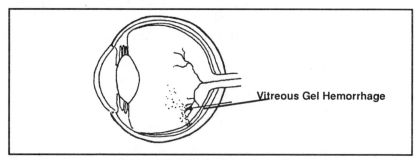

Figure 10-8. Diabetic retinopathy

Toxoplasmosis Toxoplasmosis (see AIDS chapter) is a disease caused by toxoplasma gondii. It is most frequently congenital (acquired before birth) and reactivates later in life, causing progressive damage to the retina. See Figure 10-9. The congenital form may accompany central nervous system lesions that can result in blindness, brain defects, or death.

Onchocerciasis, a worm infection, can also cause severe retinal damage. Other bacterial and fungal infections may be easily carried by the blood to the retina. A patient is more susceptible to viral infections of the retina if the immune system has been compromised by AIDS.

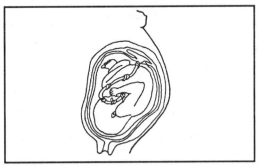

Figure 10-9. Congenital toxoplasmosis

Retinal Vein Occlusion (or Artery Occlusion) An impaired retinal blood supply can create a blockage of the central vein or artery of the retina, causing blindness. See Figure 10-10.

Hypertensive retinopathy is damage to the retina caused by high blood pressure, which narrows the blood vessels of the retina.

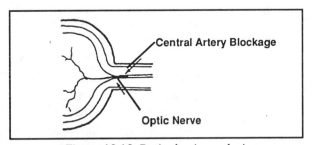

Figure 10-10. Retinal vein occlusion

Medication Certain types of medication used to treat psychiatric disorders can also damage the retina if taken over a prolonged period. Chloroquine, a medication often administered in large doses for conditions such as rheumatoid arthritis, may cause damage to the retina.

Tumors

Retinoblastoma is a malignant tumor that is usually discovered in a patient within the first three years of his or her life. The affected eye may have pupil whiteness and strabismus, or squint (an eye turn or deviation that the patient cannot control), often develops. See Figure 10-11. Other tumors are primary site (ocular) or metastic, in which transfer occurs of disease from one organ or part of the body to another not directly connected with it. Tumors from other body sites such as the lung, breast, or liver may also sometimes migrate to the eyes.

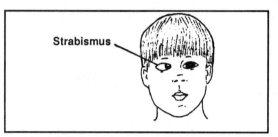

Figure 10-11. Retinoblastoma

ADAPTIVE TECHNIQUES IN MAKEUP AND BASIC GROOMING

The following information was compiled with the assistance of instructor Shireen Perry, who teaches personal living skills to the blind and visually impaired. She is a consultant to professionals dealing with AIDS patients going through vision loss. Ms. Perry received her B.A. in Home Economics, and M.A. in Clinical Rehabilitation, Orientation, and Mobility at San Francisco State University.

In this section, you will learn about working with patients who are blind or newly visually impaired, the equipment and supplies you will need to teach grooming skills, and how to organize and conduct the teaching sessions. You will be given a step-by-step guide to assist you in providing cosmetic therapy and other esthetic services to visually-impaired patients.

For a blind or visually-impaired patient, it is very important to make a conscious effort to follow a grooming routine. Any individual, regardless of his or her disability, makes a statement to others through self presentation. A patient who is well groomed tells the world, "I think highly of myself."

Persons who are newly blind will need to learn to visualize their appearance and try to recall different aspects that need attention. Because they will no longer be able to casually glance into a mirror on the way out the door to determine if they have lint on their dark clothing, or if their shoes are run down, or they have a run in their stockings, patients will need to master a non-visual systematic routine of imagery with which to double check and ensure that their entire physical appearance is in order. The sightless patient cannot always depend on a sighted person to offer the necessary feedback on all aspects of personal grooming.

There is no right or wrong way for a clinical cosmetician or cosmetologist to approach a sightless patient. Each person will react differently to you depending on his or her personality and the way in which he or she interprets the value of your service. Patients will generally be more comfortable with you if you are comfortable with them. As you become less preoccupied with the visual disability, you can begin to concentrate on what you can do to help the patient gain confidence in his or her own ability to manage the necessary procedures for personal care.

Strong communication skills will be necessary to instruct newly blind patients in adaptive grooming techniques. The esthetic professional will need to be extremely well organized so as not to confuse the patient. Working with a sightless patient can be one of the most rewarding challenges you will ever face, but you will need a great deal of patience, not just with the person who is visually impaired, but with yourself. Most importantly, you must be flexible. Some patients will readily adapt to your instruction, while others may struggle with every little detail of a procedure.

Blindness is a disability, and as with any disability it must be taken into consideration when preparing the patient's lesson plan. As an instructor, you need confidence in your ability to transmit information so that the patient will be able to comprehend it. This inner confidence is essential in order for you to feel immediately at ease with an individual who has lost the ability to see. A positive attitude is crucial because it will strongly influence the patient's reaction to you. Your positive attitude will also influence the patient's ability to perform the techniques you will be teaching. Regardless of the severity of the patient's vision loss or your emotional reaction to it, it is vital that you approach the sightless patient as professionally as you would any individual, without pity or condescension. The patient has been referred to you to learn certain independent grooming skills, not to be analyzed or pitied.

Why Would Women Who Are Blind Want to Wear Makeup?

Many women express themselves through makeup, hairstyling, and the style of dress. Why should a newly blind woman who has always worn cosmetics stop doing so? For such a patient, wearing cosmetics might make the statement to herself and to others that she is self-assured and that she has the freedom to be who she wants to be, regardless of her sight impairment.

Each patient will bring to cosmetic therapy an individual mix of emotions and physical abilities based on life experiences. The best way for the patient to discover what she is actually capable of doing is to experiment. By taking the responsibility to identify the patient's strengths and weaknesses, you can help her recognize which of her previous skills she can incorporate into the lesson plan.

Before you begin the session, you will need to ask the patient about her recreational interests, hobbies, and current or former place of employment. You will also need to know her former grooming habits. Pay keen attention to the patient as she shares this information with you. It is extremely important during this interviewing process that you focus on everything the patient says and does. Listen carefully to what the patient is really revealing and the way in which she presents the information to you. Watch the patient's facial expressions and body language. To control the dynamics of this exchange, you must concentrate on the patient's interests and skills, especially those that will help your training. At the same time, identify positive personality traits the patient has — such as a good sense of humor, attention to detail, and creativity. Prior knowledge of this information will make the education process easier for both of you. Take notes during the interview so that you can later review them when you make your assessment.

Next you will want to explain the general principles of your therapy. Once you have reviewed with the patient the requirements of the grooming procedure you will be teaching, ask the patient if he or she has any questions or immediate concerns. A patient who is newly blind may feel intimidated by the entire process and may question whether he or she will be capable of performing the grooming techniques independently. It is likely the patient will be encouraged if you maintain a positive attitude and let him or her know you will be working together as a team.

Adaptive techniques involve habit changing. For most of us change invokes fear, primarily the fear of failure. An important attitude to maintain throughout the session, regardless of circumstances that may arise, is: "How can we approach this task," not, "This can't be done."

You will need to establish what the patient expects from the session. For example, regarding the cosmetic grooming session, some patients may not want nor will they need to wear makeup foundation, while others may not require eye cosmetics because they wear glasses with darkly tinted lenses. Such patients may only be interested in enhancing other exposed facial areas. The patient's feedback will greatly influence his or her attitude toward the instruction. Always focus on the patient's goals for treatment. If you continually keep what the patient is trying to accomplish in mind and refer to it frequently throughout the session, the patient will be twice as likely to stay focused on the information you are imparting, because he or she will know that the original objective will ultimately be reached.

Before you begin, be sure to explain to your patient that he or she will be performing the procedure. You will need to reassure the patient after making this statement that throughout the session you will be offering constructive verbal feedback; you are a verbal mirror. Because work simplification and time management principles are important factors when instructing the visually impaired, you will need to clarify all your instructions so that you will present the patient with simple, step-by-step procedures.

Closely observe the patient's responses when giving instructions to insure that he or she is processing the information correctly. See Figure 10-12. Do not hesitate to re-phrase directions if necessary. The clinical cosmetician or cosmetologist should never be afraid to give the patient verbal feedback. The patient may be having problems mastering a specific technique, and your help may be required to devise a new, creative approach. Remember when pointing out to a patient that he or she is performing a technique incorrectly to reassure the patient that all that is needed to become more proficient is practice.

If the patient knows braille, encourage him or her to take notes on the techniques that he or she will be learning. Patients who do not know braille should be advised to bring a tape recorder and record the session. If possible, recording equipment should be available to provide the patient with a cassette as a practice tool.

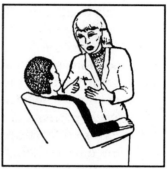

Figure 10-12. Observe the client's responses when giving him or her instructions

Materials

The following is a list of materials that you will need for the teaching sessions.

Suggested Labeling Ideas

TOOL	WHERE TO PURCHASE
Velcro	fabric store
rubber bands	supermarket, stationary store
textured sandpaper	hardware store
buttons (various sizes and shapes)	fabric store, dime store
fabric craft puff paint	fabric store
cosmetic tray	beauty supply, hardware store, thrift store
braille identification labels	contact your local center for the blind

Equipment

EQUIPMENT	WHERE TO PURCHASE
table	beauty/equipment supply, office supply
chair	same as above
lighting system	see cosmetic therapy chapter

waste receptacle	hardware store, supermarket
tape recorder	electronics store, department store

Disposable Items

ITEM	WHERE TO PURCHASE
cotton balls, cotton squares, cotton swabs	pharmacy, beauty supply, cosmetic distributor
tissue	same as above
paper bags	same as above
makeup remover	same as above
cleansing cream or lotion	same as above
moisturizing cream or lotion	same as above

Cosmetics

ITEM	WHERE TO PURCHASE
large selection of base foundations	pharmacy, beauty supply, department store, cosmetic distributor
colorless translucent setting powder	beauty supply, department store
cream and powder blushers	same as above
eye shadows (suggested colors: beige, cream, taupe, light peach)	same as above
mascara (black and brown)	same as above
eye-liner pencils (suggested colors: blond, brown, dark brown, auburn, taupe, gray, black)	same as above
lip liner and lip pencil	same as above
pencil sharpener	same as above
lipsticks (variety of shades)	same as above
brushes/sponge tip cosmetic applicators	same as above

brush cleaner	beauty supply, pharmacy, cosmetic distributor
sponges (variety) for easy identification (round, square, triangle)	beauty supply, pharmacy
tweezers	beauty supply, medical supply, pharmacy

Hairstyling Tools

TOOL	WHERE TO PURCHASE
curling iron	beauty supply, department store,
blow dryer	same as above

Men's Grooming Tools

TOOL	WHERE TO PURCHASE
mustache scissors (4 ½ inch)	beauty supply, pharmacy

Manicure or Pedicure Tools

TOOL	WHERE TO PURCHASE
cotton balls	beauty supply, pharmacy
tissue	same as above
waste receptacle	same as above
paper bags	same as above
tape	same as above
alcohol	beauty supply, pharmacy
emeryboard	beauty supply, pharmacy
nail clippers	same as above
pump spray bottle	same as above
emery board	same as above
nail brush	same as above
hand towel	same as above
nail polish	same as above
nail polish remover	same as above
empty nail polish container (as practice tool)	same as above

hand cream	same as above
orangewood sticks	same as above
small container for liquid soap bath	same as above
clear nail polish	same as above
nail polish remover (in tube)	same as above
nail buffer	same as above
buffing cream	same as above

Cosmetic Therapy for the Blind

Organize all cosmetic items prior to the session. Every item needs a "little home," and it must be returned to its predesignated place when the patient is finished using it. This will alleviate a lot of stress and frustration. A tray (cafeteria size) is the best way to organize everything the patient will need. See Figure 10-13. It should be the fixed focal point. The placement of adhesive Velcro with the rough loops on the tray and the soft loops on the cosmetic containers will keep all the items in place and will prevent them from sliding off the tray. The velcro strips should be positioned parallel to each other on the tray.

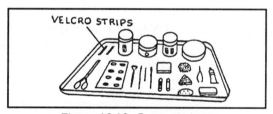

Figure 10-13. Cosmetic items

Containers will be required for brushes, cotton balls, cotton swabs, makeup sponges, eye and lip cosmetics, and makeup removal cloths. You will need both wet and dry towels and a waste container. Brushes should be in different sizes; it is important that the patient knows the uses of the different sized brushes. (See cosmetic therapy chapter for illustration of the various brushes.) Also have on hand a variety of makeup sponges in different shapes; the following sponges are recommended for cosmetic application: triangular sponge for applying foundation, circular for applying blush, and square for the application of eye shadow. You will also need makeup foundations, blushers, translucent colorless powder, black and brown mascara, eye liner, eye shadows, and lipsticks. Remove all items that you will not be using in the session from the patient's work station and place on the tray only those items that the patient will need to apply makeup.

The patient's work space should be set so that he or she can easily locate all the necessary tools for the cosmetic application. All the cosmetic items the patient will be using should be stored in special containers and placed on the tray. The patient should systematically trail her fingers around the perimeter of the tray to familiarize herself with the location of the various objects.

Labeling

The patient will identify an object on the tray by its location and by the container in which it is stored. See Figure 10-14. You can help the patient familiarize herself with the shape, size, texture, and contents of the various containers on the tray.

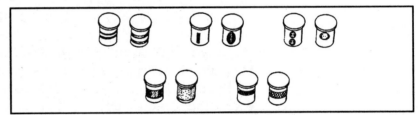

Figure 10-14. Differentiate containers

To help the patient differentiate between two containers that are the same size or shape, use the following labeling methods:

1. Place rubber bands in a variety of different widths around the container, or use more than one rubber band.

2. Make a mark on the outside of the container, such as a straight line or circle. This can be done with fabric craft textured paint, which can be found in fabric stores.

3. Buttons in a variety of different shapes and sizes can be glued to the outside of the containers to represent different items.

4. Different textured sandpaper can also be glued onto a container. The coarseness and fineness of sandpaper is determined by the "grit." The lower the number, the coarser the paper; the higher the number, the finer the paper; thus, 16 grit is very coarse, and 220 grit is very fine.

5. Soft and rough looped strips of Velcro can also be used for identification through texture.

All of the methods mentioned are considered non-braille systems for marking. If the clinical cosmetician knows the standard braille alphabet, he or she can mark the items and their containers with embossed adhesive masking tape.

It is important that each patient participate in devising his or her own unique system for labeling, because he or she is the one who will use it. You can suggest several labeling methods for the patient to use at home.

For additional information, or to order materials contact:
American Foundation for the Blind
15 W. 16th St.
New York, NY. 10011
(800) 232-5463 (outside New York)
(212) 620-2147 (inside New York)

Search Methods

Once the containers have been labeled, place them on the tray in the order in which they will be used. See Figure 10-15. The patient must be able to define a particular item by its texture and location. Give the patient plenty of time to touch all the objects being described. The following information will help you to assist the patient in this process:

1. The patient should be instructed to extend the fingertips and have them slightly curled.

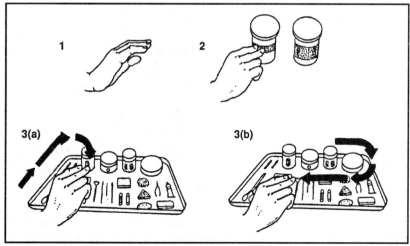

Figure 10-15. Place containers on the tray in the order in which they will be used

2. Suggest that the patient keep the palms of the hands close to the surface with her fingertips relaxed and slightly curved. This will prevent her from knocking something over as she slowly moves her hands over the items on the tray.

3. Have the patient lightly move her hands around the perimeter of the area, first from side to side, and then from top to bottom in a grid-like pattern.

4. Instruct the patient to move her hands in circular motion over all the objects on the tray. She should start by making small circles at first, slowly graduating to larger ones. By using this search method the patient will quickly locate specific objects, and she will be able to conveniently replace items or locate objects that have accidently fallen from the tray.

Makeup Application

Before the patient begins applying any cosmetics, encourage her to explore her bone structure and identify the shape of her facial features by slowly moving the tips of her fingers over her entire facial area. See Figure 10-16.

Next, the patient's skin is prepared for cosmetic application.

- Wash your hands before touching the patient.
- Drape the patient for the makeup application by covering the clothing with a makeup cape. Protect the patient's hair by pulling it back with a headcover or with a headband.
- Teach the patient to prepare the skin properly for the makeup application by assisting her with the following cleansing process: See Figure 10–16.

1. Pour a small amount of liquid cleanser into the palm of the patient's hand.

2a. Ask her to dip the pads of her fingers in the creamy cleansing solution.

2b. Apply it to the skin, working downward over the forehead, between the eyes, across the bridge of the nose, onto the cheeks, around the mouth, onto the chin, down to the jaw, and onto the neck, using delicate, circular movements to thoroughly massage it in.

3. Have the patient remove all traces of the cleanser with moistened cotton squares, starting at the top of

the forehead and working down toward the neck. She should repeat this process until she can no longer feel any residue left behind on her skin from the cleansing solution.

4. After the patient has finished rinsing the skin, offer a hand towel and suggest that she pat, not rub, her skin dry. Have her follow up the cleansing procedure by applying a toner. The toner can be poured from a plastic container with a spout onto a cotton square, or it can be stored in a purse sized plastic spray bottle and lightly spritzed over the patient's entire face and neck area. If the patient prefers the sprayer, have her close her eyes, and lightly spritz her face with the mild toning solution.

5. Instruct the patient to gently apply either a light moisture lotion or a rich lubricating cream, depending on what her skin type dictates. To moisturize and protect the patient's skin, pour a small amount of the liquid moisturizer into the palm of the hand; or use a spatula to remove the cream from the container.

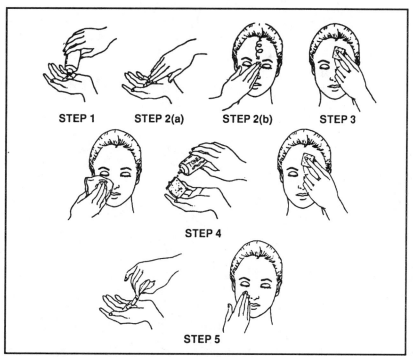

Figure 10-16. Preparing the skin for the makeup application

Applying the Foundation

Follow the standard procedure for selecting a foundation color. Refer to Chapter 7, Corrective Makeup. See Figure 10–17, steps 1 and 2.

3a. Place the foundation onto the cosmetic tray in its pre-determined position. Before the patient applies the foundation, she should pre-mix it by shaking up the makeup container.

3b. Remind her to always be sure that the cap to the makeup container is tight before she does this.

3c. Have the patient unscrew the cap and place it on the tray face up, not on its side where it would be more apt to roll off.

3d. Ask the patient to dip a clean, disposable cotton swab approximately halfway down into the container. Use a clean cotton swab for re-dipping into the container. See Figure 10-17.

4. Have the patient dot the foundation onto the following six areas: the center of her forehead, over

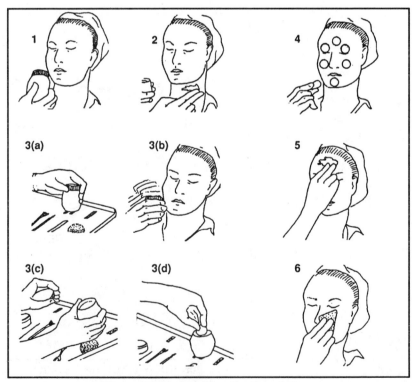

Figure 10-17. Applying the foundation

the closed left eyelid, over the right eyelid, onto the left cheek, onto the right cheek, and onto her chin area. As soon as the patient is finished using the makeup, the container should be recapped and returned to its original position on the tray.

5. Returning to the forehead, instruct the patient to make a small circle, moving her fingers in a slow, circular, upward motion, stopping at the hairline, and gently blending out the edges of the foundation with the fingertips. Have her continue doing this until she has blended the foundation into all six areas. Instruct her to use a light touch, especially when applying makeup around the delicate eye area.

6. Even if she no longer feels the moisture from the makeup, suggest that she continue blending it with a triangular make- up sponge to remove any excess foundation, and as a precautionary measure to ensure that the foundation is evenly distributed.

Translucent Powder

Store the powder in a container with holes in the top similar to a salt shaker. Have the patient shake the powder into the palm of her hand. See Figure 10-18. Recommend that the patient dip a large powder brush into the palm of her hand, taking up some of the powder with the brush bristles. (Powder puffs are not recommended because they

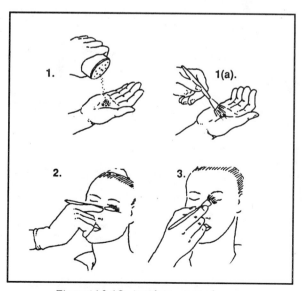

Figure 10-18. Applying powder

become soiled and also give a cakey look.) Have her tap the brush lightly and gently blow on it to remove any excess powder. By learning this simple technique, she will prevent powder from falling onto her clothing.

Instruct the patient to close her eyes and dust the powder onto her entire face in a downward motion, starting at the top of the forehead, brushing down to the jawline in a systematic way.

Instruct the patient to go back over her face with the powder brush (without re-dipping it into the powder) to buff out the application.

Eyebrow Care

To apply color and define her eyebrows, the patient can either use an eyebrow pencil or a brush on eyebrow powder with a brush applicator. Instruct the patient to smooth her fingers gently across her brows. See Figure 10-19. Have her repeat this process until she knows exactly where her eyebrows begin and end. Once her hands get used to feeling the shape and location of her eyebrows, it will become easier for her to determine exactly where to apply the brow color.

Using her index finger (if the patient is right-handed have her use her left index finger, if left-handed, her right) to position the brush properly, have her follow the finger with the brush or the pencil. This will keep the marking on the eyebrow and prevent her from applying color below or above it. Suggest very light, feathery strokes.

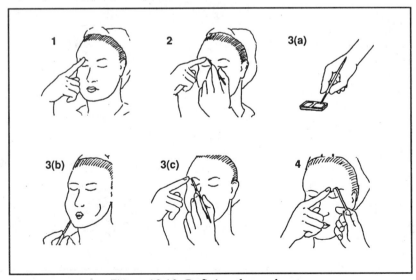

Figure 10-19. Defining the eyebrows

If the patient prefers using the brush method, instruct her to very lightly stroke the brush across the powder cake twice, repeating this process for each eyebrow so that the same amount of color will be deposited on either side by the brush applicator. Before applying the brush to her brows, she should lightly tap and blow on it. This will prevent her from having too much powder on the applicator. Remind the patient that if she feels that she has not applied the eyebrow color correctly she can always use a cotton swab dipped in cleansing solution to remove the brow color, and then begin again.

The patient should always follow this procedure by using a clean cotton swab dipped in toner to insure that she has completely removed the film residue left behind from the cleanser.

Instruct the patient to complete the process by gently brushing the eyebrows (with an eyebrow brush or a child's toothbrush) upward and back to remove any excess powder and to smooth out obvious pencil lines.

Eyebrow Arching

Eyebrow arching most likely will be too complex a procedure for most patients to perform independently; however, a friend or family member can properly arch the patient's eyebrows, or you could recommend that she have her eyebrows professionally arched. Excess hairs between the eyebrows can easily be tweezed by the patient. You can help her to accomplish this by instructing her in the following method: To remove just the hairs between her brows, have the patient place her index finger over the edge of her brow to prevent pulling out the wrong hairs, and with the other hand use a pair of tweezers to remove only the excess hairs that fall in between the two eyebrows. See Figure 10-20.

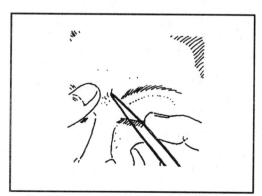

Figure 10-20. Tweezing the eyebrows

Color

The best method to use when describing eye shadow, rouge, blusher, and lipstick color to a newly blind patient is to compare cosmetic shades to colors found in nature. This will help the patient form a word association with certain cosmetic shades based on colors she already knows. For example, when defining red shades, point out that a cranberry red is more of a blue red, and a tomato red is more of an orange red.

Subtle colors such as earth tones are appropriate for newly blind patients or patients who are learning to apply makeup for the first time. These earthy color tones will easily complement the patient's natural coloring without looking too harsh or obvious.

Once the patient has more confidence in her ability to apply cosmetics, and her skill at doing so improves, she can expand her cosmetic color options by experimenting with more vibrant cosmetic shades.

Eye Shadow

Because it will draw attention to the eyes, eye shadow may not be flattering on all patients, particularly those with severe irregularities in or around the eyes. (See the eyewear section in this chapter for camouflage alternatives.)

Eye shadow should be applied subtly and carefully; only the slightest suggestion of color is needed. The lightest eye-shadow shades should be applied to the brow bone just under the eyebrows; the darker, more intense shades should be applied closest to the eyelashes. Eye-shadow shades such as off-white, cream, or light peach are suggested for the brow bone area; richer, more intense shades, such as soft brown, taupe, mauve, and rose, can be applied to the skin closest to the eyelashes to slightly enhance and define the color of the eyes.

Eye-shadow Application Method

1. Instruct the patient to apply eye shadow to the brow bone first, using one of the suggested neutral shades to highlight this area. Recommend that the patient use one of the following applicators: a fluff brush, a sponge-tip applicator, a disposable cotton swab, or the index finger.

   With a small plastic spatula, scrape a small amount of the eye powder off of the cake of eye shadow into a shallow container. This procedure need not be repeated by the patient at home, but must be followed for sanitary reasons by the camouflage therapist during a professional treatment.

Ask the patient to dip the applicator into the powder twice. (At home during her practice sessions, the patient can substitute this method with stroking the applicator gently across the cake of eye shadow twice). Remember, by having the patient lightly tap the applicator and by instructing her to gently blow on it, she can remove any excess powder. See Figure 10-21.

Have the patient apply the eye shadow to the brow bone area by stroking the shadow lightly over the

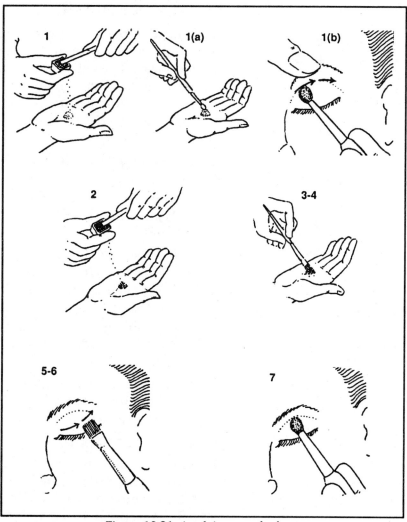

Figure 10-21. Applying eye shadow

skin just under her eyebrow, starting from the inner corner of the eye and working outward to the outer edge of her eye.

2. Select a second eye shadow that will complement the patient's eyecolor. This eye shadow should be darker and richer in color than the shade that was previously applied over the brow bone. Using the same method to remove the shadow from the cake, sprinkle a small amount in the palm of the patient's hand.

3. Instruct the patient to use another eye-shadow applicator to apply the new eyecolor. She can use any one of the following applicators: a clean cotton swab, a disposable sponge tip eye-shadow applicator, or a fluff eye-shadow brush.

4. Repeating the same process as before, the patient should be instructed to press the applicator into the eye-shadow powder twice, tap the applicator, and blow on it to remove any excess powder. This process should be used when applying eye shadow to the other eye to ensure that the same amount of eye shadow was applied to both eyelids.

5. Ask the patient to close the eye she will be applying the eye shadow to.

6. Instruct the patient to smooth on the color along the eyelashes extending it out to the corner of the lid, blending it upward toward the eyebrow, never going higher than the first crease of the eyelid except to camouflage deep set or prominent eyes

7. For further softening and blending, recommend that the patient lightly dust the eyelid with a clean, sponge-tip applicator, or she can lightly dust colorless translucent powder over the eye shadow to soften the color.

8. Repeat the same procedure on the other eye. Be sure to remind her when applying eye shadow to the other eye to use a clean eye shadow applicator.

The Fingertip Application Method

1. Some patients will find it easier to apply eye shadow with the fingertips instead of an applicator. The following method is recommended: Instruct the patient to press the tips of both of her ring fingers

into the eye shadow at the same time, using the same amount of pressure. See Figure 10-22.

2. Direct the patient to place the fingertips at the innermost corner of the eyelids and very gently stroke on the shadow over the eyelids, moving outward. If the patient has long fingernails, she should not use her fingers to perform this process.

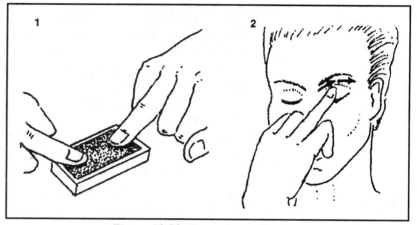

Figure 10-22. Fingertip application

Eye Liner Pencil

1. Advise the patient to position the pencil close to the edge of her eyelashes. Recommend that the patient make a series of tiny dots as close to the lash line as possible, about one quarter of the way in from the inner corner working outward (for a more conservative makeup look, keep the corner line even shorter). See Figure 10-23.

2. Have the patient smooth out the liner by smudging the line of dots together. To do this, ask the patient to gently rub a cotton swab or a sponge tip eye-

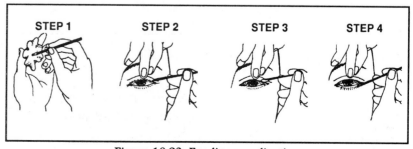

Figure 10-23. Eye liner application

shadow applicator lightly back and forth over the dots until she has completely blended them into one line. Repeat this same process on the other eye, using a clean applicator.

3. If desired, follow the same procedure for the lower lid.

Coloring the Eyelashes

For patients who have difficulty applying mascara, recommend a professional eyelash tint (see chapter on cosmetic therapy). The entire procedure (both eyebrows and eyelashes) takes approximately twenty minutes, and the dye remains on the lashes for a period of four to six weeks.

To instruct the patient in how to apply mascara, use the following method.

Be sure that you have plenty of disposable mascara wands on hand for patients to use in treatment. To prevent the mascara from becoming contaminated with bacteria, never allow a patient to re-dip the wand back into the container. See Figure 10-24.

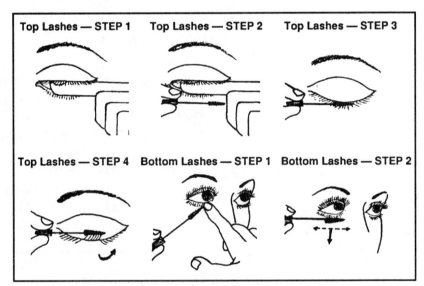

Figure 10-24. Applying mascara

Use these steps to apply mascara to the top lashes:

1. Ask the patient to look straight ahead and lower the eyelids a little, draping the eyelashes over the left index finger.

2. With the right hand instruct the patient to bring the mascara wand to where the finger is. This will help the patient guide the mascara wand right to her eyelashes.

3. Instruct the patient to replace her finger with the wand, placing it just underneath the lashes. Prompt her to gently blink her eye so that her eyelashes touch the wand.

4. Instruct the patient to stroke the eyelashes with the mascara wand by brushing in an upward and outward motion along the entire length of the lashes, slowly moving the wand away from the lashes. Remind the patient to allow the first coat to dry before applying a second.

To apply mascara to the bottom lashes, follow these steps:

1. Instruct the patient to look up toward the ceiling. Place the index finger onto the lower eyelashes and bring the wand to the finger so as to place the wand on the lashes.

2. Advise the patient to use only the tip of the mascara wand to apply color to the lower lashes. Ask the patient to sweep the mascara wand gently back and forth, and then apply downward stokes, holding the mascara tube perpendicular to the face.

Cheek Color

Follow these steps to teach the patient how to use powder blush.

1. Remove the powder blush from the container by scraping a small amount from the cake with a spatula and placing it in a small, shallow container. Instruct the patient to apply the blusher powder with a medium sized blusher brush. See Figure 10-25.

2. Direct the patient to hold the brush in the right hand and sweep it gently in the powder blush, back and forth, until the bristles of the brush are well coated.

3. Advise the patient to tap the brush a couple of times to remove any excess, and gently blow on the brush. This will also prevent the colored powder from falling onto the lower part of her face and sprinkling her clothing.

4. Ask the patient to smile and have her reach up and locate her cheek bone. Have the patient press down lightly with the right hand on this area to familiarize herself with her bone structure. She must be able to locate the top of her cheek as well as the center (sometimes referred to as the apple).

The center of the cheek is located directly beneath the center of the eye (when looking straight ahead it is about two finger spaces away from the nose and about two finger spaces below the bottom of the eye). With the patient's left hand, ask her to reach up measure this distance. She will begin to apply the blusher at this point, brushing it in the direction of her ear and out toward her hairline. The blusher should be placed at the height of the cheekbone and blended out toward the patient's hairline in an upward direction.

5. The patient can lightly dust the area with a makeup sponge to gently remove any of the excess powder.

6. This same process should be repeated by the patient to add color to the other cheek.

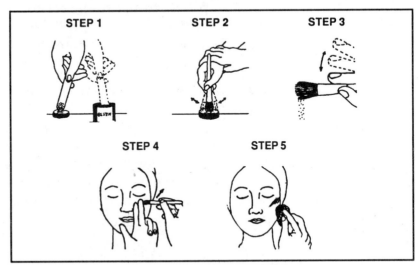

Figure 10-25. Applying blush

Use the following steps for cream rouge.

1. Cream rouge should only be worn by patients with extremely dry or mature skin. Remind the patient to apply it sparingly. Use the same instruction method

described above with the patient to assist her in defining her bone structure and in determining where to place the rouge.

2. Have the patient dot a small amount of the cream rouge onto her cheekbone area. Instruct the patient to blend in the rouge with her fingertips or with a wedge sponge, blending it outward toward her hairline. See Figure 10-26.

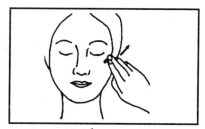

Figure 10-26. Applying rouge

Applying Lip Color

It is possible for a sightless patient to properly apply lip liner; however, it will require a fair amount of practice. Therefore she must be a willing candidate, because she is bound to make mistakes before she will be able to master this technique. If the patient appears to be enthusiastic about performing this technique, you should proceed with the following lesson plan:

1. Suggest that the patient familiarize herself with the shape of her mouth by running her fingers over the natural outline of her lips. The patient's lip should be closed in a natural position as she performs this process. Instruct the patient to use her left index finger to trail the edge of her lip. See Figure 10-27.

2. Recommend that she start at the center of her upper lip and work outward.

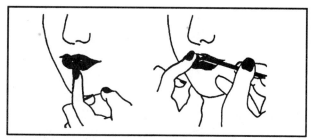

Figure 10-27. Feeling the shape of the mouth

3. Instruct the patient to hold the pencil in the right hand and follow the left index finger, trailing around the edges of the lips with the lip pencil. Repeat to define the lower lip.

To teach the patient to apply lipstick, follow these steps:

1. Remove a small amount of lipstick from the tube with a spatula and place it on the back of the patient's left hand. Ask the patient to replace the lipstick container in its original position on the tray. Fresh lipstick should never be applied over old lip color. See Figure 10-28.

2. The patient can use a sponge-tip applicator, a lip brush, or fingers to apply the lip color. If the patient wishes to use her fingers, instruct her to dip the pad on the tip of her middle finger of her right hand into the lip color.

3. Advise her to open her mouth, and, starting from the outer corner of her upper lip, press down onto the lip with the pad of the finger working inward toward the center, following the natural contour of the lips. Repeat this process on the other side of her upper lip and again on the lower lip.

4. Advise the patient to press her lips together, this will spread the color evenly over the entire lip area.

5. To instruct the patient how to use a brush or sponge-tip applicator, ask the patient to dip it into the lipstick. The patient should relax her mouth and close her lips. Have the patient begin by filling in half of her upper lip first,

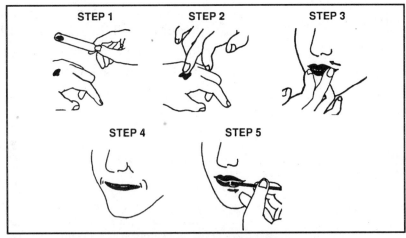

Figure 10-28. Applying lipstick

starting from the center, and working outward toward the outer edge. She should repeat this process on the other side and then on her lower lip.

A similar method is taught for applying lip gloss.

1. A sponge-tip applicator is an excellent cosmetic tool for applying lip gloss. Remove a small amount of lip gloss from the container with a spatula, and place it on the back of the patient's left hand. Ask the patient to return the container to its proper position on the tray. See Figure 10-29.

2. Instruct the patient to dip the applicator into the gloss and smooth it over one half of her upper lip, starting in the center and working outward.

3. Advise her to re-dip the applicator into the gloss and repeat the process on the other half of her upper lip. This same technique should be repeated on the lower lip.

4. If the patient wishes to use fingers instead of the sponge-tip applicator, the same gentle patting technique that was recommended for lipstick can be used. Just be sure to remind the patient to be careful not to accidentally rub the gloss outside of the lip line.

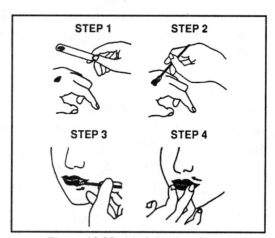

Figure 10-29. Applying lip gloss

EYEWEAR

Eyewear can do a lot more than improve vision; for patients who have scar tissue in or around their eye area, glasses can provide camouflage with which to conceal irregularities or to mask a prosthesis. Cancer patients who have had tumors that required facial surgery may have lost an eye or part of their features. In an orbital restoration, an anaplastologist/ocularist (maker of facial prostheses) designs a shell that fits over the atrophied eye, covering the scar tissue, that resembles an eye. The ocularist makes an artificial eye first and then embeds it in silicone that has been molded to fit the orbit and tinted to match the patient's skin. The prosthesis is held in place with an adhesive. Wearing glasses over the prosthesis makes it look less conspicuous. For these patients eyeglasses with interesting frames can detract attention from their appliance.

Some patients may be required to wear special prescription sunglasses or protective tinted lenses because they are ultrasensitive to any form of light, and, as a result, their eyewear ends up being a permanent facial accessory. Since eyewear is an significant part of a patient's appearance, it is important that the eyeglass frames are compatible with the individual's bone structure and the size of his or her facial features. The color of the frames should also complement the person's hair and complexion. For most patients with severe irregularities around the eye area, the alternative that eyewear can provide will be far more beneficial than most cosmetic solutions.

Because there is such a large selection of different styles to choose from, trying to select the right style of eyewear can become confusing. The following information will provide you with general guidelines to assist patients in selecting the most attractive frames and lenses.

Important Considerations in Selecting the Appropriate Eyewear

When choosing eyewear, you need to consider the following factors: patient's lifestyle, size and shape of the patient's face, patient's facial features, patient's natural coloring, color of lenses, and application of eye makeup.

Patient's Lifestyle

The right eyewear can make a man or a woman appear either authoritative or ineffectual. Be sure that the eyewear style you help the patient select will reflect his or her personality and will project the impression that he or she is trying to project.

Size and Shape

Advise the patient to stand in front of a full length mirror to try on eyeglasses. This will give you a correct sense of the patient's facial proportions. Balance and proportion are imnot suggest small eyeglass frames for a man or woman with a large body structure or large frames for a small, petite person with delicate facial features.

To determine the correct eyeglass frame size, make sure that the frame is as wide as the widest part of the patient's face. The glasses should fit securely on the patient's nose and not clasp too tightly to the sides of his or her head.

The patient's face shape is another important factor in determining the right frames to select. The following information will provide you with general guidelines with which to choose the appropriate eyewear for patients. See Figure 10-30a and b.

Square Face: A wide, firm jaw is the most visible characteristic. Angular frames emphasize the boldness, and round or oval shapes will soften it. If it balances, an unusual frame shape or color will go even further to make a square facial contour less noticeable.

Round Face: Soft-contoured frames will keep a rounded appearance; bolder shapes and more striking colors will make the face appear longer. Aviator-style frames are a favorite.

Long, Narrow Face: This facial type is overly long in proportion to the width of forehead and chin. To balance, choose relatively large frames with horizontal lines. Soft corners or curving lines will prevent these frames from calling too much attention to themselves.

Oval Face: The oval shape is ideal, permitting the widest of frames to match it. Whether petite or oversize, severe or creative in style, nearly all frames are a happy match for the oval face. Only very heavy frames are unsuitable.

Heart-Shaped Face: Select from styles that have oval lines at the top and bottom of the frames.

Diamond-Shaped Face: Eyeglass frames should be wider at the top than at the bottom and should have a definite upsweep.

Pear-Shaped Face: The frame should be heavier and wider on top and oval on the bottom and slant slightly upward.

Facial Features

Close-Set Eyes: If the patient's eyes are set too close together, a clear bridge (transparent) combined with strong upper frame corners will create the illusion that the eyes are spaced further apart.

Wide-Set Eyes: Patients with eyes that are set far apart should avoid styles with emphasis on the outer edges of the frames. Instead recommend frames with a low-position, thick, or dark bridge.

Short Nose: If the patient's nose is short, assist him or her in selecting eyeglasses with a short or rounded bridge near the top of the frame. The patient's nose will appear longer if he or she wears eyeglasses with a high bridge.

Long Nose: A long nose can be visually shortened if the patient wears frames with a low, thick, or straight bridge.

Cheekbones: When eyeglasses rest on the cheeks they leave marks. Advise patients to avoid styles that droop down onto the face; they will pull the face down and make the patient's face look somber.

Eyebrows: The eyeglass frames should follow the outline of the eyebrows but never cross over or under it. The top of the frame should stop at the base of the brow without any portion of the brow appearing in the lens. Exception to this rule would be oversized fashion frames or if the frame of the eyeglasses were deliberately placed over the area where the eyebrows would normally be to camouflage sparse or missing eyebrows. The color of the frame should either match or be color coordinated with the patient's natural eyebrow color.

Eye Makeup for Eyeglass Wearers

Eyewear provides a dramatic frame for the eyes, which is why eye makeup often needs to be altered when glasses are worn. The characteristics of the specific eyewear (frames and lenses) will dictate what advice you will offer to patients regarding the application of eye cosmetics. For example, the type of lenses that are used to correct near-sightedness will make the eyes appear smaller. Makeup techniques to enlarge the appearance of the eyes can correct this problem by creating the illusion of larger eyes. Lenses that correct farsighted-

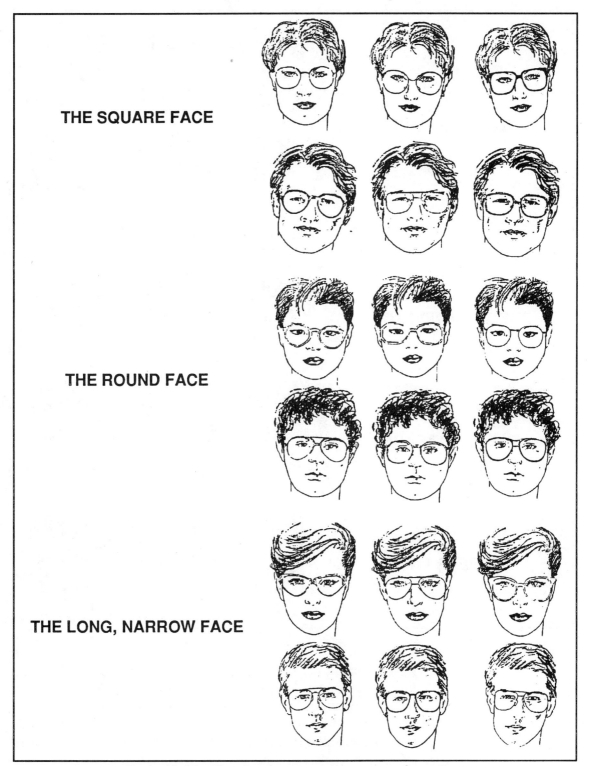

THE SQUARE FACE

THE ROUND FACE

THE LONG, NARROW FACE

Figure 10-30a. Choosing the appropriate eyewear for patients

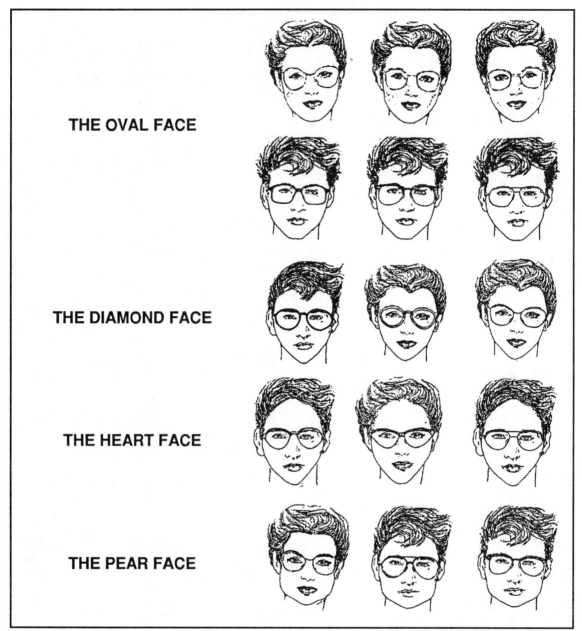

THE OVAL FACE

THE DIAMOND FACE

THE HEART FACE

THE PEAR FACE

Figure 10-30b.

ness will magnify the appearance of the eyes and make them look larger. Darker frames will require a stronger tone of lipstick to balance color. Blush should never disappear under eyeglass frames; it should always be applied slightly lower so the color will be visible. Eye makeup should be applied sparingly to prevent the eyes from appearing overly made-up. Darkly tinted lenses will require a heavier application of eye makeup to lessen the contrast between the shade of the lenses and the patient's natural coloring.

HAIRSTYLING

A patient may approach you and ask for professional advice on styling his or her hair. The best hairstyle for a patient who is blind is one that is easy to manage, fits the patient's personality, and flatters his or her facial features.

If you are a licensed cosmetologist and you trim or style a patient's hair, make sure that you allow extra time in the session to review the styling process with him or her. Try to suggest simple, uncomplicated techniques that visually-impaired patients can easily master. As you describe in detail the styling technique, allow the patient an opportunity to try doing it, and offer him or her verbal feedback about how well he or she is progressing. Suggest a second session for the patient to address any problems he or she may have encountered when trying to manage the new style independently.

A patient who has recently lost his or her vision may be having problems with his or her hair. Something as simple as making a part in his or her hair may be difficult for the patient to do at first. Advise the patient to comb his or her hair back while it is still wet, and, as it drys, suggest that the patient gently push his or her hair forward slightly from the crown and let the hair fall into its natural part. This process is a lot easier for the patient than having to struggle with making a straight part with a comb. This type of simple suggestion can help a newly blind person adapt to personal grooming skills.

If the patient wants to use a curling iron but is afraid of burning, suggest that he or she practice first with a cold curling iron until he or she becomes proficient using it. Once the patient feels comfortable manipulating the curling iron, he or she can begin to practice with it on the lightest setting. The patient must be cautioned to always allow sufficient time and never rush through the procedure. It takes time to learn to use this styling tool properly, and the patient must be willing to practice. As the patient moves the curling iron through the strands of hair, he or she will begin to sense the heat near his or her fingers.

TRIMMING MUSTACHES AND BEARDS

The clinical cosmetician or cosmetologist may be asked by a patient to trim his beard or mustache, or he may request a simple technique that he could use to perform this procedure independently. The following information will assist you in offering the patient an efficient method with which to trim his facial hair. Recommend to your patients that they use very small scissors to trim the moustache or beard. The patient should be instructed to work one side of the mouth at a time, moving from the outer corner of the mustache inward toward the center. Hold the scissor blade against the lip with the moustache hairs hanging over the edge of the blade. Tilt the scissor blade at a 45 degree angle outward, and cut the hairs with one stroke. Repeat this procedure on the other side, starting at the center of the mouth, working toward the outer corner of the mouth. See Figure 10-31. He should run his fingers over the top of his moustache to feel for stray hairs, trimming them as he goes along.

The patient can use either scissors or electric razor, depending on what he is more proficient using. He must be systematic and very careful. Using only downward strokes, he must make sure that the scissors are open wide enough to catch any of the hairs he is trying to trim. He should use the left index finger (if he is right handed) to guide the scissors along.

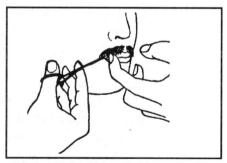

Figure 10-31. Trimming a mustache

NAIL CARE

Hands are one of the most expressive parts of the human body; they are on permanent display. Nail care for the patient need not be elaborate. Professional manicures and pedicures should be suggested for those patients who choose not to or have trouble mastering the following manicuring techniques. The clinical cosmetologist or manicurist can instruct the patient to independently perform a simple manicure by using the following guidelines:

Before the session begins have everything the patient will need displayed on a tray. Place all the manicuring tools in the order that they will be used, and label them just as you did the makeup items for the cosmetic session.

Cover the top of the tray with a clean hand towel, and line up the following: alcohol (for disinfecting your hands), an emery board, a nail brush, nail clippers, a small container filled with liquid soap and warm water, a nail brush, a hand towel, several pre-made cotton tipped orangewood sticks, a nail buffer, tissue, cotton balls, nail polish remover in a tube, nail polish, and hand cream. You will also need a small waste receptacle (a small paper bag can be attached with tape to the side of the table that the tray is setting on.

Ask the patient to review all the objects on the tray in the same manner as you would a patient receiving cosmetic instruction.

A key in shaping the nail is to conform to the natural curvature of the finger tips. Discuss with the patient the most natural nail shape, and advise him or her to file his or her nails accordingly. Have the patient begin by filing the nails of his or her left hand, starting with the little finger and working toward the thumb. Instruct the patient to use the emeryboard on the outer part of the nail, filing inward toward the center, using the tip of his or her finger as a guideline, moving from right to left and from left to right. Remind the patient that by filing outward with the growth of the nail it will avoid splitting the nail. Using the tip of the patient's finger as a guideline, recommend that he or she position the emeryboard at a 45 degree angle. Use two quick strokes and one long sweeping stroke on each side of the nail. The patient should be reminded to never file deep into the corners of the nail, because it will weaken it.

Once the patient has finished filing his or her nails on both hands, ask the patient to soak the fingers on the left hand in the warm soap bath. After two minutes or so have the patient remove his or her hand and wipe it dry and with a clean hand towel and push his or her cuticles back.

If the patient wishes to cut his or her nails, the best tool is a nail clipper. Make sure that you instruct the patient to put his or her fingernail in the nail clipper with the base of the clipper even with the underside of the finger. The nail should not be tilted up or down. The patient can use this same technique for his or her toenails as well. Note: A diabetic, an AIDS patient, or a patient undergoing cancer therapy should never clip his or her own nails because of risk of possible infection.

Have the patient take a small amount of cotton and wrap it around the tip of a orange-wood stick. Instruct the patient to dip the cotton-tipped wood stick into the soapy water. Working from the center toward the edge advise the patient to clean very gently under the free edge of the nail.

Before the patient attempts to polish her nails, you can recommend that she practice first with water or a clear nail polish until she feels comfortable with the following technique. Instruct the patient to dip the brush into the polish and gently wipe off any excess by pressing the applicator gently against the sides of the nail polish container. See Figure 10-32.

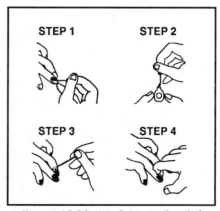

Figure 10-32. Applying nail polish

Advise the patient to use the tip of his or her ring finger on the hand that is holding the brush to locate the tip of the finger to be polished, and then lower the brush on the nail and slide it back until it barely touches the cuticle. Use two to three strokes to apply polish. The more the patient does this (motor memory) the more control she will eventually have. Repeat this process until the patient has polished all their nails on both hands. Advise the patient to allow the nails to dry; this will take five to ten minutes. If the nail is "slick to the touch and not tacky" the nails are dry.

When finished with the polish, the patient should hold the container horizontally and replace the brush in the bottle. Do this by sliding the brush across the top of the bottle with slight pressure until the brush goes into the bottle. Instruct the patient to re-cap the nail polish container and place it back in its pre-designated position on the tray.

Alternatives to this type of nail polish are brushes that automatically dispense nail polish when brushing onto the nail. Nail polish remover also comes in tubes that resemble marking pens, making nail polish removal easier for the patient.

The patient can locate any excess polish outside the nail by tracing the area around the cuticle and the nail edges with the pads of his or her fingertips to feel for dried polish.

To remove all traces of excess polish, instruct the patient to carefully apply a cotton-tipped orangewood stick immersed in polish remover around the cuticle and the edges of the nails.

Once the patient's nails have completely dried, he or she can massage in a hand lotion or cream starting at the wrists and massaging it gently onto their hands using a gentle kneading action.

Some patients (especially male patients) will not want to polish their nails, even with clear nail polish. These patients can use a nail buffer and buffing cream in place of polishing to give their nails a bright or a low-key luster. This is also a good method for increasing blood circulation in the fingertips, making the fingers a little more sensitive.

REVIEW

You should now be familiar with:

- the various diseases associated with blindness.
- adaptive blind techniques in makeup and basic grooming.
- materials needed to perform adaptive blind techniques.

11 Dermatology

INTRODUCTION

Lewis Tannenbaum, M.D.

Dermatology is the medical and surgical specialty that deals with the skin. It is a very broad field and encompasses the structure and function of the skin in both normal and abnormal conditions. It includes dermatologic surgery and pathology, as well as the diagnosis and treatment of a myriad of skin conditions ranging from common conditions such as psoriasis, acne, and warts, to the uncommon, such as leprosy and neurofibromatosis (Elephant Man disease), as well as the often deadly malignant melanoma.

While the dermatologist's main purpose is to improve the function and maintain the integrity of the skin, an equally important role of the dermatologist is to improve the skin's appearance. In most instances these goals can be achieved simultaneously. However, to do this, dermatologists must begin to bridge the gap between the cosmetologist/esthetician and the dermatologist/cosmetic surgeon. Dermatologists are familiar with pharmacological formulations and are thus able to sort out those ingredients in cosmetics that are needed, harmful, or merely "hype." With this background, it is not surprising that some dermatologists have begun to work more closely with estheticians to provide the optimum environment for skin care.

Dr. Lewis Tannenbaum is a board-certified dermatologist. He received his medical training at Downstate Medical Center in New York, completed his internship at the University of California at Irvine, and his residency at Harvard Medical Center.

After being in practice for more than ten years, I realized that the results my patients were getting from estheticians in the community were inconsistent. In some instances there was a definite benefit from the facials and deep pore cleansing administered, while in others the skin-care line used was inappropriate. My frustration with this type of result led me to hire an esthetician to work full-time with my patients. I now have two estheticians working with me on a full time basis. In addition to providing deep-pore cleansing to patients with acne and related complexion problems, the esthetician in a dermatologist's/cosmetic surgeon's office has other roles.

With cosmetic surgical procedures, it is invaluable to have the esthetician meet with the patient preoperatively to emphasize what the appearance of the skin will be immediately following surgery and to educate the patient about what measures can be taken to minimize "down-time" and get back to a normal life. Often we will schedule a treatment for corrective makeup immediately after the surgery. This is most important in that it helps the patient better accept the appearance of his or her skin immediately after surgery. It is also less traumatic if patients know that steps have already been scheduled to improve their appearance, even before full healing is completed.

Besides facial skin treatments and pre- and post-operative consultations with corrective makeup, another area of importance for the esthetician is to review skin-care products and cosmetics with patients and make recommendations for change in these areas. This is often an overlooked area for most busy dermatologists.

Dermatologists, plastic surgeons, and cosmetic surgeons are finally beginning to recognize that their patients have certain questions that may be better answered by an esthetician. A long time ago I realized that esthetic dermatology is what patients are demanding. It represents the best that the dermatologist, cosmetic surgeon, and esthetician, all working together, can offer.

DERMATOLOGY

The information contained in this chapter will give the esthetician a basic introduction to the medical specialty of dermatology, and to the various skin conditions encompassed by dermatology that can be camouflaged or improved upon through the use of aesthetic procedures.

Dermatology is a medical specialty concerned with the diagnosis and treatment of disorders of the skin, hair, and nails. The skin and mucous membranes are composed of epidermis, dermis, subcutaneous tissue, and the appendages of the skin. Dermatologic medical conditions include the physical signs of sun damage (aging), cherry spots, pigmented lesions, skin growths, hair and nail disorders, acne, eczema, psoriasis, viral, bacterial, and fungal infections, parasitic infestations, and skin cancer. Treatment encompasses topical and systemic medications, as well as surgery, laser therapy, cryotherapy (freezing), burning (cautery or electrodessication), and radiation treatments.

The dermatologist is a physician who in addition to the standard medical training has taken four years of graduate training in his or her specialty. Most dermatologists have passed a rigorous examination leading to board certification.

DISORDERS OF THE SKIN

Although there are important exceptions, as a general rule skin diseases are not life-threatening. They can however be severely debilitating and cause psychological problems.

Viral Infections Viral infections of the skin include common and German measles, varicella (chicken pox), herpes zosters (shingles), herpes simplex (cold sores), molluscum contagiosum (shiny, pearly white papules on the skin's surface), and warts. See Plate 1.

Bacterial Infections Bacterial infections include impetigo (a highly contagious, usually staphylococcal disease that can occur when bacteria enter the skin through a broken area such as a cut, cold sore, or an opening caused by eczema), boils, cellulitis (generally caused by streptococci, which may enter the skin through a wound), and erysipelas (usually a streptococci on the face). See Plate 2.

Fungal Infections Superficial fungal infections or tinea include skin disorders often referred to as athlete's foot, jock itch, or ring worm, depending on their location. On the feet they cause scaling and thickened skin. On the body they often appear as circular patches with prominent edges that itch. See Figure 11-1.

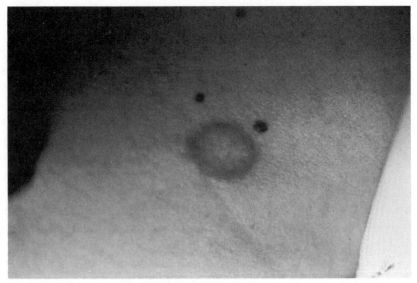

Figure 11-1. Tinea Corporis. *Courtesy of Timothy Berger, M.D.*

Parasitic Infestations Scabies, lice, insects, and marine animals can all attack the human integument. See Figure 11-2.

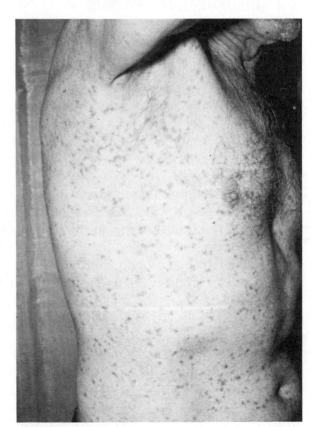

Figure 11-2. Scabies. *Courtesy of Timothy Berger, M.D.*

Dermatitis Dermatitis and eczema are synonymous and may be genetically determined as in atopic dermatitis; caused by irritant or allergic reactions to detergent, medications, jewelry (nickel), and plants, among other things. Itching is common in virtually all forms of dermatitis. Redness, blistering, swelling, and scaling may be seen. See Figure 11-3.

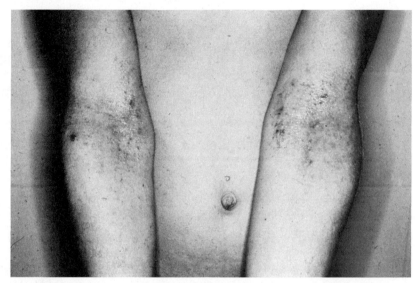

Figure 11-3. Atopic Dermatitis. *Courtesy of Timothy Berger, M.D.*

Psoriasis Psoriasis is characterized by large, thickened, red patches with scaly surfaces and sharp borders. These patches appear because new skin cells are being produced up to ten times faster than normal. Heredity, medication, and infections may cause or worsen psoriasis. One to three percent of the population is affected. See Plate 3.

Acne Acne is caused by the action of the androgens on the hair follicles and sebaceous glands in a susceptible person. Acne begins when a hair follicle produces cells that stick together so tightly that they cannot be shed. These cells mix with other skin materials, such as pigment and bacteria, and stick to one another, forming a plug. This blocks the pore. This lesion is called a comedone. Bacteria are trapped and multiply. The sebaceous gland continues to produce sebum (oil). Frequently the follicle bursts or leaks, forming a papule or pimple. As the follicle releases its contents into the surrounding tissue, inflammation occurs. This is why the surface surrounding the pimple is reddened and swollen. White blood cells enter the tissue, causing it to liquefy, forming pus. Acne vulgaris consists of four types of blemishes: pustules (pimples with pus at the top), closed comedones or comedos (whiteheads), open comedones or comedos (blackheads), and deep cysts or abscesses. These blemishes may or may not occur at the same time. Acne vulgaris in its worst form can cause scarring. See Plates 4 and 5.

Rosacea (Acne Rosacea)

Acne rosacea is associated with redness of the face (especially the nose, cheeks, chin, and forehead), accompanied by telangiectasia (fine capillaries) and pimples. It is common in persons of northern European extraction. Rosy cheeks and easy blushing may be the earliest form of rosacea. See Plate 6.

The Office Management of Acne Vulgaris, a Personal Approach

Theodore A. Labow, M.D.

Acne vulgaris is, unquestionably, the most common skin condition affecting those in the age group that extends from the early teens to the mid-thirties. Though rarely associated with any significant systemic manifestations, acne can have devastating emotional repercussions on those affected by disfiguring forms of the disorder.

No single method of treatment is the best approach for all patients with acne. Therapy must be individualized according to the type and severity of the disease, and often must be modified as one observes the response to the prescribed regimen.

Most patients with acne are best served by a multi-phasic approach to treatment. This may include topical and systemic medications as well as office treatment employing various physical modalities. One type of the latter is sometimes referred to as acne surgery, the essential component of which is extraction of comedones and incision and drainage of pustular and cystic lesions. In my estimation any patient who

exhibits open or closed comedones, pustules or cystic lesions is a candidate for acne surgery.

I should like to give you just a few of my reasons why acne surgery has been a immeasurable value in many of my acne patients:

1. Comedone (blackhead) formation is at the heart of the pathological changes that take place in the skin in acne. Removal of comedones will not only improve the appearance of the skin, but will prevent progression of inflammatory lesions. Additionally, topically applied medications can more readily gain access to the emptied follicle.

2. Early drainage of inflammatory lesions may prevent them from evolving into cystic lesions with a potential for scar formation.

3. Properly performed acne surgery makes it easier to dissuade patients

Theodore A. Labow, M.D., is retired Clinical Professor, Department of Dermatology, College of Physicians and Surgeons, Columbia University, New York, New York.

from picking their own "pimples," which often, in my experience, turns a simple comedo-pustule into a veritable disaster. Improperly applied and/or excessive pressure can cause rupture of the follicle and a resultant inflammatory reaction. In other cases patients may excoriate their skin, leading to superficial ulcerations, which often heal with scarring.

4. The patient benefits psychologically from observing the immediate positive effects of the treatment. They appreciate the fact that there is a team approach to their problem.

Through the years, our assistants have come to us with a variety of backgrounds. Some acquired their skills in Europe where, at least in the past, formal training courses were offered. Others had been registered nurses working in dermatology in the former Soviet Union. Many came to us with a background in cosmetology. All received additional instruction in specialized techniques under our supervision.

In order to give the reader an overview of what I regard as the proper management of acne, I should like to detail my approach to the new patient who presents with this condition.

One must begin by taking a careful history with emphasis on the chronological progression of the condition, any possible relationship to stress, diet, externally applied substances, and, in the female patient, hormonal factors, including the menstrual cycle and oral contraceptive therapy. Prior treatment and the response to it must be carefully reviewed. A complete medical history should be taken. One should not treat skin diseases; one should treat patients with skin disease, and knowledge of the patient's complete medical background is essential.

Listen carefully to the patient to see if there are any pre-conceived ideas about the cause of the condition that will need to be talked about, and perhaps modified, in the course of the subsequent discussion with the patient. Try to get a handle on what emotional effects the condition is having on the individual. In this regard remember to be both tolerant and understanding. Remember, feelings are not right or wrong; feelings ARE!

Only at this time should one proceed to the examination of the skin. The distribution of the eruption is observed and then a determination is made as to the types of lesions present. These may include comedones of both the open and closed type, comedo-papules, pustules, cysts, and scarring. Pay careful attention to the patient's basic skin type as this will dictate the forms of topical therapy which will be best tolerated.

At this point we usually begin the acne surgery treatment. We explain to the patient the nature of the treatment to help allay the apprehension that some patients may have.

We begin by cleansing the patient's face with a liquid soap preparation such as Tincture of Green Soap, carefully removing any makeup. A thin coat of cream is then applied. We most commonly use the following formula which can be prepared by any pharmacist:

Burow's Solution	10.0
Aquaphor	20.0
Ungt. Aqua Rosae	30.0

Burow's solution contains aluminum subacetate, which has an astringent effect and is normally well tolerated. Occasionally, in the patient with a very sensitive skin, by history or examination, the following formula will be substituted:

Aqua Distill.	40.0
Aquaphor qs ad	100.0

In thick and oily skin, if one desires to produce a degree of peeling, a full or half-strength of Whitfield's Ointment may be utilized.

In the next step, the patient's face is steamed for an eight-to-ten minute period. The purpose of the steaming is to hydrate and soften the keratinous debris within the blackhead and facilitate its removal. I explain this to patients with an analogy, pointing out how much easier it is to cut fingernails or toenails after soaking in a hot bath. We use floor model electric steamers with the patient lying on the treatment table in the supine position. The excess cream is then gently wiped off.

At this point, in what is the most important part of the treatment, comedone extraction and evacuation of pustules is carried out. I do not like the use of the surgical instrument called a comedone extractor for a variety of reasons. My objection to their use is best understood in terms of the physical laws governing the application of force. The handle of the instrument acts as a lever multiplying the force applied by the operator's hand. This magnified force is then applied to the skin by the relatively narrow rim of the tip of the instrument, which surrounds the blackhead, and is sufficient in some cases to injure the tissue. Furthermore, one is attempting to push the comedone up by pressing down of the surrounding normal tissue, certainly an unphysiological approach.

In our approach, the two forefingers of the operator are covered with a freshly laundered or disposable surgical towel. One finger is placed on each side of the comedone. The skin is elevated just a bit by the fingers and pressure is applied gently between the two fingers in a slight upward direction. Pressure is gradually increased as needed until the blackhead pops out without trauma to the surrounding skin.

When they have demonstrated their competence, we allow our assistants to use a scalpel with a #11 blade on selected lesions. This is a blade with an angular point. The sharpness and angle of the point vary from one manufacturer to another. The tiny incision that is created will permit less traumatic treatment of the lesion, which then should heal better than if left untreated. Patients sometimes express concern that acne surgery will produce scarring. It is important to emphasize to them that, to the contrary, the treatment should minimize the scarring that can result from inflammatory disease.

During this stage of treatment, the assistant consults the physician if there are any unusual or severe lesions and latter may elect to drain these himself and/or use intralesional cortisone injections to reduce the inflammatory component. We do not allow our assistants to perform these injections.

The next stage of our treatment is usually the application of dry ice slush. We prepare this by pulverizing solid dry ice in a large mortar and pestle and then adding acetone. If solid dry ice is not available, it is possible to prepare it from a carbon dioxide cylinder fitted with a chamois bag which is roughly triangular in shape. The wide end is open, but closed during filling with a clamp. The narrow end is fitted to the cylinder. When the valve of the tank is opened, the rapid expansion of the carbon dioxide causes cooling and the formation of dry ice "snow."

We use large cotton applicators, which we prepare, to brush the super-cooled acetone over the face. Care must be taken not to overtreat or to allow any small particles of ice to remain in contact with the skin. Improper technique can result in the equivalent of first, and even second-degree burns. If dry ice prepared from a tank is utilized, it is best to form it into a small ball, which is then wrapped in large, opened, gauze sponges which are twisted closed, dipped in acetone, and brushed over the face. The usually desired endpoint is a very slight transient blanch from freezing. However, in fair, sensitive skins, even a lighter application is preferable until one has had the opportunity to judge response.

The treatment is concluded with the application of a masque, which is allowed to dry and then gently removed with iced water. Here again, some individualization of methods is in order. Although a mild mask of powdered kaolin mixed with water can always be used, we may opt to use a more astringent mask also containing menthol and bentonite if the patient has oilier and thicker skin.

Upon conclusion of the treatment, the patient is offered an oil-free makeup if desired. Again, depending upon skin type, there may be some transient post-treatment erythema and mild edema, which should be explained to the patient.

At this time it is my policy to take the patient back into my consultation room and discuss the acne process in detail with an emphasis upon what is known about its pathogenesis. The explanation should be in reasonably simple terms. I have found the use of drawings illustrating the progression of lesions from early comedone through cysts to be helpful. I like to explain how each prescribed medication affects the disease process. There is little doubt in my mind that a well-informed patient will be a more compliant one.

The home-care routine will be individualized according to the type of acne, the patient's skin type, and past response to therapy, if the patient has had prior treatment. I am not a devotee of scrub cleansers or abrasive sponges. I have seen little evidence that rubbing away the stratum corneum does much to reduce comedone formation. Furthermore, irritation can result that will cause the skin to be less tolerant of topicals such as retinoic acid and benzoyl peroxide. Ordinarily, cleansing with a mild soap will suffice. If the skin is quite oily, an astringent may also be used.

It is my policy to initially prescribe oral antibiotics only for patients with a significant pustular, nodular, or cystic component to their disease. I would add those cases which have shown a poor response to what I would regard as an adequate program of topical measures. Other oral medications which may be useful include nonsteroidal anti-inflammatory agents, prednisone, estrogens, and Accutane. The indications for use of these drugs is beyond the scope of this discussion.

Useful external therapeutic agents include topical antibiotics, benzoyl peroxide, salicylic acid, sulfur, resorcin and the occasional judicious use of topical steroids where there is superficial inflammation. The latter should be used only on a limited basis and may be more effective if applied after a gentle steaming of the face.

In female patients, the use of cosmetic products should be discussed. A number of years ago it was found that some cosmetic ingredients would induce comedone formation when rubbed into the rabbit ear. Such ingredients were labeled comedogenic, i.e., "capable of inducing blackhead formation." It has become fashionable to screen cosmetic products using this test and label those which do not cause blackheads as non-comedogenic. The relevancy of this test to humans was recently substantiated in a study using the fluorescence of comedones created by their bacterial contents. The two tests showed close correlation. Although the role of cosmetics in exacerbating acne is far from clear, if the patient is going to use makeup, I do suggest "non-comedogenic" products.

At this point I will give the patient the opportunity to pose any questions they may have. I also like to be certain that they understand their home-care directions, which I write out for them. Although pre-printed instruction sheets are time savers, they may leave the impression of a mass production line approach to the treatment and may leave less of an impact. I like to conclude this initial visit on a positive note. These patients do need reassurance that there is hope for their skin problems, and that they can do something other than to wait to outgrow their pimples. However, they must be reminded that they must be consistent with the home management and that it takes time to see a response. Even after there is decided improvement, occasional flares, perhaps related to stress or menses, are not usual and must not be a cause for despair.

I hope this outline will be helpful to the reader. In closing, I should like to emphasize that this represents my personal clinical approach and some of the views expressed may not necessarily be shared by other dermatologists. It is intended to convey my conviction that the dermatologist working hand-in-hand with nursing assistants who have a background in cosmetology make the ideal team to treat acne. I should like to stress the fact that this is not designed to be a "do-it-yourself" manual. Reading this article cannot alone teach you to do acne surgery any more than reading the section in this book on clinical dermatology can suffice to enable one to treat diseases of the skin. It is intended only to give the reader some insight into acne management.

Prickly Heat

Prickly heat (heat rash, miliaria) is a skin disorder that occurs with exposure to heat and is associated with an irritating rash. It is caused by a blockage of the sweat glands. See Figure 11-4.

Skin Injuries

Skin injuries include cuts, abrasions, burns, and animal bites. (For burn injuries see chapter on burns.)

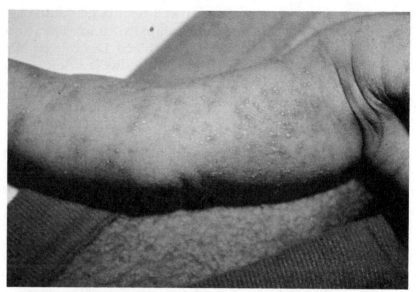

Figure 11-4. Miliaria (heat rash). *Courtesy of Timothy Berger, M.D.*

Autoimmune Disorders

Connective tissue diseases are the largest group of autoimmune diseases and include lupus erythematosus (a chronic disease that causes red, often scarring plaques, hair loss, and sometimes internal effects); dermatomyositis (skin rash and muscle weakness); scleroderma (hardening of the skin and other tissues). This large group of disorders are all caused by the body's immune system reacting against its own tissues, causing damage. Vitiligo, pure white patches caused by the destruction of pigment cells (melanocytes), and alopecia areata (patchy hair loss, see end of this chapter) may also be autoimmune disorders. See Plate 7.

Xanthelasma

Xanthelasma are yellow, plaque-like patches on the eyelids. These patches are a result of a disposition of cholesterol and fat. Xanthelasma are more common in the elderly and in persons with elevated blood cholesterol. See Figure 11-5.

Tumors

A tumor, also known as a neoplasm (new growth), occurs when cells in a specific area multiply excessively. Tumors are either benign (noncancerous) or malignant (cancerous). Moles (nevi) are benign tumors. Seborrheic keratoses are also benign tumors. They may be yellow or brown, sharply marginated, round or oval raised lesions. Malignant melonoma is a serious skin cancer that arises in moles or in the pigment cells (melanocytes) of the skin. They appear as small brown or black patches, or large, multi-colored patches, plaques, or nodules (bumps) with irregular borders. They may crust on the surface or bleed. Discovered in its early stages melanoma may be cured. However, left untreated melanoma can be fatal. See Figure 11-6.

Basal cell carcinoma is a malignant, raised, translucent, pearly, nodule that may crust, ulcerate, or bleed. It is rarely life threatening. Basal cell carcinoma is the most common cancer, with over 250,000 cases diagnosed yearly in the United States. See Plate 8.

Squamous cell carcinoma is a malignant, raised, pink, opaque nodule or patch that frequently ulcerates in the center. See Plate 9.

The three malignant tumors listed above are the most common types of skin cancer. With the widespreading AIDS epidemic, a once rare form of skin cancer is now appearing more frequently. Kaposi's sarcoma is a condition characterized by skin tumors and most often afflicts AIDS patients. The tumors, blue-red in color, appear anywhere on the body. In AIDS patients these tumors frequently involve the internal organs (see chapter on AIDS).

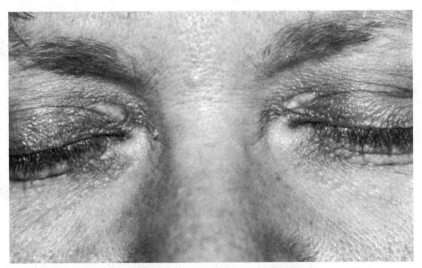

Figure 11-5. Xanthelasma. *Courtesy of Timothy Berger, M.D.*

Impaired Blood Supply

Poor drainage of blood can cause superficial and deep varicose veins. Impaired arterial flow can result from hardening of the arteries (atherosclerosis). Leg ulcers may occur and are particularly common in the elderly. Eczema or dermatitis frequently complicates disorders of the veins of legs. Spider veins may be associated with poor drainage, but commonly occur in women with normal circulation.

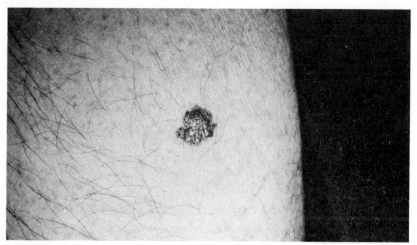

Figure 11-6. Malignant Melanoma. *Courtesy of Timothy Berger, M.D.*

DERMATOLOGIC EXAMINATION

A dermatologic examination is the means by which a dermatologist arrives at a diagnosis. The examination is performed in two phases: obtaining the patient's history and the actual physical examination.

Patient History

The first thing a dermatologist does when he or she meets the patient is document the patient's medical history. Since many skin diseases are hereditary, documenting the patient's family history is important. Next the doctor listens to the patient describe his or her symptoms. The patient is questioned concerning any discomfort, such as pain, aching, or itching. Because the skin is constantly exposed to the environment, the patient is also asked where he or she has traveled, what substances he or she has ingested, applied to the skin, or been exposed to.

Physical Examination

After the doctor documents the patient's history he performs a physical examination. First the dermatologist examines the patient to see what unaltered primary lesions are present. These may include macules (flat areas of skin with differing color), patches (flat areas greater than one centimeter in diameter), papules (elevated bumps less than one centimeter in diameter), plaques (flat elevated areas greater than one centimeter in diameter), wheals/hives (transient plaques), nodules (elevated bumps greater than one centimeter in diameter), and raised, fluid-filled lesions called vesicles (less than one centimeter in diameter), pustules (containing thick yellow pus), bullae (greater than one centimeter in diameter), elevated due to edema (swelling). Observing even the most minute details of the skin is vital to the dermatologist attempting to reach a correct diagnosis.

The dermatologist will look for secondary lesions, scales, scratches or crusts. When a scale is present it is a sign that there is an abnormality in the keratinization process, and that the epithelial layer is not shedding properly. Scales are usually white, gray, or silver in color, and dry. Crusts are associated with acute disorders. Crusts (scabs) result from an accumulation of serum, cells, and foreign matter. Crusts are moist, black, yellow, or honey colored. An erosion is a superficial loss of the skin. Left untreated an erosion can become an ulceration (a hollowed out deeper defect in the skin).

DERMATOLOGIC THERAPY

There are three ways a dermatologist can administer medication to the patient: systemically, topically, or through a physical modality. Topical medications are applied directly to the skin surface. Systemic medications are administered into the body, beneath the skin surface, either orally, by injection, or by inhalation. Physical modalities encompass ultraviolet light, laser, electrosurgery, and x-rays.

Topical Medications

Since the skin is easily accessible many medications can be applied directly to the skin in the form of topical preparations. Categories of topical medications include anti-infectives, anti-inflammatories, keratolytics, caustics, emollients, sunscreens, and photo sensitizers. Appropriate topical therapy requires that the dermatologist first make an accurate diagnosis. The success of a topical medication depends in part on the base. A base is a vehicle that contains the active ingredient. The following is a list of the most common bases used in dermatologic topical medication:

Ointments: The most well-known ointment is petrolatum (vaseline). Ointments are greasy but they lubricate and protect the skin. They are spreadable bases that soften and smooth the skin, and act as barriers against irritants.

Creams:
: Creams are made from fats such as almond oil or mineral oil mixed with paraffin (white wax). The purpose of a cream is to make the skin feel softer and smoother and to reduce roughness, cracking, and irritation of the skin. When any oil is applied on skin that is roughened, the scaly surface is coated with a film, cementing down the dry flakes. Creams vanish when applied to the skin and are easier to spread.

Lotions:
: Lotions are pourable liquids in which a medication is dissolved or suspended in water, alcohol, or propylene glycol. Lotions dry on the skin and cool it as they evaporate, leaving a film of medication.

Wet dressings:
: Wet dressings includes baths, soaks, or compresses. Wet dressings are used to dry, cleanse, and relieve itching. Anti-infective agents can be added to the water, which is the main active ingredient in wet dressings. This type of topical therapy is used on eruptions that are crusted, vesicular, weeping, and bullous.

Powders:
: Powders are solid materials ground into very fine particles. Powders absorb moisture. Talcum powder is an example of a moisture absorbent base. Antifungal preparations are often added to powders to treat conditions such as athlete's foot.

Pastes:
: A paste consists of zinc oxide, starch, and petrolatum. Pastes protect the area where applied and induce a drying effect on the skin. Pastes are most often applied under dressings.

Tinctures/ Paints:
: Tinctures and paints are substances dissolved in alcohol, acetone, or an organic solvent. Tinctures and paints evaporate quickly. When applied to the skin tinctures and paints produce a cooling, drying effect. An example of a tincture is iodine.

The following is a list of topical medications used to treat dermatologic disorders.

- **Corticosteroids** are anti-inflammatory cortisone derivatives. They are used to treat inflammatory disorders such as dermatitis. Corticosteroids used in excess may cause thinning of the skin, dilated blood vessels, and, if applied inappropriately to the face, rosacea.

- **Psoralens and Coal Tar** are photoactive drugs. When applied to the skin and exposed to ultra-violet light a therapeutic photosensitve reaction is produced. Photoactive medication is most commonly used in the treatment of psoriasis and vitiligo.

- **Tretinoin (Retin-A):** This vitamin A derivative is used for the topical treatment of acne vulgaris and to retard the physical signs of aging. For years Retin A was used for the treatment of acne before it was recognized as an anti-aging drug.

In the treatment of acne in which comedones, pustules, and papules are present, Retin-A is effective because it prevents comedone formation and suppresses keratin proliferation. Additionally, tretinoin stimulates mitotic activity (mitosis division of a cell) and increases the turnover of follicular epithelial cells (cells lining the follicle), causing extrusion (the "pushing-out") of comedones. Retin-A can be formulated in gel, cream, and liquid.

Tretinoin creams have received much attention as a therapy for wrinkles. Since early 1988 tretinoin is the first therapy clinically proven to reverse some of the signs of aging caused from photodamage (prolonged sun exposure). In this day and age as population ages, Retin-A has been touted as a "fountain of youth."

Some side effects of Retin-A are severe local erythema (redness) and peeling at the site of application. Medicated or abrasive soaps and cleansers, soaps and cosmetics that have a strong drying effect, and products with high concentrations of alcohol, astringents, spices, or lime should be used with caution because of possible interaction with tretinoin. Patients should be particularly cautious when using preparations containing sulfur, resorcinol, or salicylic acid with Retin-A. Patients should also avoid exposure to sunlight and sunlamps.

Because of the increasing consumer usage of Retin-A it is important for the clinical cosmetician to know if the client is using this topical medication. Facial treatments should be designed towards hydrating the epidermis because of the drying effect of Retin-A.

- **Antimitotic** (chemotherapeutic) agents are used in the treatment of skin tumors. Fluorouracil in cream form is used to treat actinic keratosis and occasionally basal cell carcinoma. This drug causes inflammation of the skin. Vinblastine can cause Kaposi's sarcoma to regress when injected into the lesion, or given intravenously.

- **Anti-infectives** are often used topically in the treatment of acne or impetigo. Benzoyl Peroxide, cleocin, and erythromycin are used in acne; mupiricin (Bactroban) is used to treat impetigo. Elimite cream and gamma benzene hexachloride (kwell, lindane) are used to treat scabies and lice.

- **Caustics and vesicants** are topical medications used to treat certain benign skin tumors, such as warts.

Systemic Medications

There are four main types of systemic medications: antibiotics, antihistamines, immunosuppressive agents, and steroids. The following is a list of the different types of systemic medications that a dermatologist may prescribe for various skin conditions.

Antibiotics: Antibiotics are substances that have the capacity to stop the growth of or kill microorganisms. They are frequently used in the treatment of acne. The following is a list of the most commonly used antibiotics.

Tetracycline: Tetracycline is an antibiotic that is used in treatment of acne. It can discolor developing teeth and therefore is not prescribed for children. It also should not be taken by pregnant women.

Clindamycin: This antibiotic is occasionally used to treat serious bacterial infections that are resistant to more commonly used antibiotics. Since clindamycin may cause serious diarrhea, it is often used topically when possible.

Erythromycin: This antibiotic is used to treat infections of the skin; however, resistant staphylococci may increase. It may be prescribed for patients with acne.

Minocycline: This tetracycline derivative may be used in low doses to treat acne. It is more effective than tetracycline, but is very expensive.

Penicillin:
: Derivatives such as dicloxicillin are commonly used to treat skin infections. Allergic reactions are common.

Isotretinoin: 13 Cis-retinoic acid
: Isotretinoin (Accutane) is a major breakthrough in the treatment of severe nodulocystic, scarring acne and is prescribed when other drug therapies have proven ineffective.

Accutane is related to Retin A and vitamin A. Accutane inhibits sebaceous gland function and keratinization. Accutane is available in 10 mg, 20 mg, and 40 mg capsules.

Generally, a single course of therapy has been shown to result in a substantial and prolonged remission of cystic acne.

Accutane has serious side effects; therefore, all patients must sign a patient information/consent form. There is an extremely high risk that a deformed infant will result if pregnancy occurs while taking Accutane in any amount. Therefore, Accutane must not be used by women who are pregnant or who may become pregnant while undergoing treatment. Some other side effects may include: cheilitis (painful peeling of the lips, dryness and peeling of the skin), predominantly on the face, palms, and soles; nose bleeds; sore gums; musculoskeletal aches and pains; and increased sun sensitivity.

Skin care treatments for patients on Accutane should be designed to hydrate the epidermal layer. Rich emollient creams and conditioning masks should be used. Avoid the use of abrasive products such as scrubs, peels, and drawing masks since these products will worsen the dryness the patient is already experiencing.

Antihist-amines:
: Antihistamines are frequently prescribed to relieve itching. They work best for hives. Most cause drowsiness. Commonly used ones are chlorpheniramine, diphenhydramine (Benedryl), and Atarax (Vistaril). Seldane and Hisminal are newer, more expensive, and non-sedating.

Immuno-
suppressant
Agents: This type of systemic drug therapy is useful in treating psoriasis and some autoimmune diseases. The function of the immune system is to respond to invading organisms or injury. Immunosuppressive agents suppress antibodies or sensitized white blood cells that are part of the immune response. Autoimmune disorders occur when the body reacts against its own cells and tissues. This produces disorders such as lupus erythematosus, dermatomyositis, and scleroderma. Cyclosporin is an immuno-suppressive drug used to suppress the body's natural defense against abnormal cells. It is also used to decrease the risk of tissue rejection. Methotrexate is a folic acid (vitamin B) derivative used to treat psoriasis.

Physical Modalities Ultraviolet light, radiation, and x-rays are considered physical modalities and used in the treatment of skin diseases. The primary source of ultraviolet light is the sun, but ultraviolet light can be artificially produced by quartz lamps or fluorescent fixtures. Ultraviolet radiation is beneficial in the treatment of psoriasis and other conditions. PUVA (Psoralen Ultraviolet A-Light), a form of phototherapy, is used in the treatment of vitiligo and psoriasis. The skin is made sensitive before exposure to ultraviolet light by topical or systemic psoralens, which increase the effect of the UVA (Ultraviolet A-Light). Coal tar can also be used as a photosensitizer in psoriasis and occasionally in eczema. Liquid nitrogen is commonly used to treat warts and solar keratoses (pre-malignant, scaly, red spots).

DERMATOLOGIC INSTRUMENTS

The following is a list of commonly used dermatological instruments.

Biopsy Punch A biopsy punch is an instrument that rotates, producing a circular cut. It is used to remove skin lesions and in hair transplantation. See Figure 11-7.

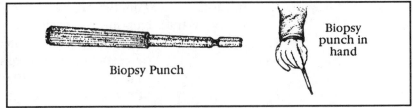

Figure 11-7. Biopsy punch

Comedo Extractor

A comedo extractor is an instrument used for acne surgery. One end of the extractor has a blade, which is used for puncturing a closed comedo; the other end of the instrument is in the shape of a small ring. Once it is punctured, the comedo is positioned in the center of the small ring. Pressure is applied, and the debris trapped inside the comedo extrudes. There are various extractors available; this describes only one type. See Figure 11-8.

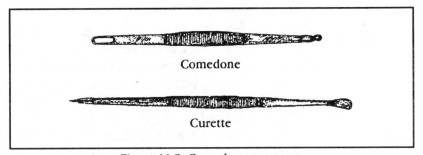

Figure 11-8. Comedone extractor

Skin Currette

A skin currette is sharp instrument used to remove both benign and malignant skin tumors such as warts, basal and squamous cell carcinomas, and keratoses. See Figure 11-9.

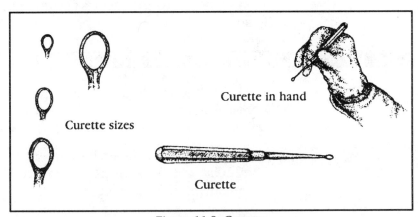

Figure 11-9. Curette

Iris Scissors   Iris scissors are used in skin surgery. These sharp scissors snip off skin tags and excise larger lesions. See Figure 11-10.

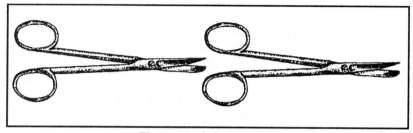

Figure 11-10. Iris scissors

Scalpel   A scalpel is a blade used in surgery to remove benign and malignant skin lesions. See Figure 11-11.

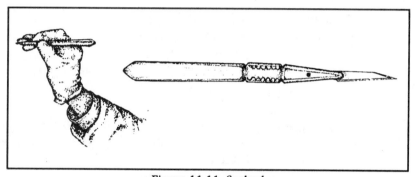

Figure 11-11. Scalpel

High-Frequency Desiccation   A high-frequency current is used to destroy dilated capillaries and skin tumors by a sparking process. This process is called desiccation. It is also used to stop bleeding. A heated loop (cautery) can be used for similar purposes. Patients frequently refer to these methods as "burning." See Figure 11-12.

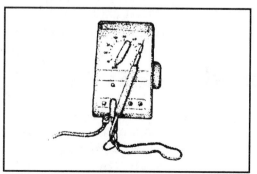

Figure 11-12.
High-frequency dessication

DERMATOLOGIC PROCEDURES

The following is a list of common dermatologic procedures.

Cryotherapy

Cryotherapy is the therapeutic use of cold. Liquid nitrogen is the most commonly used agent. Liquid ethyl chloride, freon, and solid carbon dioxide may also be used. Direct application and spraying are the usual methods of use. Superficial freezing is used to remove warts and actinic keratoses. Lesions are frozen with liquid nitrogen that is either applied directly with a cotton tip applicator or sprayed on. The lesion is frozen until it becomes white. A blister forms, crusts, and then sloughs off within ten to fourteen days. Deep freezing is a treatment for cutaneous malignancies.

Curettage and Electrosurgery

A curette is a sharp, spoon-shaped instrument used to scrape off a lesion, followed by electrosurgical destruction of tissue (an active electrical current is transmitted by needle, bulb, or disk). This is most commonly used to treat basal cell carcinoma.

Mohs Surgery

Mohs surgery is a microscopically controlled excision used for treating more serious or recurrent skin cancers. It has a high cure rate. Careful serial excisions and mapping of the tumor allow complete removal.

Radiation Therapy

Radiation therapy in divided doses is used in the treatment of basal and squamous cell carcinoma and Kaposi's sarcoma.

Dermabrasion

Dermabrasion is the removal of the surface layer of the skin. This procedure is performed by a fast-revolving abrasive wheel creating a high-speed sanding effect. It is used to reduce pitted acne scars, unsightly raised scars, and to remove tattoos. Healing takes a few weeks.

LASER SURGERY/VASCULAR LESIONS

Vascular lesions (portwine stains) are among the most common of the conditions which can be successfully camouflaged with corrective cosmetics. The following contribution by Dr. Lovic Hobby goes into extensive detail describing this condition and treatment.

Plastic Surgery and the Treatment of Superficial Vascular Lesions

Lovic Hobby, M.D.

"Plastic" comes from the Greek word "plastikos," which means to shape or to mold. Plastic surgeons are concerned with the reconstruction of deformities due to birth defects, trauma, and disease. The goal is to restore the particular problem area to its normal anatomical state. These are considered functional procedures. Plastic surgeons also work to improve the normal state. This includes reducing the effects of aging, sculpting areas of increased body fat, changing the shape of noses, enlarging breasts, etc. These are called esthetic procedures. This section will focus on what plastic surgery can do to improve various pathological conditions involving superficial blood vessel abnormalities. This work is functional, not esthetic. Certain plastic surgeons, opthalmalogists, ENT's, and dermatologists perform these types of procedures.

A commonly encountered superficial vascular lesion, and also the most obviously abnormal, is the portwine stain. These stains are dramatic deformities that are present at birth. These tumors occur early in the first trimester of pregnancy, but nothing is known about their cause. They are not considered to be hereditary. They may be originally pale pink to dark red. As the individual grows older, the lesion is progressive. The pale hemangiomas darken, while the darker lesions develop a protrusive sponginess and often have individual hemangiomas within the overall tumor. In some extreme cases, this progresses to a terribly deforming "cluster of grapes" type of tumor. This sponginess or bubbling ("cobblestoning") represents hypertrophy of the lesion itself, and is called lesional hypertrophy. The darker, thicker lesions, which involve certain anatomical structures such as the lips, nose, eyelids, and ears, will frequently cause abnormal growth of these structures in addition to the lesional hypertrophy. This is called structural hypertrophy. This type of involvement will lead to asymmetry of facial features and can cause devastating disfigurement. In addition to lesional and structural deformities, patients afflicted with portwine stains have systemic problems, usually associated with additional hemangiomas located internally. Unfortunately, sometimes these can be in the brain.

Portwine stains are referred to as intradermal capillary hemangiomas. "Hemangioma" means blood vessel tumor. "Capillary" designates the type of blood vessel, and "intradermal" means, at least in the beginning, the lesion is contained within the dermis. These tumors consist of capillaries that are more concentrated, more dilated, and more superficial than normal.

These congenital anomalies have been recorded since the beginning of medical literature. They are quite dramatic and were described originally by the term "nevus flammeus." When England began to import wine from the Portuguese city of

Lovic W. Hobby, M.D., is a Board Certified Plastic Surgeon in Atlanta, Georgia, practicing at Piedmont Hospital since 1967. He has held teaching positions as Instructor for the Department of Surgery, Division of Plastic Surgery, Columbia Presbyterian Medical Center in New York and has taught Laser Courses for the Plastic Surgery Educational Foundations symposiums and national meetings.

O'Porto in 1690, the word "portwine" was introduced into the language. During the next 200 years, the obvious similarities between the red-purple wine and the infamous nevus flammeus were duly noted. By the late 1800s, the term "portwine stain" was firmly entrenched in both the lay and medical literature.

In the past many forms of treatment were used. No entirely satisfactory treatment was available. Among those methods used were dry ice, carbon dioxide, radiation, sclerosing agents, cortisone, dermabrasion, cryosurgery, ultraviolet light, electrolysis, and tattooing. Within the specialty of plastic surgery, conventional surgical methods were used such as excision and grafting; excision and rotation and advancement of local and distant flaps; and excision with the assistance of tissue expanders, etc.

In the late 1970s, the first major advance in the treatment of this problem emerged. This was photo-coagulation surgery, done with laser light. The word "laser" is an acronym for Light Amplification by Stimulated Emission of Radiation.

Each laser, according to its lasing medium, produces a specific wavelength. Most of the tissue structures in the body absorb specific wavelengths. These tissue targets are called "chromophores." For instance, the pure blue-green light produced by the excited argon gas particles within the argon laser is readily absorbed by the color red, the dominant color of all vascular lesions. When the laser light from the argon laser is directed on anything with a red color, the red absorbs the blue-green light, and this light energy is converted to heat energy.

This can be demonstrated readily by drawing red lines across a white piece of paper and directing the laser beam at right angles across the lines. Nothing happens to the white paper, but each time the laser crosses a red line, there is an absorption of energy, a creation of heat, and a hole burned where the red was on the paper. This can be demonstrated even more dramatically by blowing up a red balloon inside of a white balloon. The laser can be directed at the balloons, and the inside red balloon will pop while nothing happens to the outside white balloon.

Clinically, this can be applied to the treatment of portwine stains. When the laser light is directed at the portwine stain or other superficial vascular lesion, the light moves through the epidermis with no effect. It even goes through the wall of the abnormal vessel with no effect. When the red of the blood inside the vessel absorbs the laser light, the light energy is transformed into heat energy. Thus, the heat source originates within the very vessel that we are seeking to destroy.

Argon laser therapy is usually administered under a general anesthetic due to the pain involved, particularly if the lesion is of any significant size. When the appropriate energy is delivered, the treated area becomes gray-white immediately. This is the equivalent of a superficial second-degree burn. After completion of the therapy, there is very little discomfort.

The wound may blister, or weep, and will usually scab within the first four to five days. The scab should be kept dry and should be left alone until it falls off, usually seven to eight days after its formation. When the scab first comes off, the treated area is red, because it is a recently healed burn. Over the next twelve months the lesion will continue to fade. Occasionally retreatments are indicated.

In the late 1980s yellow-light lasers emerged. They brought with them a wavelength that was absorbed even more selectively by the red of the blood (oxyhemaglobin) and was absorbed less by other chromophores such as brown (melanin) and yellow (xanthophile) in the body. This more specific absorption enabled the surgeon to begin treatment of vascular anomalies in the pre-pubertal age group without fear of scarring. As experience with this new technology has developed, it has become obvious that there are three significant advantages: by treating the affected person early, psychological damage from peer groups, even in kindergarten, may well be prevented; the lesion, of course, will be considerably smaller, offering increased ease in treatment; and finally, early treatment may prevent the later structural hypertrophy and facial asymmetry that are so difficult to treat.

Yellow-light laser therapy follows a different clinical course than argon laser therapy. This is particularly true of the flashlamp-pumped pulsed dye laser. Immediately after the delivery of a pulse of energy, the treated area becomes blue-black. This is a bruise. Close inspection of the epidermis reveals no burn, however. The bruise usually lasts six to seven days. There may be some slight crusting, in which case antibiotic ointment should be applied. During this time makeup is prohibited. The treated area can be wet, but should be gently patted dry. When the bruise clears, the treated lesion has essentially the same color as pre-operatively. Fading takes place for this form of therapy over a period of some two months in children and three months in adults. At the end of this time the lesion is retreated. Retreat-ments continue until no color remains or until no further improvement is obtained. The fact that almost always multiple treatments are required is a disadvantage to this type of therapy. However, it seems to be the price to be paid in exchange for the advantage of almost no scarring. General anesthesia is required for young children. Older children may or may not tolerate the procedure without anesthesia. Almost all adults are done with no anesthesia.

The present state of the art seems to indicate that both the argon lasers and the newer yellow-light lasers will have their appropriate places in the treatment of vascular defects. The thicker, darker, adult-type lesions will still respond best to argon laser therapy. The pale, flat, childhood-type lesions can be treated now with the more "gentle" yellow-light lasers.

Although some cases show remarkable improvement, the final result of treatment usually falls short of complete removal. Terms like "remove," "do away with," "get rid of," "erase," and "eradicate" are too sensational and invoke in the patient unrealistic expectations. A conservative estimate of improvement provides the patient with the most reasonable goals and the least chance for disappointment. This is not meant to detract, however, from the excellent results obtained with photocoagulation surgery. Almost all patients should expect a very significant reduction in color with very little chance of scarring.

Some patients, however, have advanced tumors with high blood flow, deep color, and thickness. The problem can no longer be satisfactorily solved with laser therapy alone. Usually these patients benefit from use of the laser in order to devascularize the tumor as much as possible, but then additional conventional plastic surgery is required. In extremely high blood flow tumors, after being devascularized with laser, the blocking of feeder vessels with small plastic pellets, known as selective embolization, may be required. This is followed by excision of the lesion with conventional plastic surgery methods. Sometimes this is done with a new technique using a laser that actually touches the tissue as it cuts. This is called contact laser surgery and is completely different from photo-coagulation surgery. A Nd YAG laser with a sapphire tip is used. This excision may be facilitated or augmented by using skin flaps, skin grafts, and tissue expanders. Plastic surgeons treating all types of portwine stains should be well aware of the capabilities offered by laser surgery as well as conventional surgical procedures.

The photocoagulation properties of lasers are applicable to almost all other superficial vascular lesions. The most common of these is the telangiectasia, or spider angioma. This lesion consists of dilated capillaries in the trunk and extremities. These lesions respond particularly well on the face and neck. They are totally unpredictable on the trunk and arms and are almost uniformly unresponsive in the lower extremities. Flat lesions respond best to treatment with the yellow-light lasers, whereas those that have a raised, central papule will respond better to the argon laser. Again, yellow-light lasers offer very little risk of scarring; the argon laser may provide a more definitive one-time treatment, but may have a small possibility of scarring.

Many other skin lesions are responsive to photocoagulation surgery. These include multiple varieties of hemangiomas, which can occur in the mouth or on the vermilion of the lips or on the skin. They include also acne rosacea, rhinophyma, cherry hemangiomas anywhere on the body, and other vascular tumors such as angio-keratomas and angiofibromas. In order to select the appropriate laser, each lesion must be individually evaluated. Those that are pale and flat will respond to the yellow-light lasers; those with more color and, certainly, those that are three-dimensional may respond better to the argon laser.

Photocoagulation surgery can be performed on tattoos also. The argon laser has been used for this since the late 1970s. The Q-switched ruby laser is now being used for tattoos. It appears to be particularly effective on homemade blue and black tattoos and less so on commercial tattoos with other colors. This ruby laser produces an excellent result with almost no scarring, whereas the argon laser, although it can remove the tattoo successfully, always produces some degree of scarring.

Lately, there has been a great deal in the news media concerning the use of cutting lasers in the performance of conventional aesthetic plastic surgical procedures such as eyelid lifts (blepharoplasty) and face lifts (rhydidectomy). This media romance surrounding lasers had led to a state of "laser worship" among the lay population. A myth has been created, resulting in the fantasy that any procedure done with the laser is automatically better than the same procedure done without it. In the only scientific study the authors found no advantage over conventional plastic surgery performed with scalpel. They concluded that there was, however, significant increase in danger to the patient, time in surgery, cost of equipment, and the need for additional personnel. It was noted also that, in order to provide the most acceptable scar, any skin incision made with laser requires scalpel re-excision of the edges prior to closing.

A significant reduction in the color of superficial vascular lesions, especially portwine stains, enhances the ability of the cosmetologist to improve the patient's appearance. Whatever the technique used, application of the makeup is done in much less time, much less opaque material is required, and more natural result is obtained. The final result of this combination of laser surgery, conventional plastic surgery, and cosmetics is usually most encouraging, resulting in a more healthy patient, mentally and physically.

Almost incomprehensible advances have been made in the treatment of superficial vascular lesions, especially portwine stains,

over the past ten years. The principle of photo-coagulation surgery offered an entirely new concept. It served to completely outdate conventional methods of treatment in many lesions and augmented greatly these same methods in others. Now the ability to extend this technology to treatment of children seems even more miraculous. The field of laser science is one of the most rapidly expanding frontiers in medicine. Developments must be constantly monitored in order to keep abreast of new technology as it becomes clinically applicable. On the other hand, enthusiasm over laser technology must be tempered by experience, knowledge, common sense, and the moral ability to resist the temptation to ride the laser bandwagon.

Sclerotherapy

This procedure can be used to treat small spider veins on the thighs and legs, but the incidence of recurrence is high. Hemosiderin (a breakdown product of hemoglobin) deposits in tissue, which could result in permanent brown staining and scarring from the injection.

Collagen Injections

Zyderm and Zyplast are the trade names for injectable collagen. Collagen is derived from purified animal collagen. Because it is very similar to human collagen it is readily accepted by the body and the surrounding tissue. Injectable collagen is effective in smoothing lines around the lips and in corners of the eyes. For deeper depressions, such as furrows that form after many years of smiling and frowning, Zyplast collagen is used. It may also be used to improve certain types of scars.

Injectable collagen has not proven useful in the treatment of small, superficial lines located directly under the eyes; or for certain scars, namely "ice-pick" acne scars, or scars with sharp edges.

Prior to administration a skin test is performed to determine any possibility of an allergic reaction. Individuals with a history of autoimmune diseases or serious allergic reactions, or people who are allergic to lidocaine, are not considered suitable candidates for collagen treatment.

As with any procedure there are risks involved; the needle could be accidentally placed through a blood vessel, which could result in a scab, scar, or temporary discoloration. Injection into a blood vessel could also cause a blockage of blood flow and loss of circulation to nearby sites; however, this is extremely rare.

DERMATOLOGIC CONDITIONS

The following skin conditions are the most common dermatologic disorders that a clinical cosmetician may be asked to camouflage.

Hypopigmentation

Hypopigmentation occurs when skin abnormally loses some (hypo) or all of its pigment. Patches of pale skin occur in various skin disorders such as pityriasis alba, a form of hypopigmentation that results from mild eczema; mainly in children and often appearing on the cheeks. Hypomelanosis (white markings) is a condition found on older skin, mainly on the arms and legs. Albinism is an extremely rare, inherited disorder caused by melanin deficiency. The skin is pale, hair is light, and the person is extremely sensitive to sunlight. Hypopigmentation is a common complication of cryotherapy. See Plate 10.

Medical Treatment: Dermatologists treat pityriasis alba with topical cortisone medication. Doctors recommend that once the irritation and dryness subsides, the treated area should be exposed to sunlight to stimulate the return of pigment. There is no effective treatment for guttate hypomelanosis or albinism, but sunscreens are advised.

Cosmetic Treatment: Hypopigmentation can be minimized with the use of cover creams that match the patient's skin tone. To disguise the hypopigmented areas recommend that the patient apply an opaque cover cream solution directly to the affected area, blending out the edges. A second application (only on the borders) may be necessary only if the borders bleed through. For a more natural look the patient can apply a second coat of makeup with a lip brush or artist's flat brush. Skin dyes such as Vitadye, Dy-O-Derm, or bronzers work best to camouflage hypopigmented body areas and can be obtained from a pharmacist. Several coats must be applied to achieve the correct shade.

Vitiligo

Vitiligo is a condition in which the destruction of melanocytes (cells responsible for producing skin pigment) results in patches of complete depigmentation, sometimes having a hyperpigmented border, and often enlarging slowly. Vitiligo occurs most commonly on the face, hands, armpits, and groin. The affected skin is extremely sensitive to sunlight because of the absence of melanocytes. Repigmentation occurs in about 30 percent of the cases. The cause of vitiligo is unknown. It occurs in all races. Vitiligo is more of a problem in people with dark complexions because the disease is more apparent. Vitiligo starts with a few small patches. Its course is unpredictable. It may remain in one area, or it may spread and involve large areas of the body. See Figure 11-13.

Medical Treatment: Treatment for vitiligo may include either topical or systemic psoralens or both, combined with ultraviolet light therapy (PUVA). Creams containing corticosteroid drugs may also be prescribed to patients with vitiligo. Rarely, in severe cases, chemicals are used to remove all the remaining pigment to give the person a uniform white color.

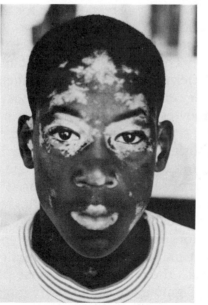 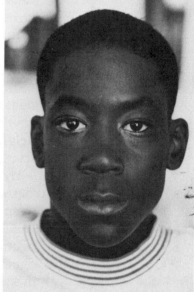

Figure 11-13. Vitiligo — before and after camouflage makeup is applied

Cosmetic Treatment: Dark complexioned vitiligo patients often experience prejudice from within their own culture, making this disease very distressing not only physically but emotionally. Light complexioned vitiligo patients, on the other hand, will be able to minimize the appearance of vitiligo by covering it with a light cream base foundation such as a pan-stick, or a makeup that offers a total finish to the complexion. Patients with darker skin require heavier coverage because the color difference between the vitiligo areas (white) and the pigmented areas is so great. Theatrical makeup or opaque, waterproof, cover creams can be used to mask vitiligo. After the initial application instruct the patient to go back and re-apply a second coat of makeup with an artist's flat brush along the borders, where demarcation is more evident. Select cover creams that contain sunscreen, sunblock, or both. Skin dyes such as Vitadye or Dy-O-Derm will be more effective on hands, feet, or body areas where makeup would easily come in contact with clothing and rub off. The dyes must be applied in several coats until the correct color intensity is achieved. These dyes can be purchased from a pharmacist. Vegetable or henna eyelash or eyebrow dye can also be used on facial hair to restore color. These can be obtained through a beauty supply store.

Hyperpigmentation

Hyperpigmentation is abnormally increased pigmentation of the skin. The cells responsible for this are found in the basal layer and are called melanocytes. These are the cells that manufacture the pigment of the skin and are involved in tanning. They do this by producing a chemical compound called melanin. In the beginning the melanocytes look similar to other cells, flat with a dark spot in the center, but as the melanocytes mature they develop hollow arms with extenders that project from the sides. These extensions reach out to neighboring cells and provide them with melanin, which results in coloration of the skin. See Plate 11.

Hyperpigmentation may occur as a result of the following factors: chronic inflammation or injury, hormonal disturbances from oral contraceptives or pregnancy, psoriasis, and tinea versicolor (pityriasis versicolor). Hyperpigmentation may also occur from using perfumed cosmetics in the sun, because the chemicals they contain can cause photosensitivity. Changes in skin pigment are significantly more common in persons of medium skin pigment (Asians, Hispanics, light-skinned blacks).

Medical Treatment: Hyperpigmentation may be treated with Retin-A and bleaching creams that contain hydroquinone. There are many treatments for tinea versicolor (hyperpigmentation), including sodium thiosulfate, selenium sulfide, dandruff shampoos, zinc pyrithione, topical antifungal creams, and oral ketoconazole.

Cosmetic Treatment: Cover creams will successfully mask the uneven pattern of dark blotches caused by hyperpigmentation. Recommend that the patient use either theatrical makeup or opaque cover cream that matches his or her skin tone. If the cosmetic solution bleeds through it could alter the color of the camouflage makeup. To avoid this either use a thicker application or apply a thinner coat first and set it with powder, then re-apply a second coat. Remind the patient when he or she is concealing hyperpigmentation to pay special attention to the darker borders; it may be necessary to go back over them to make sure the spots are completely concealed.

Dark Circles Cause is unknown but usually associated with allergies (hay fever, sinus trouble).

Medical Treatment: NONE

Cosmetic Treatment: If the dark circles under the eyes are melanin deposits, recommend that the patient protect his or her under-eye area from sunlight by wearing polarized sunglasses and a cover cream that contains sunscreen. Suggest that the patient use an under-eye concealer, either a pigment in a oil-based moisturizer or a water-resistant cover stick. The color of the cover-stick or concealer should be half a shade lighter than the patient's skin tone. Apply the cover stick over the dark circles and around the entire eye area to camouflage discoloration. Opaque cover creams can also be used to camouflage dark circles, but because of the opaque cover cream's thicker consistency it tends to draw attention to the fine lines under the eyes. To avoid this problem suggest that the patient use an artist's flat brush (a #4 or a # 6) to apply the cover cream directly under the eyelashes and around the eye area. A cotton swab dipped in translucent powder can be used to roll on setting powder to keep the makeup from gradually sinking into the fine lines and creases. See Plates 12, 13, and 14.

Melasma/Chloasma

Melasma is a Greek word that means "black spot." Melasma (or chloasma as it is commonly called) is of unknown cause in some cases but is influenced by hormones and exposure to sunlight. This condition appears most commonly in dark-haired, dark-skinned women. Pregnancy or use of birth control pills can lead to melasma (chloasma). If melasma is caused by pregnancy or by birth control pills it can take up to five years to disappear or can last indefinitely. The resulting hyperpigmentation can affect any or all of the following facial areas: the forehead, cheeks, nose, upper lip, and chin. See Plate 15. Wearing perfume or certain cosmetic facial preparations in the sun can also worsen melasma.

Medical Treatment: Hydroquinone is prescribed to help fade the mottled liver spots caused by melasma. When combined with Retin-A hydroquinone is very successful in depigmenting discoloration caused by melasma. Sunscreens are also used to prevent repigmentation. Freezing with liquid nitrogen or dry ice can also lighten pigment. Electrosurgical destruction or a mild acid is an alternative form of treatment that has been used to eliminate melasma.

Cosmetic Treatment: Patients should be encouraged to apply a total sunblock to the affected area daily to prevent further discoloration. This should be done twenty minutes before the patient applies an opaque cover cream solution to conceal the discoloration. Opaque cover creams with total sun protection (SPF of 15 or more) will cosmetically camouflage the hyperpigmented areas, and at the same time provide the patient with additional sun protection. Patients should be instructed to apply a thick application of cover cream so the discoloration will not bleed through and alter the color of the makeup, giving it a grayish cast. A terracotta or pink powder blush can be applied lightly to counteract this problem and will prevent it from looking muddy.

Nevus/Nevi

A nevus is any congenital lesion of the skin; a birthmark. Nevi begin to form when a person is conceived, in the womb or during developmental stages. A nevus may be flesh-colored, brown, blue, or black. They may be smooth, flat, or slightly raised, hairy or rough in texture. Lay persons refer to brown lesions as moles, but medical professionals use the term nevus. See Figure 11-14. A freckle contains an increase in melanin in the basal layer and may appear in early childhood. A lentigo is a pale or brown spot that looks like a freckle. It may also be confused with a mole. It arises in later years and is probably caused by overexposure to the sun. In rare cases moles can become cancerous. One third of melanomas, the most serious type of skin cancer, occur in preexisting moles. Blue nevi most frequently appear on the backs of hands.

Medical Treatment: Some nevi should be excised because of their malignant potential. Nevi may grow lighter or darker or completely fade away with time; or nevi may grow larger and more obvious during puberty or pregnancy. The vast majority of these moles are benign, but if they change in size, shape, color, texture, sensitivity, or if there is irritation, discharge, bleeding, itching, or pain, it could indicate malignancy. In such cases medical advise should be sought immediately. Nevi can be removed by shaving them off at the skin's surface and destroying the base with an electric needle. Surgical excision and skin grafting may be necessary with larger nevi.

Cosmetic Treatment: If a nevi has been excised some slight scarring may result. The extent of this scarring will depend on the size and the shape of the nevi. The unsightly appearance of a nevi can be minimized with the use of eyeshadows or lipsticks. Depending on the nevi's location these can be used to draw attention away from the nevi and create another point of interest. An opaque cover cream can also be applied over the nevi to conceal it.

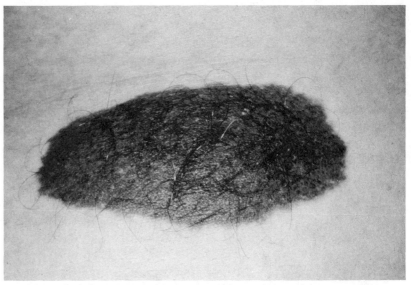

Figure 11-14. Congenital Nevus. Courtesy of Timothy Berger, M.D.

Telangiectasia

Telangiectasia refers to small, dilated, blood vessels. Spider angioma of the legs may develop on anyone; with women they often develop during pregnancy, generally diminishing after delivery; however they may never completely disappear. The cause is usually not apparent. Genetic factors may be important. Facial telangiectasias may be related to sun exposure or rosacea. See Plate 16.

Medical Treatment: Electrodessication usually eliminates facial telangiectasia. Sclerosing solutions such as hypertonic saline may be used to treat spider veins of the legs. Argon and pulse dye lasers may be used for some lesions.

Cosmetic Treatment: To help the patient camouflage telangiectasias suggest that he or she apply a green color corrector to tone down the red or purple undertones in the skin, set it with translucent powder, and wait ten minutes for it to stabilize before attempting to apply a thicker, more opaque cover to the area.

Rosacea

Rosacea is a chronic skin disorder that involves dilated central facial blood vessels with redness, or redness combined with papules and pustules. Patients with rosacea may have prolonged facial flushing and numerous telangiectasias. Both men and women suffer from rosacea. See Plate 17.

Medical Treatment: Antibiotics such as tetracycline or topical metronidazole (metrogel) are the most effective treatment for this skin disorder. Hot drinks, alcohol, and spicy foods should probably be minimized. Occasionally Accutane (isotretionoin) is used for severe cases.

Cosmetic Treatment: Abrasive exfoliants, scrubs, face masques, or peels can severely aggravate rosacea. Patients should be cautioned to avoid using extremely hot or cold water on their skin when cleansing. To properly instruct patients on the most effective way to camouflage rosacea, advise the patient to first apply a green color corrector, which will neutralize the red and tone it down. Caution patients to avoid trying to completely conceal this condition with thick, oil-based foundations because they will completely rob the skin of its natural coloring and make it look mask-like. A light application of a water-based foundation or a light oil base will make rosacea less obvious and will provide the best camouflage solution.

Cherry Hemangioma

Cherry hemangioma, or cherry spots, are purple or brilliant small red blemishes caused by localized overgrowth of blood vessels. They can be flat or raised and appear anywhere on the body.

Medical Treatment: Cherry hemangioma can be removed by electrosurgery, shave excision, or both.

Cosmetic Treatment: Because of the small size of the lesion a lip brush should be used (instead of finger application) to discreetly apply the matching camouflage cover cream to this minuscule area.

Portwine Stains (PWS)

Portwine stains are discussed above under Laser Surgery/ Vascular Lesions.

Cosmetic Treatment: To conceal the appearance of a portwine stain a thin coat of corrective makeup must be applied and set with a light application of translucent powder. Repeat this process with an additional application of cover cream to prevent discoloration from bleeding through. Again, set with sealing powder. Allow the application to stabilize for a few minutes, and then dust off excess. If the portwine stain is extremely dark you can use a green color corrector first to tone down the redness. See Plates 18 and 19 for before and after photographs.

Acne

Acne is an eruptive and common skin disease that is brought about by the plugging and inflammation of the hair follicle. It manifests as papules, pustules, or comedones on the face, chest, and back. In certain instances acne can produce severe scarring. See Figure 11-15.

Acne vulgaris is, unquestionably, the most common skin condition affecting those in the age group that extends from the early teens to the mid-thirties. Though rarely associated with any significant systemic manifestations, acne can have devastating emotional repercussions on those affected by disfiguring forms of disorder.

Medical Treatment: Treatment does not cure acne, but it can control the symptoms, allowing the body time to heal itself. The treatment given to patients for acne is antibiotics to retard bacterial growth and prevent comedo, papule, and pustule formation. If the acne is severe, cysts will develop. Cysts can be injected with cortisone. Treatment of acne depends upon the type of acne the patient has. Mild cases are treated with topical benzoyl peroxide, antibiotics, or tretinoin (Retin-A). Patients with severe acne may be treated with isotretinion (Accutane), a derivative of vitamin A. Dermabrasion, punch graft transplantation, and collagen injections are options available to patients with acne scarring.

Cosmetic Treatment: Unfortunately, the pitted acne marks that are left behind from acne are difficult to disguise with makeup. Cover creams can be useful if they are applied sparingly to the areas that are discolored by scarring. Oil-based, opaque makeup should never be used on patients with active acne because it is greasy and can interfere with topical medication, not to mention its bacteria-attracting qualities. Only water-based makeup should be recommended by the camouflage therapist to patients who are seeking a cosmetic solution to cover their acne. Patients' need to be forewarned that they may be disappointed in the final cosmetic result because the thin application of a water-based foundation when applied to the skin will not provide as much coverage as an opaque cover cream. The most that patients can expect is a minimal result that will somewhat diminish the redness and inflammation that accompanies acne scarring. See Plate 20.

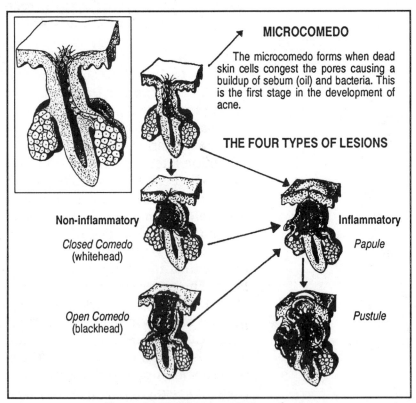

Figure 11-15. The progression of acne

Discoid Lupus Erythematosus (DLE) Discoid lupus erythematosus is an autoimmune disorder that is chronic and causes superficial inflammation of the skin. DLE begins as raised, reddish-brown or purple, circular, thick plaques with crusted edges, developing into flat, hypopigmented patches covered with scales, which eventually fall off and scar. If the scalp is affected, permanent hair loss may result. See Plate 21.

DLE is more common in females that in males and is more likely to develop in blacks than in whites. Discoid lupus is triggered and worsened by ultraviolet exposure, especially UVB.

Medical Treatment: Because there is no cure, treatment for lupus is aimed at alleviating inflammation and other symptoms associated with lupus. Patients may be given topical steroids, oral corticosteroids, antimalarial medication, and nonsteroidal anti-inflammatory drugs to combat other symptoms, such as joint pain. Patients must not expose themselves to ultraviolet light and must constantly protect their skin from the sun by wearing high SPF sunscreens and protective clothing, such as long sleeves and wide-brimmed hats.

Cosmetic Treatment: Because lupus can be chronic, cosmetic therapy must be coordinated with the patient's medical treatments. Contact should be made with the patient's physician before any cosmetic treatment is given. Since the application of a protective sunscreen or sunblock is mandatory, and the sunscreen must dry on the skin for twenty minutes before corrective makeup can be applied, the patient should be advised to arrive at the session with his or her skin thoroughly cleansed, toned, and moisturized with a sunscreen. Cosmetically the camouflage therapist should anticipate using cover creams to conceal erythema, hypo-pigmentation, or hyperpigmentation. Also, temporary or permanent hair replacement may need to be discussed with the patient.

Scleroderma Scleroderma is chronic hardening and thickening of the skin. It is a rare condition that can affect many organs and tissues of the body, especially the skin, arteries, kidneys, lungs, heart, gastrointestinal tract, and joints. The disease is more likely to appear between the ages of forty to sixty and is twice as common in women as it is in men. The severity of the symptoms varies. Scleroderma produces changes in the skin that make the face and fingers, in particular, wax-like, shiny, tight, and thick.

Medical Treatment: There is no cure for scleroderma. Treatment is designed to relieve symptoms and associated problems. The severity and number of symptoms vary. The following is a list of some of the drugs prescribed to treat scleroderma: vasodilator drugs (prescribed to widen the blood vessels by relaxing the muscles within the walls of the vessels), antihypertensive drugs (prescribed to treat high blood pressure that can lead to kidney damage or stroke), and corticosteroid drugs to reduce inflammation. Physical therapy allows the patient to regain his or her mobility, and dialysis is used to support kidney function.

Cosmetic Treatment: Because of the effect scleroderma has on the skin and arteries, camouflage makeup instruction is extremely beneficial to patients with scleroderma. Abnormal pigmentation and telangiectasias are characteristic of this medical condition. Discoloration and redness can easily be concealed with the application of cover creams. Often, specific areas such as the hands and feet have a tendency to appear white, red, or blue. Keep the cosmetic therapy simple for the scleroderma patient because while his or her skin appears mask-like, it is also very tight, and the patient may have problems performing complicated camouflage procedures.

Dermatitis (Eczema)

Dermatitis is a broad term used to define many scaly red, sometimes vesicular, reactions of the skin. Often the cause of dermatitis is not known. Listed below are the most common forms of dermatitis.

Contact Dermatitis

Contact dermatitis is an irritant or allergic response of the skin caused by direct contact with some irritant or allergen such as poison oak, poison ivy, paints, or detergents. Most cosmetics are uncommon causes of contact dermatitis. Resulting skin eruptions can appear as small, slightly inflamed, flat spots on the skin or as dark red patches covering larger areas of the body. When the white blood cells in the body attack an allergen the skin becomes red, inflamed, itchy, and sensitive. See Plate 22.

Medical Treatment: Topical and systemic cortisone derivatives relieve many of the symptoms of an allergic reaction by reducing inflammation.

Cosmetic Treatment: In rare instances repeated contact dermatitis can cause scarring. Camouflage makeup can be useful in concealing this type of scarring, but the camouflage therapist must be aware of the possibility that the patient may be allergic to one or several of the ingredients in the makeup. All products used on sensitive skin patients should be patch tested prior to application. The cosmetician should place a small amount of the cover cream solution on a gauze square and then tape it to the inside of the patient's forearm. The test patch should be left in place for forty-eight hours and examined for reaction one or two days later. In order to decrease the possibility of skin irritation caused by the corrective makeup, recommend that the patient purchase cover creams only in small quantities to insure freshness and to prevent prolonged exposure to bacteria.

Atopic Dermatitis

Atopic dermatitis, also known as eczema, is an inherited skin condition. Individuals with a family history of asthma, hay fever, or dry skin seem to be more likely to develop (it is not contagious) this form of dermatitis. Atopic dermatitis causes itching, erythema, inflammation, fine scaliness, irritated papules, and crusty erosions.

Medical Treatment: There is no cure for atopic dermatitis. Most cases resolve as patients enter adulthood. Anti-inflammatory medications such as corticosteroids, both topically and systemically, may be prescribed by dermatologists to relieve the symptoms of this skin condition. Antihistamines are also prescribed because they may be effective in temporarily controlling itching. Antibiotics may be used in secondary infection.

Cosmetic Treatment: Patients afflicted with atopic dermatitis may be benefited by the use of camouflage techniques after the weeping, crusted, erythematous (red) patches heal. Hypo- or hyperpigmentation may result. Corrective makeup should be applied over a moisturizer because patients with this type of skin disorder generally have dry skin. Light, creamy cover creams will provide the best coverage, as opposed to thicker, more opaque cover-ups that would emphasize the skin's tightness and look unnatural. Makeup should be free from fragrance, waterproof, and resistant to sunlight.

Seborrheic Dermatitis

Seborrheic dermatitis most commonly affects the central facial and scalp areas, which proportionally contain a greater number of oil glands. It is characterized by dry, scaly patches. It is most frequently seen on the forehead, on the front and sides of the hairline, on the eyebrows and eyelids, in the facial creases, on both sides of the nose, above and behind the ears, on the scalp, on the chest and back, under the armpits, and around the groin. Seborrheic dermatitis in its mildest form is called dandruff. Dry, cold weather and lack of sun all appear to aggravate the problem, triggering flare-ups. It is more common in certain neurological disorders and in HIV infection. Certain normal yeast organisms may be contributory. See Plate 23.

Medical Treatment: The general method of treatment is topical corticosteroids (cortisone) or anti-yeast medication. Mild coal tar or zinc pyrithione shampoos are used frequently.

Cosmetic Treatment: While patients afflicted with this form of dermatitis appear to have dry skin, in actuality they have normal or oily skin with surface scales. The clinical cosmetician must be careful not to use too thick or rich skin-care products when cleansing, toning, or moisturizing the patient's skin.

Photodermatitis

Photodermatitis, most often acute but sometimes chronic, is an inflammation of the skin due to hypersensitivity or overexposure to light or sunlight. It may be due to topical or systemic medications. The common sunburn is the most recognized form of photodermatitis. Patients who are extremely sensitive to sunlight can experience such symptoms as blisters and hives. See Plate 24.

Medical Treatment: The best treatment for this condition is to prevent it from occurring by avoiding sunlight, wearing protective clothing, and using sunscreens consistently.

Cosmetic Treatment: Cover creams will successfully conceal scarring, telangiectasias, and hypo-/hyperpigmented areas resulting from photodermatitis. A sunscreen should be applied at least twenty minutes before the camouflage makeup is applied. Corrective makeup that is waterproof and resistant to sunlight will provide additional protection from the sun.

HAIR AND SCALP DISORDERS

Hair is an appendage of the skin. It is a slender, threadlike outgrowth of the skin and scalp on the human body. Due to the absence of nerves there is no feeling in the hair. The technical term for study of the hair is trichology. The chief purposes of hair are adornment and protection of the head from heat, cold, and injury. Hair, properly groomed and cut, serves as a picture frame for the human face. It also can camouflage imperfections on the face and head. For example, correct styling can minimize round, oblong, square, and pear-shaped faces. Large ears can also be covered or minimized by correct styling.

It is important for the cosmetologist to have thorough knowledge of the hair and scalp and how to maintain healthy and beautiful hair and scalp.

Hair is chiefly composed of a protein called keratin, which is present in all horny growths, such as hair and nails. Sebaceous glands or oil glands are the little saccular structures situated in the dermis. Their ducts are connected to the hair follicles. They secrete an oily substance called sebum, which gives luster and pliability to the hair and skin.

Blood circulation also affects the general health of the hair. Hair derives its nourishment from the blood supply. Certain drugs, such as hormones, may cause problems. Hair loss or excessive hair are examples.

The secretions of the endocrine glands influence the health of the body. Any disturbance can affect the health of the body and ultimately the health of the hair.

Hair has three basic shapes. As it grows it assumes the shape, size, and direction of the follicle. Straight hair is generally round. Wavy hair is oval, and curly hair is almost flat.

The average life span of hair is from two to seven years. Factors such as age, sex, heredity, and health have a direct bearing on hair life.

The color of the hair mainly depends on heredity. The cosmetologist must understand the color and pigmentation of the hair to give color services. The cosmetologist must also understand hair texture, porosity, and elasticity.

Melanin or pigment is contained in the cortex of the hair. Graying hair results from the lack of pigment in the cortex. In most cases graying is the natural process of aging. In some instances it can also be caused by illness. In some cases localized graying can occur from an injury.

Hirsutism, or hypertrichosis, means excessive or superfluous hair. It usually occurs on women's faces in unusual amounts. This can be helped by medical or mechanical means. Medically, a reduction in hormones influences the excessive growth of hair; mechanically, electrolysis is performed by inserting a fine needle with an electrical current to kill the hair papilla. This method is done by specially trained electrologists for permanent removal of unwanted hair.

Temporary removal of hair can be accomplished by several means, such as shaving, tweezing, waxing, and depilatories. Training in all areas is important to the welfare and healthy condition of the client's skin.

Texture, porosity, and elasticity of hair are factors the cosmetologist should have full knowledge of. Hair texture refers to the degree of fineness and coarseness. It may vary on different parts of the head. This is due to the diameter or feel of the hair. Diameter refers to the coarseness or thickness of the hair. Fine hair is the finest or smallest in diameter. Wiry hair can be either coarse, medium, or fine. It usually has a hard, glossy finish caused by cuticle scales lying flat against the hair shaft. Porosity is the ability of the hair to absorb moisture regardless of texture. Porosity plays a vital part in successful chemical treatments of hair, for example, hair coloring, permanent weaving. Elasticity is the ability of the hair to return to normal form without breaking. Normal to dry hair can be stretched about one-fifth of its length. Wet hair can be stretched 40–50 percent of its normal length.

Dandruff

Dandruff consists of small white scales that flake off the scalp. The medical term is pityrissis. The causes of dandruff is shedding of the epithelial cells, which instead of falling off individually accumulate on the scalp, falling off in clumps.

Dandruff is usually associated with flaking and sometimes itching. Special medicated shampoos and topical medications are beneficial.

Alopecia

Alopecia is the technical term for any abnormal loss of hair. Contributing factors can be hormonal changes in the body, menopause, ponytails, or braids pulled too tight continually and in some cases following pregnancy.

Alopecia senilis refers to baldness that occurs in old age.

Premature alopecia refers to baldness occurring anytime before middle age. It is usually a slow process starting with receding frontal hairline and loss of hair on the top of the head (vertex). Alopecia areata in its mild form (one or a few patches) usually spontaneously resolves. In a small percentage of cases total scalp alopecia (alopecia totalis) or total body alopecia (alopecia universalis) occurs. Other causes of focal or diffuse hair loss are syphilis, endocrine disorders, cancer and cancer treatment, sudden weight loss, severe illness, and medications.

There are also many unproven treatments currently on the market that claim to stimulate hair growth.

Alopecia areata is baldness in spots or patches. See Figure 11-16. The cause is unknown. Some artificial methods to correct hair loss of the scalp, eyebrows, eyelashes are the following:

Rogaine (minoxidil 2 percent) — Rogaine 2 percent is a topical prescription medication that is somewhat effective for male pattern baldness of the vertex (top or crown of the head). Patients must commit themselves for four months or longer before there is evidence of hair growth. Possible side-effects of Rogaine include irritant and allergic contact dermatitis.

Scalp — wigs, hairpieces, and toupees properly sized and styled can enhance beauty and build self-esteem for premature baldness. New models of ventilated human hair wigs and

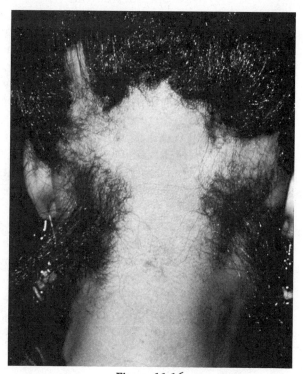

Figure 11-16
Alopecia Areata. Courtesy of Timothy Berger, M.D.

hairpieces can be undetectable and a boost to the ego. More permanent remedies as hair transplantation are becoming very common. Hair plugs are surgically taken from areas that are thick with hair and transplanted to the bald pattern spots. Though this is often a painful method, it is probably the most effective and satisfactory.

Eyelashes — artificial strip lashes or individual lashes can be glued on temporarily with good results.

Eyebrows — can be penciled in with a colored pencil that matches the hair or with pressed colored powder, applied with a brush.

Permanent eyebrows, eye liners and lip liners are making dramatic inroads in the cosmetology industry. This is done by tatooing. Hair lines and color are tatooed into the skin matching the color of the hair. This method should only be done by someone who is artistic and knowledgeable about color mixing and competent in makeup techniques. Once applied, it is permanent. References and credentials prior to having this service performed should be investigated. See the chapter on micropigmentation.

Fungal Infections (Tinea)

Tinea is a medical term for ringworm. Ringworm is caused by a fungus. All forms are contagious. Tinea can be transferred from one person to another. It is carried by scales or hair containing fungus. It usually appears as small, itchy, red, scaly patches. These clients should be referred to a physician for treatment.

Tinea capitis — ringworm of the scalp. This condition is common in children but rare in adults. Symptoms are red patches or spots on the scalp. The patches spread, and the hair becomes brittle and dull. The hair will break leaving a stump.

Animal Parasites

Pediculosis capitis — a highly contagious condition caused by the head louse, infesting the hair of the scalp. As they feed on the scalp itching occurs. Scratching can result in bacterial infection. They can be transmitted from one person to another by contact with combs, brushes, or by touching. Several remedies on the market can treat this. Talk to a pharmacist, and follow manufacturer's instructions.

**Non-Contagious
Disorders of the Hair**

Canities is a term used for gray hair. The cause is loss of natural pigment in the hair. There are two types:

1. Congenital canities exists at or before birth. They occur in albinos and occasionally others.

2. Acquired canities may be due to old age or premature graying in adult life. Other causes of acquired canities may be prolonged illness, heredity, and wasting diseases.

Dyes used to treat premature graying are a common cause of allergic reactions on the scalp, face, or neck. Dye reactions usually do not result in hair breakage or loss. Straighteners, in contrast, cause burns on the scalp if not properly applied. Hair breakage and hair loss are common after burns from hair straighteners.

REVIEW

You should now be familiar with:
- disorders of the skin.
- dermatologic diagnosis.
- topical and systemic drug therapies.
- dermatologic procedures.
- the medical and cosmetic treatment of dermatologic conditions.
- hair and scalp disorders.

12 Camouflage Therapy and the Burn Patient

INTRODUCTION

Jerold Kaplan, M.D.

There is no more severe form of trauma for a human being than a major burn injury. The victim of a major burn sustains both physical and psychological trauma far in excess of other injuries. The initial hospitalization is frequently measured in terms of weeks or months, and the patient may face literally years of reconstruction or rehabilitation. Even with the optimal care provided by modern medicine, the burn patient frequently has permanent physical and psychological scars.

Optimal management of a burn patient in the 1990s and beyond demands a team approach to care. This team includes the physician, nurses, occupational and physical therapists, dietician, psychologist or psychiatrist, social workers, and now, a new and valued member of the team, the camouflage therapist. One of the most common effects of a second-degree burn injury (even though the skin may heal well) is hypo- or hyperpigmentation, or variegation in pigmentation. There is no medical or surgical means of totally correcting this disfiguration, and therefore camouflage therapy offers the only help to the patient of reasonable normalcy. Skin grafts, no matter how skillfully performed, leave some variation in pigmentation or appearance

Dr. Jerold Kaplan is Medical Director of the Burn Center at Alta Bates Hospital in Berkeley, California. In addition, Dr. Kaplan is a consultant in burns for the San Francisco East Bay Emergency Medical Services, Chairman of the Pain Control Committee for the East Bay Cancer Program, and serves on the Advisory Board for the California Health Review. His many professional associations include the American Burn Association, The International Society for Burn Injuries, and the Bay Area Fire Protection Forum.

at the periphery in conjunction with normal skin; camouflage therapy can eliminate or minimize this disfiguration.

Camouflage therapy, like all areas of burn care, requires a skilled and dedicated individual to support both the physical and psychological aspects of rehabilitation. It is necessary to be able to provide the patient with a realistic assessment of what can and what cannot be done, and with the ability to provide a long-term outlook. While there are many makeup preparations that are available "over the counter," only the skillful application of these products can result in a successful outcome. It is here where the instruction and guidance of a skilled camouflage therapist is mandatory.

For patients with severe burn injuries, it is sometimes the unfortunate fact that even with all that modern medicine, surgery, and camouflage therapy has to offer, there will be residual scarring that cannot be completely hidden. In these instances, it is extremely valuable to the patient to have appropriate counseling by someone who is knowledgeable in "making the best of a bad situation." Suggestions as to color and clothing selection, hair styling, the use of a wig or false eyelashes, or a false mustache and beard can be a valuable aspect of the patient's long-term rehabilitation.

POST-BURN PATIENTS

Unlike people who have grown up with congenital lesions, post-burn patients are continually confronted with difficulties associated with the healing of their scars and the repeated surgical efforts to alter them. Even after years of reconstructive surgeries, the burn patient is often left with a distorted physical appearance.

The camouflage therapist is vital in helping the person who has been scarred by a burn rediscover his or her sense of self. The primary goal of the camouflage therapy session is to return to the burn patient a feeling of control over his or her body. To understand how much a person's life is altered by a severe burn injury, we must examine what happens to the patient from the time he or she is burned until the time of entry into camouflage therapy.

SEVERITY OF BURNS

Injury and death from burns have reached epidemic levels in this country during the last quarter-century. Burns can be caused by scalds from hot liquids, fabric ignition, cigarettes, exposure to chemicals, and electrical fires. The extent of the burn is determined two ways: by its depth and by the amount of body surface involved.

The depth is determined by degrees: first, second, or third. See Figure 12-1.

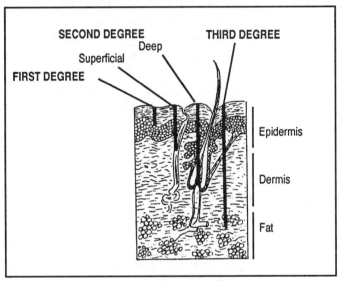

Figure 12-1. Degrees of burns

A *first-degree burn* is considered very minor. A good example would be a sunburn. Treatment for this type of burn is generally pain medication and the patient is released from the hospital after a few hours.

Second-degree burns, or partial-thickness burns, occur when damage extends to the outer dermal layers. These burns are characterized by blisters and typically heal without surgical intervention if they are kept clean and free from infection. If the second-degree burn is deep, all but the appendages of hair follicles and sweat glands are affected. Epithelium (the cells occurring in one or more of the skin layers that cover the entire surface of the body and that line most of the hollow structures within it) are replaced from the hair follicles and sweat glands to restore the surface area. In some instances, skin that has healed from deep second-degree burns may be poor quality tissue that not only restricts movement but also looks unsightly. In such instances, skin grafting may be needed to restore function to the extremity.

Third-degree, or *full-thickness burns,* destroy all the elements of the skin, with damage extending into the subcutaneous fat. Even the nerve endings are destroyed, preventing the patient from experiencing pain. Skin grafts are usually required on third-degree burns for wound coverage. Sometimes a burn is classified as fourth-degree when even more destruction has occurred, extending to the muscle, tendon, and bone. These burns are treated in much the same manner as third-degree burns.

The degree of damage from a burn is also estimated by the amount of body surface area involved. This measurement is always made in relation to the total body area. Although many different ways can be used to obtain this measurement, the most frequently used method is the "Rule of Nines." This is the method used on adults. It divides the body area into nine parts, with each area attributed a multiple of 9 percent. Thus, the head and neck area are considered 9 percent, each arm and hand are another 9 percent, each leg and foot are considered 18 percent, the back and buttocks are 18 percent, the chest and abdomen are 18 percent, and the perineum (the region between the thighs, bounded in the male by the scrotum and anus and in the female by the vulva and anus) is measured as the remaining 1 percent. See Figure 12-2. In the case of smaller burns, the size of the patient's hand is equivalent to 1 percent of the total body surface area.

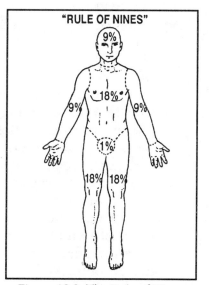

Figure 12-2. The Rule of Nines

The Lund-Broder chart is another method, utilizing a more detailed breakdown of body surface area, taking the victim's age into consideration. It makes allowances for the changing proportions of the body surface from infancy to adulthood. The head of a baby, for example, is considered 20 percent of the total body surface, whereas in an adult the head is considered only 7 percent. See Figure 12-3.

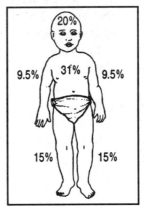

Figure 12-3. The Lund-Broder chart

The American Burn Association, on the other hand, classifies the severity of burns by placing different types of burn injuries in categories of minor, moderate uncomplicated, and major.

Minor burn injuries are second-degree burns that cover less than 15 percent of the total body surface area in adults and less than 10 percent in children if less than 2 percent are third-degree burns. Minor burns do not include burns that affect the facial area, eyes, ears, hands, feet, or perineum. This classification also does not include electrical burns, inhalation injuries, fractures due to burn, or poor-risk patients such as the elderly, very young children, babies, and those already suffering from some other medical condition.

After the burn, patients are transported to a local hospital for the examination of their wounds and then released. The emergency room visit would be followed up with the appropriate medical care until the patient has completely recovered from the injury.

Moderate, uncomplicated burn injuries are second-degree burns of 15 to 25 percent of body surface in adults, and of 10 to 20 percent in children if less than 10 percent are third-degree burns. This classification does not include burns to the face, eyes, ears, feet, or perineum. It also does not include burns from electrical injuries; nor does it include more complex injuries such as fractures, burns that involve the respiratory system, or burn injuries incurred by poor risk patients.

Persons suffering from moderate burns would be transported immediately to a nearby hospital equipped with the appropriate care facilities for uncomplicated burn injuries.

A major burn injury is a second-degree burn involving 25 percent of the total body surface in adults, 20 percent of the body surface in children, all third degree burns encompassing 10 percent body surface or more, all burns involving the face, eyes, ears, hands, feet, and perineum, all inhalation injuries, electrical burns, and complicated burn injuries involving fractures and major trauma. Poor risk patients are also treated as major burn injury patients. Persons with major burn injuries are immediately transferred to a burn unit or a hospital facility where they receive immediate care. These patients are treated for shock and given intravenous fluid therapy. Patients with smoke inhalation are given appropriate respiratory support. Major burn injury rehabilitation includes a series of corrective surgeries for functional movement and for cosmetic purposes.

BURN CARE FACILITIES

There are two types of burn facilities: a burn center and a burn unit. A burn unit is located in a designated area within a hospital. A burn center is more specialized than a burn unit and is equipped to handle all the needs of burn patients. For a burn center to be recognized, it must treat burn patients exclusively. It must have a minimum of six beds and treat at least fifty patients a year. Burn centers have special rehabilitation areas, as well as training and research departments. Larger burn centers also have an intensive care section within the facility. The director of the center is usually a general or plastic surgeon who is board certified, with an additional year of experience in burn patient care. A burn nurse is a bachelor's degree registered nurse with several years of patient care in a burn facility. Physical and occupational therapists must be registered, have a minimum of three months training, or at least six months' burn facility experience. A licensed dietician must also be on staff.

Patients with minor burn injuries can be treated in hospitals that have burn programs. The program is run by a board certified surgeon, generally a physician with at least three months of training in burn-injury care. A burn program will have an ICU and a cardiac unit, and the nurse in charge must be registered and have a minimum of six months' ICU experience, and preferably at least three months' burn nursing training.

Hospital emergency departments can provide treatment for persons with minor burn injuries as well. The emergency room must have a physician on duty who is knowledgeable in cardiopulmonary resuscitation and intravenous fluid technique, and who is experienced in treating minor burn wounds.

Emergency care at the site of the accident is provided by trained medical emergency technicians or firefighters who have completed a certified training course on burns, including chemical and high-voltage burn injuries. These professionals have a basic knowledge of fluid and wound therapy.

BURN CARE

There are five main objectives in treating patients with burns: adequate fluid resuscitation, prevention of bacterial contamination to the wound, nutritional support to assist the body in repairing itself, physical rehabilitation to prevent functional limitations, and psychological rehabilitation to assist the patient in the emotional adjustment phase.

Before a wound can be covered, all non-viable tissue (dead skin) must be removed, leaving the wound healthy. This can be accomplished in one of the following ways: full thickness wound excision — the removal of debris down to fat or muscle; tangential excision — the shaving off of layers of dead tissue on the surface of the skin down to the viable tissue; acute epluchage or piecemeal removal of separating eschar — manual removal of slough from the burned tissue; and enzymatic removal — the use of a topically applied chemical to break down and dissolve dead tissue. The surgeon performing one of these types of excisions must be careful not to destroy healthy tissue by accidentally removing it, which would cause unnecessary scarring and prolong rehabilitation.

The closure of a wound can be delayed because of infection. As long as the wound remains open it stays in the inflammatory stage of healing. Prevention of infection decreases tissue and function loss. The burn wound is cleansed daily, either by immersion in a bath or spraying with a fine mist of water. Either process will remove serum and non-viable tissue and decrease risk of infection.

After the wound has been cleaned down to the living surface (raw, red tissue), or to a capillary bed that is ready to be grafted, the wound is prepared for closure. Minor burns will heal spontaneously, but major wounds will have to be grafted. The goal is to cover the area with healthy tissue (epithelium) that is both functional and esthetically acceptable. Each skin graft contributes to additional scarring because the skin has to be taken from another area of the body, called a donor site.

There are two different types of skin grafts, a full thickness graft (tissue that is taken from the dermis) and a split graft (tissue that is removed from the epidermis and only a portion of the dermis). See Figure 12-4. A careful plan must be developed before a decision is made to graft skin. If only a small wound needs to be closed, skin can be taken from the buttocks. By using this area as the donor site the patient can hide the scar with clothing.

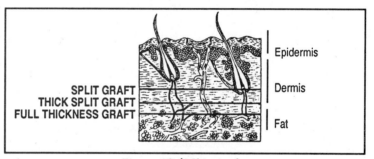

Figure 12-4. Skin grafts

Because full-thickness grafts allow the best pigment match they are generally used on areas such as the face. Facial skin grafts are taken from donor sites in the "blush" areas above the nipple line or the upper thigh. This epithelium provides a better color match than skin taken from the buttocks area. Certain parts of the body must be made functional before esthetic appearance can be considered. The face, especially the eyelids, the neck, the hands, the feet, the axilla (the arm pit), and the popliteal fossa (the depressed area behind the knee), all must be grafted to insure mobility first. Patients who have burns that cover over 50 percent of the body surface will need repeated operations. If a donor site has to be reused for grafting sessions, the possibility of depigmentation will increase as the quality of donor skin decreases. Hypopigmentation is a real concern for dark-skinned patients, whereas hyperpigmentation is a very common problem resulting from skin grafting on Caucasians.

After the skin has been grafted, the area must be immobilized so it can heal. Healing begins when the graft, which is fed by plasma, links up with an ingrowth of capillaries. Motion is discouraged in this area to give the graft time to take. Approximately fourteen days post-graft the burn patient will begin wearing pressure garments. Pressure garments are tight-fitting clothes that prevent collagen from producing hypertrophic (red, raised) scars while the wound is healing. During this recuperation phase, pressure garments are worn constantly for six months to two years, depending on the age of the patient. It is important to note that while wearing these garments patients must not use moisturizers containing mineral oil because it will break down the garment fibers.

Once the pressure garments have been fitted, the patient is ready for physical rehabilitation. Physical and occupational therapists work with the patient to measure and record range of motion. Joints are exercised to increase function. This allows both the patient and the burn team an opportunity to evaluate the healing progress. It is during this stage of recovery that judgment is made concerning the patient's discharge date.

Before the burn patient can leave the hospital, a nutritionist must be consulted to evaluate the patient's caloric intake. Because of the burn injury, the patient's body needs more calories during hospitalization to meet its nutritional requirements. When the patient returns home, however, the intake of calories must be reduced, or weight gain will result. Extra weight can be very harmful because of the potential outgrowth of skin grafts, and the weight would be very difficult to lose. Next the surgeon must determine if the wound has healed enough for the patient to be treated outside the hospital. The doctor's evaluation will be based on three factors: the outcome of a thorough physical examination, the patient's nutritional status and ability to maintain a healthy diet, and the patient's mental attitude.

PATIENT CARE AFTER DISCHARGE

Once a discharge plan for the patient has been approved, a hospital representative is advised. Generally, a social worker makes arrangements with community health or social agencies to provide needed services for a patient to return home. A screening process allows the discharge planner to evaluate the suitability of the patient's home and the family's ability to care for and manage the burn injury after the patient has been released from the hospital.

The role of the vocational rehabilitation counselor or the medical social worker is to design a follow-up schedule for the patient. Appointments are made, and a plan is devised for out-patient medical care. Return visits to the hospital are pre-planned, and an outline of dates is prepared for the patient for any possible future reconstructive surgeries.

Home care health-aides may be suggested. The patient's needs will determine how often a heath-care provider is to visit a patient's home. Aides are trained to assist the burn patient with simple household tasks. When needed they bathe the patient or help the patient to exercise. The health-aide then reports the patient's progress to the program supervisor.

The transition from hospital to home may be a period of great distress for post-burn patients. While at the hospital they were treated in the same manner as the other patients. The hospital staff did not stare at them or make them feel conspicuous because of their looks. Socially they were accepted by other patients, who were their peers. The hospital provided a safe environment — a protective place that sheltered them from the harsh reality of the world. For the first time since the injury the patient feels the stigma attached to people who appear physically different. Acutely aware of the need to cope with this distinction, that patient realizes that his or her differences will always lead to segregation from others who are considered normal by aesthetic standards.

Often, when the patient returns home, he or she finds his or her role in the family altered. Once possibly the head of the household or the strong one in the family, the post-burn patient is now perceived by other family members as a helpless victim in need of constant assistance. Unresolved family conflicts can add tension and cause unnecessary stress for the patient. It is during this transitional stage that the post-burn patient comes to realize that his or her life will never be the same and that he or she will have to adjust to all these new changes. Residual effects of a burn injury can cause many problems for patients and their families, problems for which there is no single solution.

Social workers have the special task of focusing on the patient's needs and difficulties during this readjustment phase. A social worker working in a medical facility usually has a master's degree or a doctorate in social work. The aim of the social worker is to assist the burn patient in re-entering society after the trauma of the burn injury. A social worker assigned to facilitate the post-burn patient's transition will locate a burn support group or supply the patient with a psychotherapist experienced in counseling burn patients, or both.

Psychotherapists are trained professionals (either psychologists or psychiatrists) who have the ability to communicate to the patient a certain empathy that lets the patient know they understand what the patient is feeling. They give advice and psychological support. The therapist is someone the patient can talk with about difficulties during the long rehabilitation process. The main objective of the sessions are to help the patient re-establish his or her values, to regain control over his or her behavior, and to resume a healthy mental attitude.

Burn support groups generally meet once a month and offer patients and their families an opportunity to get to know one another, discuss problems, and share experiences. Camaraderie within the group develops, and for a brief time patients can feel as if they are not alone in experiencing the trauma associated with their burn injuries. The common bond that emerges encourages friendships between these patients that often last a lifetime. Individuals participate and interact with one another by sharing stories of their personal victories and defeats.

The burn support meetings can provide an informative source of reference for cosmeticians who are considering working with burn patients. At these meetings you will have an opportunity to learn from the patients how they feel both physically and emotionally during their recovery period. A word of caution, however: be extremely conservative in dress and manner. I strongly encourage attending all meetings alone. Your presence in the group, especially in the beginning, may not be welcomed by all. Eventually, however, if you remain unobtrusive and sincerely interested in the welfare of the patients and their families, there is a good chance you will be accepted. Do not attempt to recruit camouflage patients by coming to the meetings. Patients who wish to inquire about your services will approach you on their own.

Patients learn to overcome emotional barriers resulting from the burn injury through a strong network of medical professionals. The health-care team provides the patient with information and services, with the hope that the patient will utilize these resources to help him- or herself.

The clinical cosmetician's role is to help the patient become more self confident by helping him or her re-establish personal identity through learning about proper skin care and learning how to camouflage his or her burn scars. This support can make a major difference in the patient's self-perception and may lead to eventual self-acceptance.

SKIN CARE

Post-burn patients experience a variety of skin problems, such as severe xerosis (dryness), itching, inelasticity, redness, ingrown hair, milia, hyper- and hypo-sensitivity, and pigmentary problems. Much of the itching a patient experiences during the post-burn period is due to dryness. A proper skin-care regimen can be designed by the clinical esthetician to alleviate much of this discomfort.

The two most important objectives that the clinical cosmetician will focus on are hydration of the skin to ease tightness and itching and the improvement of circulation to activate the skin glands and increase cell metabolism.

Skin Treatments

Before a skin treatment can be designed to meet the specific needs of the patient, the clinical esthetician must conduct a very thorough examination, by taking an in-depth personal history of the burn injury and evaluating the overall condition of the skin. It is vital that the esthetician listen carefully and that all information obtained during the consultation be recorded.

Clinical Considerations

You will need to know the answers to the following questions.

- How long has it been since the patient's burn injury occurred?
- Is the patient experiencing any sensitivity, itching, soreness, irritation, inflammation, or tightness?
- Will the patient be wearing pressure garments?
- Is the patient already following a prescribed skin care program?
- Is the patient using any topical medication?
- Does the patient have any known allergies to cosmetics?

What to Expect

Skin that has been grafted has a different appearance and feel. It may be much smoother than normal skin because it has fewer pores and hair follicles. There may be areas that are lighter or darker in pigment. The outer edges of the skin grafts may have milia present, or ingrown hairs. Scar tissue will lack elasticity, and there may be redness present. The facial skin may have a tight, mask-like appearance. There also may be signs of surface dryness and flakiness. Never work on a patient's skin if there are any open wounds or if there are any signs of infection or inflammation.

Charting

Below is a sample form for charting information about a patient.

Patient's Name _____

Referring Physician _____

Date _____

Clinical Cosmetician _____

S: (subjective)

History of the patient: What type of burn does the patient have. Date of the burn injury. Areas affected. Reason for visit.

O: (objective)

Medical documentation   Physical description and location of the potential treatment area(s), including clinical photographs or a diagram illustrating the extent of the patient's scarring, including the placement of skin grafts as well as the donor sites from which replacement tissue was taken from.

A: (assessment)

Esthetician's diagnosis   Confirmation of the patient's problem. For example: dryness, scarring, and pigmentation problems. Any problem skin areas that require special attention, and a detailed description of the esthetician's

	proposed therapy should also be included.
P: (prescription)	A detailed outline of the follow-up treatment program is prepared

Example:

1. Hydration of the skin (list patient treatment method, including skin care products).
2. Massage to flatten scar tissue (document patient exercise schedule.)
3. Any scheduled follow-up treatments.

Cleansing

The first step in the care of traumatized skin is cleansing. Cleansing the face twice a day (morning and night) will remove surface oils, bacteria, and cover creams. Anti-bacterial soaps can cause dryness and must be avoided. Commercial soap should also be ruled out as a cleansing agent because it is ineffective as a makeup remover and cannot break down the waxes in most cover creams. Choose instead for the patient a gentle, vegetable oil based cleansing lotion. Teach the patient to massage in the cleanser using moistened hands in an upward circular motion, working up a fingertip lather. This will loosen and soften any makeup, making it easier to remove. Caution the patient to keep the skin adequately lubricated during this process or the skin may dry out, resulting in friction. A soft flannel cloth or cotton square moistened with warm water can be used to remove the cleanser. This procedure can be followed up with a second cleansing using a non-irritating synthetic soap. This type of soap has less alkaline and is specifically formulated for sensitive skin types. It will not interact with hard water and therefore can cut through the greasy film residue that can be left behind after washing the face with a cleanser. A synthetic sponge with a small amount of soap applied directly on it is then immersed in warm water and gently rubbed over the entire facial area. It is very important that the patient use a synthetic sponge rather than a natural sponge because bacteria will not breed as readily in artificial fibers. The sponge should be used with plenty of water to protect the skin from abrasion. Afterward, the patient's face should be rinsed thoroughly with tepid water and blotted dry with a soft towel. If the skin is extremely dry (as is the case with most post-burn patients) omit the second part of this cleansing treatment.

Toning

Cleansing must be followed by toning. The purpose of a toner is to refresh the skin and to remove any surface residue left after cleansing. Bracers, clarifiers, or toners (as they are most commonly called) contain varying proportions of water, alcohol, and solvents. Solvents aid in dissolving dead skin cells and removing surface oils. It is the appearance of these loose stratum corneum cells on the cotton ball that many patients perceive as residual dirt left behind even after cleansing. Astringents contain much stronger solvents than toners. For that reason, astringents must never be used by a post-burn patient because the high alcohol content will cause dryness and irritation to sensitive skin. Have the patient apply the toner by saturating a water-soaked cotton square with the solution and wiping it over the face or by spraying a light mist of toner directly on the face.

Moisturizing

Cleansing and toning must be followed by moisturizing. Skin that has been grafted has very few, if any, pores or glands. Split thickness grafts and their donor sites may scale and remain dry for months after grafting. Often the only oil that is present is from epidermal lipids. Severe dehydration results when the sebaceous and sweat glands are destroyed, as is the case with deep second- and third-degree burns. With the absence of perspiration and natural surface oils, the skin lacks the ability to provide its own protective barrier. If the surface of the skin is not kept pliable, the skin can split or crack, causing a fissure, which will allow bacteria to invade and cause infection.

Moisturizers have two distinct components: humectants that draw outside moisture to the skin and occlusive ingredients that seal in the moisture already present in skin. The best moisturizer for patients with severely dehydrated skin is one that contains both humectant ingredients and occlusive agents.

Humectants such as glycerin, lactic acid, lecithin, and propylene glycol loosen dead skin cells and reduce the flaky appearance of surface dryness. The drier the patient's skin, the more humectants his or her moisturizer should contain. Creams and lotions should cling to the skin but be non-sticky.

A close examination of the patient's skin will reveal what type of lubricant should be recommended. Skin with split-thickness grafts is unable to lubricate itself until the injured sebaceous glands have been restored. As soon as the grafts have healed, patients should use a rich emollient-cream (water in oil) emulsion to prevent tightness and itching. The patient can determine if the moisturizer is rich enough by first doing a hand test. If it is a water-in-oil solution, the patient will feel a warming sensation from the oil as it is rubbed onto the skin.

Full thickness grafts will have a soft, smooth appearance. Patients with this type of graft require less lubrication because the transported tissue has all the working glands and can produce its own oil and moisture. After the graft is intact, the patient can use a light lotion (oil in water emulsion). A moisturizer that is primarily water will produce a cooling effect on the skin as it is applied, caused by the evaporation of water as it is rubbed onto the skin. Moisturizers should be nontoxic, nonirritating, and nonallergenic. Most importantly, the protective cream should contain a preservative with active ingredients that will kill bacteria and protect the cream from a variety of organisms.

Sunscreen

A sunscreen with a sun protection factor of at least 15 should be used over the moisturizer. See Figure 12-5. Tanning on grafted areas can cause permanent hyperpigmentation. Postburn patients are instructed to remain out of the sun for at least six months following the injury. Patients should use a sunscreen that contains preparations such as para-aminobenzoic acid, zinc, or titanium oxide. The patient should put the sunscreen on twenty minutes before exposure to natural light in order to ensure protection from the sun's harmful rays. Sunscreen should be re-applied frequently, even on cloudy or hazy days. In addition, protective clothing should be worn. Hats and sunglasses can be used to shield out direct

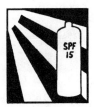

Figure 12-5. Recommended sun protection factor

sunlight and prevent hyperpigmentation. Even the area under the chin should be protected since sun reflects off of water, sand, and snow.

Massage

Massage is one of the most useful methods of physical treatment for post-burn patients. When performed properly, it can help bring oxygen to the blood by activating its distribution and encouraging circulation and cell growth. Firm, even pressure when applied to scar areas can break down fat cells in the subcutaneous layer of the skin and flatten raised scar tissue.

Following the surgery, and with the surgeon's permission, patients should began massaging the scarred areas as soon as the sutures have been removed. At first, some patients may be reluctant to perform the massage techniques because of the sensitivity of the scars, but that should decrease with time.

A non-irritating lubricating cream should always be used and re-applied as necessary. Friction can cause blistering if the skin is not kept properly lubricated. The scar itself, raised areas on the edges of the skin grafts, and the areas underneath the skin where there is hardened tissue should be massaged gently in a circular motion with the balls of the fingers. The time period for each massage session will depend on the healing phase of the burn. See the section on facial massage in this chapter. In the beginning at least ten minutes per session should be allotted to flatten out the edges of the scars and tone out the redness of the skin. A goal of one hour, divided into six massage sessions per day, will help to aid blood circulation, eliminate constriction, and decrease dehydration in the burned area.

Exfoliants

Sometimes milia occurs when oil glands and hair follicles get trapped under the top epidermal layer and above the scar tissue. The use of a mild exfoliant can unroot the dead, dry, flaky, skin cells that lead to further plugging of the pores. See Figure 12-6.

Strong exfoliating granular scrubs or abrasive cleansing pads should not be used on delicate skin tissue because they can cause severe irritation. A natural exfoliant peel (one that contains ingredients such as papaya, an active enzyme, sunflower oil, and a humectant such as honey) will reduce hyperkeratinization without irritating the skin by rubbing.

This treatment can be incorporated into the patient's skin-care regimen once a week to slough off cellular debris. Sterile cotton swabs can also be used to remove dead skin cells by gently rotating them on the face in an upward and downward motion.

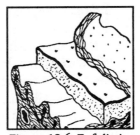

Figure 12-6. Exfoliation

Unwanted Hair Removal

The type of hair on the body and the rate at which it grows is determined largely by genetics, by the hormones produced by the ovaries, and by the adrenal glands. These glands are governed by the pituitary gland. The pituitary gland is the "master" gland and is located at the base of the brain. If a change transpires in the body and any of these three glands become affected, it can cause a change in the production of hair. Sometimes the emotional or physical stress caused by the trauma of a burn injury can activate hormonal changes in the body. Sensitive hair follicles become triggered, resulting in unwanted hair growth. Under normal conditions, hair follicles produce almost invisible hair on the body. In certain follicles, no hair is actually growing, but the follicle's ability to produce hair still exists. If the brain gives the body the wrong signal, instead of producing little or no hair, these follicles could produce thick, coarse, unsightly body hair. Excess hair on the face or body of a patient can also appear on skin tissue that has been replaced by full-thickness skin grafts.

Excessive, superfluous hair can be concealed or temporarily removed by a variety of methods such as chemical depilation, bleaching, waxing, tweezing, or shaving. See Figure 12-7. The choice of the hair removal method will depend on the amount of unwanted hair, its color, texture, location, and the regrowth period. The hair follicles can become inflamed by the use of any of these methods. Trauma to the follicles can either discourage hair growth or encourage it by stimulation. In some cases, the temporary removal of hair

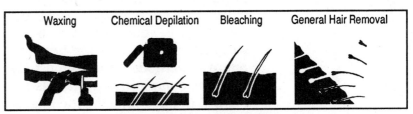

| Waxing | Chemical Depilation | Bleaching | General Hair Removal |

Figure 12-7. Hair removal methods

makes it appear more obvious because shortening it by shaving or cutting makes the hair less flexible and coarser.

Patients with partial-thickness burns may have a problem with ingrown hairs if hair follicles become trapped underneath scar tissue. The constant irritation of the follicles can eventually lead to chronic inflammation. If this occurs, the post-burn patient should be referred to an licensed electrologist for the permanent removal of this hair.

Electrolysis is the only permanent method of hair removal. A needle is inserted into the opening of the hair follicle, and an electrical current destroys the hair at the bottom of the follicle. A galvanic or high-frequency electric current is used. The galvanic treatment is a much slower technique, but there is less regrowth. Electrocoagulation (a modified, high-frequency electric current) is a process that allows more hairs to be removed at one time.

Patients should be discouraged from using home electrolysis devices. A great deal of skill is required to successfully locate the root of the hair and penetrate it enough to cauterize it. Even if the patient has the dexterity to operate such a device, he or she may not have enough knowledge to eliminate the hair properly and could cause a dermal burn. Scarring can also result from the patient improperly inserting the needle into the skin.

The best way to locate a reputable electrologist is through the dermatology department of a local teaching hospital. The safety and effectiveness of the technique will depend primarily on the electrologist's experience. The cosmetician should meet the electrologist at his or her facility before any patients are referred. This will allow you to see where the treatments will be given, to examine the office for cleanliness, and to meet with the electrologist beforehand.

Electrolysis can have a number of disadvantages. It can be a long and tedious process. It can also be uncomfortable for the patient. Treatments usually last half an hour and are scheduled once or twice a week. Because each root must be removed individually, the process can take years to remove excessive hair growth and can be very costly. Electrolysis, therefore, is generally more beneficial for the removal of facial hair. Body areas are best treated with temporary hair removal methods. Patients must also be cautioned that there could be complications, such as areas of hyperpigmentation, the risk of infection, and the possibility of scarring.

Masquing

Weekly skin-care treatments should also include the application of a facial masque. A masque will improve circulation, remove dead skin cells, and restore color tone to the skin. A treatment masque designed for dry skin can also rehydrate skin tissue by forming an occlusive covering over the skin, sealing in moisture and natural oils. See Figure 12-8.

Many different commercial masques are available. Because there is such a large selection, it might be difficult for your patient to know which one is best. A cream masque will not dry out the skin or pull at delicate tissue. A rich treatment masque will soothe and relieve some of the itching caused by surface dryness. The masque should contain simple ingredients that will not cause sensitization.

Instruct the patient to cleanse his or her skin thoroughly before applying the masque to the face and neck (avoiding the delicate eye area). The use of organic facial masques should be discouraged because there is a greater danger of microbiological contamination in cosmetic products that do not contain preservatives. The patient must be instructed to use a spatula and not place fingers into the container. The masque should remain on the skin for ten to twenty minutes. It should be removed with tepid water and followed with a toner and a moisturizer to prevent moisture evaporation.

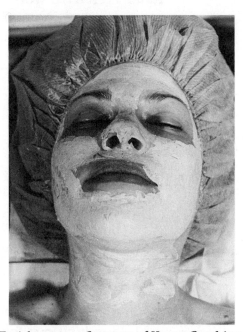

Figure 12-8. Facial masque. *Courtesy of Henry Gambino, Ph.D.,* taken from his book, *Modern Esthetics,* Milady Publishing Company.

Storage   All cosmetic products must be kept free from bacterial contamination. Skin-care products must be protected from damage caused by excessive heat and moisture, and in some cases light. Jars must be sealed after each use and stored in an area that is cool and dry.

Professional Skin Treatments   Occasionally a clinical cosmetician will be called upon to give a facial treatment to a post-burn patient. Such a treatment can be extremely beneficial. Much consideration, however, must be given to the privacy of the patient. These treatments must be conducted in a doctor's office, a hospital, or a separate area of a salon with a private entrance to prevent the patient from being exposed to other clients seeking beauty treatments. The appearance of a post-burn patient can evoke fear and disapproval from other clients, and the patient should be protected from these kinds of reactions.

THE TREATMENT ROOM

If skin-care treatments are to be performed in a doctor's office or a hospital facility such as a burn unit, a special area or treatment room will have to be designated. The basic components of a typical medical facility are the reception room, secretarial work station, physician's office, examining rooms, surgery room(s), utility or supply rooms, and laboratory. Minimal furnishings and equipment can be stored in one of the examining rooms. However, the treatment room should have the following basic furnishings:

1. An examining table
2. A cabinet for storage of gowns, towels, files, and cosmetics
3. A counter with a sink
4. A mounted mirror
5. Two chairs (one for the operator and one for the patient
6. Electrical outlets
7. A magnifying lamp
8. Adequate lighting (preferably a window)
9. A facial steamer
10. A crock pot or a warmer
11. A writing area for documentation
12. An infrared lamp (optional)

MATERIALS NEEDED FOR FACIAL TREATMENT

Patient Charts
- encounter forms
- diagrams (face and body)
- manila folders
- pen

Patient Needs
- face towels
- sheet or blanket
- synthetic sponges
- headband or head drape
- hospital gowns

Cosmetic Agents
- cleansing lotion
- cleansing cream
- massage cream
- skin toner
- moisturizer
  (for dry, normal, and oily skin)
- spray atomizer
- collagen fibre masques
- sample packets of sunscreen
- paraffin wax
- enzyme face peel
- gentle scrubbing grains

Disposables
- sanex
- cotton swabs
- cotton roll
- cotton squares
- table paper
- spatulas
- mineral water
- tissue

Medical Instruments
- comedo extractor
- manicure scissors
- lancets
- tweezers

DOCUMENTING THE PATIENT'S HISTORY

Ask the patient to fill out an information card before the treatment begins. This form should record the patient's vital statistics:

Patient's name: _____

Referred by: _____

Date: _____

Sex: _____

Age: _____

Race: _____
(Caucasian, Black, Hispanic, Asian, other)

Address: _____

Business telephone #: _____

Home telephone #: _____

Current skin care regimen: _____

Allergies: _____

Medication: _____

The date the burn injury occurred: _____

Surgery dates: _____

Many post-burn patients may have never had a facial before, so do not take for granted that they will automatically know what to expect. Make sure the patient understands exactly what is going to be done and why before you begin.

THE ANALYSIS

Facial skin undergoes a variety of changes; many of these same factors should be considered when conducting a skin analysis on a post-burn patient.

ESTHETIC CONSIDERATIONS

- climactic changes
- chronological aging (genetic traits)
- photoaging (sun damage)
- physical and emotional stress
- medications (systemic and topical)
- pre-existing medical conditions
- abnormalities on the skin
- extent of burn scarring
- pigmentation
- ingrown hairs
- milia
- dehydration

PREPARATION FOR THE FACIAL TREATMENT

Prepare the treatment room by setting up all the necessary supplies on a utility table, including cleanser, toner, massage creams, and moisturizers. Cotton wool wipes can be made into compresses by cutting strips of rolled cotton into squares and immersing them in warm water. Place implements such as tweezers, manicure scissors, and comedo extractors in a sterilizer within reach. Turn on the paraffin wax, and start the facial steamer.

THE FACIAL

1. Have the patient prepare for the facial by changing into a gown and removing jewelry.
2. Ask the patient to lie down on the facial chair.
3. Wash your hands. Put gloves on.
4. Place a clean head band or head drape on the patient to protect the hair.
5. Adjust the gown by folding it down to expose the neck and shoulder areas.
6. Cover the patient from the waist down with a sheet or a blanket.

7. Apply warm, wet towels over the patient's face.

8. Remove the cleansing cream from the jar with the spatula, or squeeze the cleansing lotion into your hands and warm it up by blending the cream between your fingers.

9. Apply the cleanser by massaging it into the skin with very light circular motions, working your way up from the patient's shoulders, up the neck, to the chin, along the jaw line, across the cheeks, onto the nose, between the eyes, onto the forehead, and sliding back down to the temples.

10. Remove the cleansing cream with moistened cotton squares.

11. Place a moistened cotton compress over each eye.

12. Thoroughly examine the patient's skin under a magnifying lamp, making special notations of any abnormalities on the skin and the extent of any scarring. All dry areas, milia, ingrown hairs, and skin discoloration must be considered before a treatment method can be established.

13. Prepare a detailed assessment outlining the skin care procedures that you will be performing on the patient during the session.

14. Turn on the facial steamer and adjust it at a distance that feels comfortable to the patient.

15. Place wet, warm towels over the patient's face.

16. After a few minutes (2 to 3) remove the towels. Apply a papaya enzyme face peel. (See the chapter on cancer for a recipe.) Leave the enzyme peel on for five minutes under the steam or the infrared lamp.

17. Turn off the steamer. Use clean, moist, cotton squares or flannel cloth to remove all traces of the peel.

Comedone Extraction Once the skin has been exfoliated it is ready for comedone extractions. Because split-thickness grafts are taken from the dermis horizontally, epithelial structures are present on the underside of the grafts. The growth of the sebaceous glands under the grafts will sometimes lead to multiple small milia. A skin lancet can be used to unroof these epithelial-lined cysts. To open and remove whiteheads that are close to the surface, make a small incision with the point of the lancet directly into the plugged hair follicle. Determine the slant of the pore by assessing the direction of the other hairs in that area. Insert the lancet into the pore opening. Wrap both your index fingers in either cotton or tissue. This will buffer pressure and provide clean contact. Very gingerly, without forcing, gently press down on both sides of the plugged pore. See Figure 12-9. If your attempt is unsuccessful, do not force it.

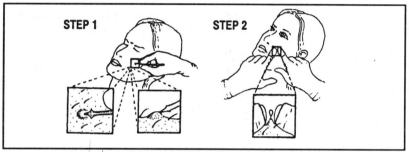

Figure 12-9. Comedone extraction

Facial Massage

After the skin has been cleansed, exfoliated, and the milia has been expressed, the patient is ready for massage. Massage will relax the patient, improve surface dehydration, and help eliminate tissue constriction.

A rich massage cream, one that contains vegetable oils, should first be applied as a lubricant to prevent friction. The lotion should be warmed in the hands before applying it. Only the middle and fourth fingers of each hand should be used. Massage gently yet firmly with even pressure, using only the pads of the fingertips in a tight, circular motion, working from the outer edges of the scars inward. Raised areas and areas where there is hard tissue should be major focal points. To increase circulation, repeat the circular movements starting at the base of the chin and working upward toward the forehead. Massage should not last more than fifteen minutes in one facial session.

Now you are ready to complete the facial treatment with either a collagen fiber masque or an herbal paraffin gauze masque to seal in moisture.

The Collagen Fiber Masque

In 1975 a special form of collagen began to appear in hospitals for the treatment of burns, wounds, and for use in heart surgery. Consisting of sterilized, translucent white sheets, the collagen, when laid over skin that needed to heal, was able to supply the organism with a protein material in the exact location that required it. Scientists discovered that the externally-applied collagen was rapidly taken up by the body and made part of its own protein tissues during the healing process.

Collagen masques consist of a network of fine collagen fibers isolated from bovine collagen under mild conditions. Native soluble collagen is freeze dried onto this network; thus the mask is basically a reproduction of the skin's structure and can be designated a second skin. When moistened, the masque turns into a gel-like material that can easily be molded to the contours of the area being treated. The intimate contact between the masque and the skin forms a barrier that seals in moisture, allowing a more efficient utilization of active substances. See Figure 12-10.

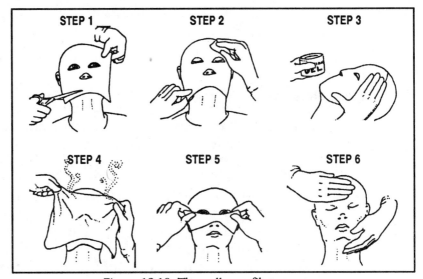

Figure 12-10. The collagen fibre masque

Before applying the masque, aCELLeration GEL (manufactured by Reviva Labs in Haddonfield, N.J.) must be massaged into the skin. This is a pure, clear gel concentrate with minerals that aid the skin in balancing the acid mantle and in retaining the moisture content. The gel contains purified water, hydroxy methylcellulose (a thickener from plants), citric acid (a neutralizer and astringent) that is used to adjust the acid mantle, and both methyl propyl and methyl paraben as preservatives to protect the product from bacterial contamination.

The gel can be applied directly over the massage cream on areas where scarring or severe dryness is evident, utilizing the following procedure:

1. Place the dry sheet of collagen onto the patient's face and neck. The bottom portion of the masque can be cut off and used on the neck area.

2. Starting at the top of the face, using wet cotton pads, moisten the collagen fibre tissue a little at a time, carefully molding it to the skin. The masque has slits cut out for the eyes, nose, and mouth. If the masque needs adjustment this is the time to do it.

3. Apply the aCELLeration GEL again over the masque onto the scarred areas.

4. Place warm, moistened towels over the masque as often as is necessary to retain moisture and promote warm heat during the treatment, or adjust a facial steamer to direct vapor mist toward the masque, making sure the heat and steam from the vaporizer feels comfortable to the patient. The masque should remain on for fifteen minutes.

5. To remove the masque, gently lift up the sheet starting at the neck area. It will not tug or pull on the skin tissue.

6. Once that masque has been completely removed massage in only a sunscreen. The gel and the massage cream should remain on the skin.

Paraffin Herbal Masque

Another type of masque that can be used for dehydrated, sensitive, burned skin is the paraffin herbal masque. Herb extracts such as comfrey, camomile, and peppermint are combined with wax to soothe and refresh the skin. The purpose of the masque is to ensure moisture retention. The warmth from the paraffin relaxes the patient. The wax forms a vacuum over the skin and forces it to perspire. The moisture is then sealed in and becomes trapped under the wax, forcing it back into the stratum corneum layer of the skin. The paraffin masque, like the collagen masque, can be applied directly after the massage. To ensure that the wax will be warm enough for the treatment, the heating pot should be turned on before the facial begins. The wax should be heated to a temperature of approximately 130° Fahrenheit or 54.4° Celsius.

To apply the paraffin herbal face masque:

1. Warm towels should be placed on the patient's face and neck area to retain the heat and prevent the massage cream from drying out.

2. The steam vapor should be directed at the towels to hold in the heat while the first paraffin strip is being prepared. This process should take no more than three minutes.

3. Holding each edge end of the sanex strip, dip the middle of the strip into the thermostatically controlled heating pot.

4. Once the strip has been coated, pull it out slowly, scraping the wax-covered portion along the rim to prevent the wax from dripping.

5. Remove the towels and place a moistened cotton wool square over each eye.

6. Wait a couple of seconds for the wax to harden.

7. Starting at the base of the patient's throat, lay the strip across the neck, working upward.

8. Apply the strips to the face in a mummy-like fashion. Cut or fold a strip to place above the upper lip like a mustache. Leave both nostrils clear for breathing. Continue to apply the strips upward on the cheeks, across the bridge of the nose and around the eye areas. Complete the application with a strip over the forehead area.

9. Continue to build the wax strips up until the neck and face area have been completely covered with four layers of the strips, one application on top of the next. The strips should remain in place and the patient allowed to relax for ten to fifteen minutes under an infrared lamp. When the masque is ready to be removed, peel back the top corners and lift off.

10. Remove the eye pads.

11. Cleanse the skin by removing the massage oil or cream with moistened cotton squares.

12. Follow this procedure with a light spray mist of skin refresher.

13. Apply a light moisturizer and sunscreen.

CAMOUFLAGE THERAPY

Any health-care professional working with disfigured burn patients will encounter special challenges. This is particularly true for the camouflage therapist, whose role is to assist the patient in regaining a sense of physical identity. Ultimately, the goal of camouflage therapy sessions is to help the patient come to terms with visible scarring and to develop self re-definition within the context of the world at large.

The post-burn patient wants to learn how to redefine features, conceal hyperpigmentation, and, if necessary, compensate for hair loss.

Camouflage options must be kept simple so that patients can confidently perform their own treatments without becoming overwhelmed by the cosmetic solution.

The patient's dexterity should be a major consideration in designing a treatment plan. Some post-burn patients, due to their age or medical condition, lack the mobility needed to perform the more technical aspects of camouflage therapy, such as application of eye liner or false eyelashes. For this type of patient, treatment will have to be simplified.

In some instances, the appearance of a burn patient may be so distorted and irregular that there is very little hope for great success cosmetically. A patient with severe scarring should not automatically be considered unsuitable and beyond the aid of camouflage therapy merely because of his or her appearance. It is important for the clinical cosmetician not to bias the outcome of a camouflage therapy session with a negative attitude before attempting to conceal severe burn scars. True professionals must be able to accept the reality that at some point they will be confronted with camouflaging scars that cannot be changed cosmetically or improved upon. To practice the art of clinical cosmetology, the cosmetician must always anticipate this challenge and be prepared. The patient's participation in the therapy is in itself rehabilitation, whether or not the result ultimately produces a cosmetic solution. Therefore, the purpose of the therapy sessions is to engage the burn patient in a problem-solving process, allowing him or her to express needs in a creative environment, which is ultimately a form of catharsis. By using various methods and techniques, many post-burn patients regain control over their physical image and start to view themselves as capable rather than unattractive.

THE ASSESSMENT

Before beginning camouflage treatment, you must first interview the patient to determine which areas you will be working on. The consultation will also give you an opportunity to analyze the patient's physical features, allowing you to assess which methods you will use. Each burn patient is unique. No two patients will have the same problem. Six basic steps will assist you in making a proper assessment of the patient's condition and help you design a suitable camouflage solution:

1. Find out as much as you can about the patient's medical history: for example, any medication the patient is taking, if the patient is under the care of a physician; any known allergies; age; lifestyle, e.g., hobbies, peer groups, etc.

2. Establish the patient's priorities. Discuss any expectations.

3. Study the patient. Use your creative imagination to visualize how you will correct or conceal the patient's scarring.

4. Since most of the scarring that results from burns is three dimensional (not flush with the skin, but raised), there are of course limitations to what can successfully be altered with corrective makeup techniques. Be sure that the patient has a clear understanding of these restrictions in advance, so that expectations for the session are realistic.

5. Design a camouflage approach to the patient's problems. If illustrating your approach would be helpful, do so by sketching out your plan on a face or body diagram.

6. Present your plan to the patient. Ask for the patient's feedback. Listen actively.

7. Set up a reasonable schedule for the treatments that includes a time period within which to accomplish the goals you and the patient have agreed upon. Decide if the patient's needs can be met in one appointment or if you will need to schedule a series of treatment sessions with sufficient time between them for the patient to practice.

CLINICAL CONSIDERATIONS

The healing stage of the scar will determine its shape and color. Burn scar tissue develops as the patient heals and may occur on the sides of the skin grafts or in areas where the grafted skin did not adhere. Pink granulation tissue grows from the exposed tissue and is eventually covered by skin that grows over the wound from the cut edges. When healing finally occurs, the granulation tissue has developed into tough scar tissue.

Unlike surrounding skin, scar tissue has a different color, usually red. Certain grafted areas will appear sallow in color, especially if the new skin has been exposed to the sun. In such instances do not attempt to match the patient's exact skin tone. Instead, apply a thin covering of color corrector first to correct the uneven skin pigment. Color correctors are tinted lotions in non-flesh colors that tone out discoloration and imperfections. When applied sparingly they will lighten discoloration and act as a primer, so that the application of the cover cream will not need to be so thick. The principle is that by neutralizing skin pigment with color correctors skin discoloration is diminished.

SKIN-GRAFT DISCOLORATION	COLOR CORRECTORS
sallow, yellow, skin tone	lavender, mauve, rose
red, ruddy, skin tone	green, aqua, blue
sallow, dark complexions	apricot

The more the facial area is grafted the more mask-like the appearance will be. A thick application of heavy, opaque, cover cream will only compound the problem, making the uneven texture of the skin more apparent. Choose instead a lightweight camouflage makeup, preferably one with more oil to assure a natural look. Remember, post-burn patients suffer from surface dryness, and this type of corrective cover will prevent the skin from looking flaky. The extent of dryness will also determine whether or not you should recommend that the patient set the application with a fixer powder. With severe dryness, it is sometimes better to omit this step because it tends to make the application look cakey and artificial.

The Face

Unlike other areas of the body, a scarred face cannot be disguised with clothing. Facial expressions are a means of communicating our innermost thoughts and feelings to others. When the patient's features become distorted that communication instrument becomes dysfunctional, and the entire transmission system to convey feelings and emotions is altered.

In terms of communication, the eyes and mouth are the two most important features of the face. Our eyes express our thoughts when we speak or when we are spoken to, and our mouths form the words with which we communicate.

Eyebrows Many facially disfigured burn patients have lost their eyebrows. The loss of eyebrows can make the eyes appear distorted.

To replace the eyebrows, you must first determine the proper dimensions. Artificial eyebrows should be placed directly on the brow bone itself, right above the eye socket.

1. Use an eyebrow pencil to measure from the side of the nose up past the inner corner of the eye (the tear duct) to determine where the front of the brow should begin. Place a dot there with the pencil.

2. Next, measure where the arch of the eyebrow should be by resting the eyebrow pencil against the cheek and pointing it straight upward so it passes the outside edge of the iris. Place a dot there with the brow pencil.

3. Angle the pencil so it touches the side of the nostril, measuring at a slant straight past the edge of the eye so that the pencil is touching the end of the brow bone to determine where to finish drawing in the eyebrow. Place a dot there as well.

4. Very lightly, using a very sharp pencil, sketch in the brow. Use small, feather-light strokes in order to avoid a painted-on look. By using more than one eyebrow pencil, you will create a more natural effect. Select the color of the pencil by matching the pencil color to the hair-color. Blondes and redheads should use a blond, auburn, taupe, light brown, or grey eyebrow pencil; brunettes should use medium brown combined with a grey pencil. Patients with dark brown or black hair should use a combination of dark brown and black eyebrow pencils. Black eyebrow pencil should never be used alone unless the patient has very dark black hair; otherwise it will look harsh and unnatural.

Crepe Hair

Crepe hair can also be used to replace eyebrows. Select two colors that compliment the patient's natural hair coloring and intertwine them. Apply medical adhesive with an artist's flat brush directly to the brow bone and attach the crepe hair to the eyebrow area with tweezers. Work with just a few hairs at first, gradually increasing the number until your artificial brow resembles a natural eyebrow. Use manicure scissors to trim away any scraggly hairs. Remember to always measure the eyebrow area first for brow placement. If the eyebrow is placed too high or too low, or made too thin or too heavy, it will appear obvious and will make the patient feel even more self-conscious about his or her physical appearance.

Eyebrow Prosthesis

Eyebrow prostheses can also be used to replace natural eyebrows. Synthetic or real hair is woven into lace and shaped to form eyebrows. You will have to trim the ventilated eyebrow to custom fit the patient. This type of artificial brow can be purchased from a wig maker or theatrical makeup store.

Micropigmentation

Eyebrows can also be replaced by micropigmentation (facial tattooing). Many cosmetic surgeons offer this service. Members of the International Association of Permanent Cosmetic Artists also perform the service. For pigment implantation to be successful, patients must have completed all their reconstructive facial surgery. Use extreme caution when recommending micropigmentation, as it is irreversible. Patients who want to change hair color in the future should be discouraged from using this type of camouflage therapy, or at least sufficiently forewarned of its permanence. Also take into consideration the fact that hair naturally tends to turn gray or white as one ages.

An appropriate hairstyle (such as bangs) can be used as a camouflage tool to conceal missing or sparse eyebrows, and thick-rimmed eyeglasses can also camouflage missing eyebrows.

Eyes

The goal is to redefine the eye area if necessary. How you contour (highlight or shadow) around the patient's eye area will depend upon his or her bone structure and upon any grafting done in that area.

The appropriate position for the eyes is one width of an eye apart. By shading (darkening) the outer edges of the eyes and highlighting the inner corners you can create the illusion that the eyes are further apart. False eyelashes can also be used on the outer corners of the eyes to reinforce the illusion.

To make the eyes appear closer together do exactly the opposite, shade the inner corners of the eyes and highlight the outer edges.

Cover any discoloration around the eye area with a cover cream before attempting to contour. A taupe, blonde, or gray eyebrow pencil can be used as a tool for this procedure, with an artist's flat brush (#4 or a #6) to blend out the edges. Start by lining the crease of the eyelid with the eyebrow pencil; this will define the eyelids (see the chapter on application). Go over the line with the brush to smooth it out until it looks like a thin shadow instead of a definite line.

Do not attempt to camouflage grafted eyelids with the application of brightly colored or frosted eye shadows. Instead apply a flat matte eye shadow that is compatible with the patient's eyes and hair color. Place the shadow discretely near the edges of the eyelids closest to the eyelashes. This will defer attention away from the surrounding eye area and draw it in toward the eyes.

False Eyelashes

False eyelashes can be applied to replace or enhance pre-existing lashes. They should be trimmed by the cosmetician before fitting them onto the patient (see corrective makeup chapter).

The Lips

The lips are the principle facial opening. This fleshy portion of the mouth is the channel through which we speak. When the lips are in motion, particularly when the patient is speaking, much attention is directed toward the mouth. Lip cosmetics such as lipsticks and lip liners can be implemented to redefine and reproportion this very focal facial area.

Lip abnormalities caused by burn injuries can distort the entire face. Altering the shape of the mouth can be tricky. If the sides of the mouth droop, the patient will look angry. If the lips are made too thin and tight, the patient will appear rigid and inflexible. But if the lips are full and have a curve at the sides the patient will appear cheerful and approachable.

The size and the shape of the lips should be in proportion with the rest of the facial features. The mouth should symmetrically balance the lower portion of the face (see corrective makeup chapter). Do not make exaggerated changes in the shape of the lips because this will cause them to appear even more obvious. Bright lipsticks should be avoided because they will draw too much attention to the patient. Recommend instead a lip liner in a subtle shade (terracotta or nutmeg for patients with gold skin tones, burgundy or mauve for patients with a pink cast to their complexions) followed with a clear gloss. The lips should be defined working from the center to the outer corners of the mouth. For male patients, no color should be used at all except a brown eyebrow pencil to redefine the border around the mouth.

Mustaches and Beards

On men the shape of the upper and lower lips, the chin, and the jawline can all be successfully camouflaged with the application of a beard or a mustache. Excellent ready-made beards and mustaches can be purchased at a hair replacement center or at a theatrical supply house (see chapter on cosmetic therapy).

Wigs

Some post-burn patients may also require additional prosthetics such as wigs (see chapter on cancer). During the initial visit, you can determine with the patient if this alternative should be investigated.

Keloid Scarring

Grafted skin lacks elasticity and tends to contract. It is thicker than normal skin. After six to nine months following a burn, scars reach their maturation stage, and then they will fade, soften, and flatten. Sometimes an excess of collagen forms at the site of a healing scar and creates what is called a keloid. The darker the patients' skin color, the more likely a keloid scar is to form. This is the most difficult type of scarring to correct unless it is located in an area where it can be hidden with hair, such as the beard area or the upper lip on a man. Recommend using an artificial mustache or beard to conceal scarring. If this alternative is not appropriate for the patient, then conceal the discoloration first with a cover cream that matches the patient's natural skin tone and then try highlighting the depressed areas on both sides of the scar, contouring the protruding areas in and around the scar. Use an artist's flat brush (#4 or a #6) for this technique.

Areas of the Body

Certain areas, such as the hands and the neck, will be more difficult to conceal because they are subject to constant friction from clothing, which can cause makeup to wear off.

For discoloration on the hands use only a light application of cover cream because the camouflage makeup will come off on anything that the hands rub against. Make sure that a fixer powder is used to set the application.

Have the patient wait a full ten minutes before brushing it off. A fixer spray will act like a hair spray to adhere the corrective cover to the skin. It can be purchased at a theatrical makeup supply store. Caution the patient that under no circumstances is this product to be used on the face.

A cover cream used to conceal discoloration or hyperpigmentation on the neck area may not be the best solution for camouflage. This body area is subjected to constant friction from clothing, which can cause the makeup to rub off. The neck area in contact with clothing, such as blouse or shirt collars, might best be concealed with scarves, jewelry, or high necklines.

REVIEW

You should now be familiar with:

- partial and full-thickness burns.
- the medical care of burn injuries.
- documenting the post-burn patient's medical history.
- esthetic treatments for burn patients.
  - a. skin-care procedures.
  - b. camouflage therapy.

13 Plastic Surgery

Ronald E. Tegtmeier, M.D.

Plastic surgery is designed to correct deformities, primarily in the skin and the structures immediately underlying the skin. The deformities may be caused by congenital birth defects such as cleft lip and palate; trauma such as automobile accidents or burns; cancer, especially cancers that destroy parts of the head and neck or breast cancer (where the plastic surgeon would perform breast reconstruction); various hand deformities such as injuries or arthritis; or cosmetic defects such as a nose that is too large, or the defects that are caused by aging, such as sagging skin.

The term *plastic surgery* comes from the Greek word "plastikos," which means capable of being molded or formed. This is why plastic materials are called plastic, because they can be molded or formed, and plastic surgery is called plastic surgery because it involves molding or reforming various parts of the human body in order to correct the types of deformities mentioned above. Plastic surgery is designed to correct deformities that, if uncorrected, would leave the individual looking or functioning abnormally, such as birth defects, injuries, cancer, or hand deformities. Reconstructive

Ronald E. Tegtmeier, M.D., is a board-certified plastic surgeon. He obtained his premedical education at Dartmouth College and received his M.D. degree from Harvard Medical School. Subsequently, he studied surgery at the University of Colorado and plastic surgery in England, as well as at the University of New Mexico. He has been in private practice in the Denver, Colorado, metropolitan area since 1976. He is the creator and author of a series of relaxation tapes designed to help patients be more comfortable with plastic surgery and enhance their results.

plastic surgery, therefore, is primarily designed to restore normalcy. This surgery may be done on an emergency basis, such as after an automobile accident, it may be done on an elective basis, or it can be scheduled ahead of time if there is no urgent rush to do the surgery.

COSMETIC SURGERY

Cosmetic surgery is undertaken to improve the appearance of what would otherwise be considered a normal portion of the body. For example, if someone sustains a broken nose, repair of the injury would be reconstructive surgery. However, if someone has a large but otherwise normal nose, reduction of the nose to improve the appearance would be considered cosmetic surgery.

THE PLASTIC SURGEON

A plastic surgeon is a doctor who is specially trained to perform plastic surgery. Any doctor who is licensed in any state in the country can perform plastic surgery, regardless of the amount of special training he or she has had. For that reason, it is important to understand the training that different types of physicians have had. Men and women who are licensed to practice as physicians or surgeons in the United States go through four years of premedical training during college, and then either go through medical school and receive an M.D. (Medical Doctor) degree, or go through osteopathy school and receive a D.O. (Doctor of Osteopathy) degree. Today people with these two degrees have almost the same training, with the training for D.O.s having a little more emphasis on manipulation of the spinal column. After receiving the M.D. or D.O. degree, these individuals then study in an internship where they learn their practice specialties. The American Medical Association and the American Board of Medical Specialists have set up a series of board certifications to ensure that individuals who become certified in different specialties have the training required to practice that specialty and have passed a series of examinations to prove that they have the necessary knowledge. The American Board of Plastic Surgery is the only "board" that is certified by the American Medical Association and the American Board of Medical Specialists to provide certification for individuals practicing plastic surgery. In order to be certified by the American Board of Plastic Surgery, a doctor not only must have an M.D. or a D.O. degree, but must also have three to four years of general surgical training, or training in another surgical specialty, followed by two to three years of specific plastic surgery training. The doctor undergoes a series of written and oral examinations documenting his or her knowledge, experience, and proficiency in plastic surgery techniques. Thus, a board-certified plastic surgeon has approximately fourteen years of education after graduating from high school.

Other specialists also perform various types of plastic surgery. For example, some ophthalmologists are trained in plastic surgery of the eye area; and many ear, nose, and throat surgeons are trained in plastic surgery of the nose and facial areas. More and more dermatologists are learning dermatologic plastic surgery in order to treat various types of skin disease and skin cancers. Dermatologists are also now trained in certain areas of cosmetic surgeries, especially chemical peels and dermabrasions.

Surgeons certified by the American Board of Plastic Surgery are trained in both reconstructive and cosmetic surgery. The theory behind this is that the more knowledge one has about reconstructive surgery, the more tools one has to correct cosmetic deformities and the more one has been trained in precise subtleties of cosmetic surgery, the better one can correct reconstructive deformities. Thus these individuals are often referred to as plastic and reconstructive surgeons. Some plastic surgeons specialize in cosmetic surgery only. These individuals may have originally trained as plastic and reconstructive surgeons, or they may have trained initially in one of the other specialties, but their emphasis is in cosmetic surgery.

THE OPERATING ROOM

While some plastic surgery is performed on an emergency basis in the emergency room, most plastic surgery is performed in the operating room. See Figure 13-1. The operating room is special in two ways: It is supplied with all the equipment needed for surgery, as well as for various types of anesthesia; and it is a clean environment. The equipment includes cardiac monitors as well as medications that would be needed to treat any type of allergic reactions or other emergencies such as shock or heart problems. There is a very remote chance of any of these occurring, since, in most cases, plastic surgery is performed on healthy patients who do not have other major medical problems. Nevertheless, every safety precaution is taken to assure the safety of the patients. The room itself is cleaned on a regular basis to minimize the bacteria, viruses, and fungi that could cause infections. The area where the operation itself takes place and the area immediately surrounding it are known as the sterile field. Everything in this field that comes in contact with the incision is sterile, including the sheets, the instruments, and the gloves and gowns of the surgeon and assistants. These may be sterilized either by autoclave (which is a high-pressure steam sterilizer) or by gas sterilization, in which items are exposed to ethyl oxide in a special container. Either of these methods kills all germs. Everyone in the operating room also wears a clean surgical scrub suit and mask to minimize the possibility of any germs passing from the mouth, nose, or other parts of the body into the room.

1. Intravenous fluid for transmission
2. Clocks
3. X-ray screen
4. Surgeon
5. Assistant
6. Tray of instruments
7. Antistatic table cushion
8. Operating table
9. Padded patient support
10. Pedal for raising table
11. Spare gas cyclinder
12. Movable anesthetic apparatus
13. Anesthetic gas flow rate monitor
14. Patient pulse and cardiograph monitor
15. Piped anesthetic gases
16. Operating room technician
17. Anesthesiologist
18. Shadowless operating lamp

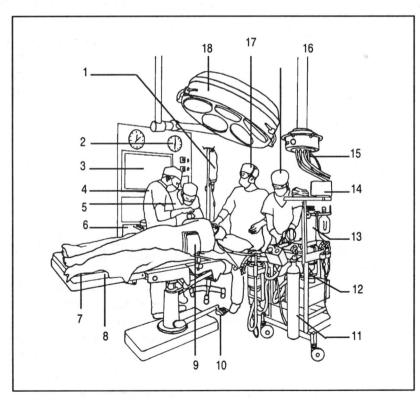

Figure 13-1. An operating room

During an operation, the patient lies on the operating table in the center of the room, covered by sterile sheets, with only the area of the operation exposed. The area may be discolored brownish or yellowish due to the antiseptic used to sterilize the skin. The surgeon and assistant, or assistants, stand close to the table wearing sterile gloves and gowns with masks and caps to prevent hair from falling into the sterile field. The scrub nurse, who is the primary nurse at the operating table, has a small stand, usually called a Mayo stand, upon which he or she places the instruments that are being used at the time so that they are conveniently close to the incision. The scrub nurse also has a sterile back table where other supplies and instruments that may be needed later during the operation are kept. It is important that all other people stay away from the sterile area so as not to touch and contaminate anything. Usually there is a circulating nurse who does not have on sterile gloves or gown. That nurse's job is to provide sutures or other needed equipment that may be outside of the room, or in cabinets inside the room but outside the sterile area. At the head of the table is usually the anesthesiologist (a physician who specializes in anesthesia) or the nurse anesthetist (who also specializes in anesthesia). The job of these specialists is to monitor the patient and regulate the anesthetic. Close to them is the machine that is used to administer anesthesia and that contains all the necessary equipment in case of an emergency. Overhead is a special operating room light that provides optimal lighting near the incision.

EQUIPMENT USED IN PLASTIC SURGERY

Instruments commonly used in plastic surgery (see Figure 13-2) include:

Scalpel — A surgical knife. Most modern scalpels have disposable blades so that a new blade can be placed on the handle any time the old blade becomes dull. This is done at the beginning of every operation and often a number of times during the operation. The scalpel is used not only for making the incision but also for carving cartilage, dissecting one tuft of tissue from another, or precisely cutting any tissues.

Dissecting scissors — A dissecting scissors is generally blunt at the tip and is used in dissecting or separating tissues; for example, separating skin from the underlying fatty tissue or muscle so that the skin can be moved like a flap, or so that it can be tightened, as in a face lift. It is also used to uncover nerves and tendons so that they can be repaired.

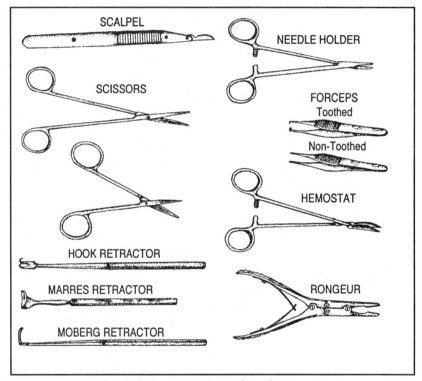

Figure 13-2. Instruments used in plastic surgery

Sharp cutting scissors — Used to trim the skin and sharply cut tissues.

Retractors — Various types of retractors are used to hold the skin away from other structures so that they can be exposed and worked upon. Retractors can also hold the skin away from underlying muscles and fatty tissue so that the surgeon can operate on the underlying tissues. Small, long retractors can be used to hold the skin of the nose away from the underlying cartilage and bone so that the underlying bone and cartilage can be sculpted during a rhinoplasty.

Hemostats — Hemostats are clamps used to close blood vessels so that they do not bleed. The blood vessels can then be tied with sutures or electrocoagulated (treated with an electrical current so they will not bleed), after which the clamp is removed.

Forceps — Forceps, which are similar to tweezers, are used to hold tissue so that it can be cut or sutured.

Needle holders — Used to hold the needle when it is attached to the end of a suture, so that the suture can be more accurately and easily placed in various tissues or in the skin to close an incision.

4 x 4s — Gauze pads four-inches-by-four-inches, commonly referred to as "sponges." These are used to soak up or wipe away any blood or other fluid that make it difficult to see the area that the surgeon is operating upon.

Sculpting instruments — Special instruments somewhat like rasps, chisels, or small scoops (called curettes) or rongeurs. Rongeurs are biting instruments used to bite away bone or cartilage in order to sculpt and reshape the framework of the nose or various portions of the facial skeleton. These can also be used to work on the bones of the hand to correct deformed bones.

Sutures — Various types of sutures are used to approximate tissue or close incisions. There are two basic types of sutures. Non-absorbable sutures may be made of silk, nylon, or synthetic (plastic polypropylene), which is similar to fishline. These sutures are commonly used in the skin. They do have to be removed after the initial healing has taken place (usually between three and seven days) but leave less scarring. The other type of suture is the absorbable variety. These sutures can occasionally be used in the skin behind the hairline or in other areas where it does not matter if there is a little more scarring, but are more commonly used underneath the skin to keep an incision closed after non-absorbable sutures have been removed from the skin itself. These sutures will dissolve generally over a period of one to four months.

IMPLANTS

Even though plastic surgery is not directly related to the use of plastic materials, plastic materials are commonly used in plastic surgery in the form of implants. Each year nearly 200,000 implants are surgically placed. The most common is the breast implant. Surgical implants are used to enlarge the chin contour or to fill in defects in the skull. Penile implants have been used to help impotent men. Implants can also be used as artificial joints in the hand and other areas. Most of these implants are made out of silicone. Silicone has been used in over two million patients over the last thirty years and has proven to be relatively safe. It is well-tolerated and has never been rejected in the way a kidney or heart transplant might be rejected. The site around an implant may become infected, and the implant may have to be removed while the infection is treated, but then can usually be replaced. If this were to happen, however, it would usually happen during the early healing phases after surgery. Infection is seldom a problem after initial healing has taken place. Once an implant is put in position, the body forms a layer of scar tissue around it holding the implant securely in place. Within a few weeks, generally, patients report that the implant feels like it is part of them.

MACHINES

The most common machine used in plastic surgery is the electrocautery machine. This machine generates a special type of electrical current and transfers it to the tip of a hand piece where it is used to coagulate blood vessels to stop them from bleeding. The current can be modified slightly so that it produces what is called a cutting current. With a cutting current, the tip of the handpiece can be used like a scalpel to cut tissues, and at the same time it coagulates some of the smaller blood vessels that it encounters.

The suction-assisted lipectomy aspirator is a suction machine that generates high-powered suction necessary to perform suction-assisted lipectomy procedures. A plastic suction tube is run from the aspirator to the suction cannulas, or tips. These tips are introduced through small incisions into various parts of the fatty layer of the body to remove parts of the fat and improve body contour.

A laser generates a very intense light of one limited frequency. Ordinary light bulbs generate all colors of the rainbow and therefore appear mostly white, but lasers produce only very discrete colors. The Argon laser produces a blue-green color and is commonly used to treat blood vessels or lesions such as hemangiomas. The CO_2 laser generates a color that is outside the visual spectrum and hence cannot be seen by the naked eye. This laser is used like a scalpel to cut deep tissue or to vaporize tissue on the surface, and hence destroy skin lesions or remove unwanted extra growths. Laser light is very high frequency, very precisely controlled and focused, and it can be used very accurately. (See dermatology chapter — laser surgery/vascular lesions.)

MEDICATIONS

Several medications are commonly used by plastic surgeons. Retin-A is used to treat keratosis or wrinkling; Efudex (5-FU) is used to treat skin damage or keratosis; hydroquinone is used to bleach brown areas; and cortisone is used to treat keloids or hypertrophic scarring. Chemical peel solutions most commonly contain active ingredients of phenol or trichloracetic acid. Often used are various types of pain medication, which are usually narcotics, most commonly morphine and Demerol, as well as various types of codeine or synthetic codeines. Also used are lesser pain medicines such as Darvon and Tylenol.

Antibiotics are used to treat infections in wounds or boils. Commonly, antibiotics are also used prophylactically; that is, they are given to patients prior to an operation, before any infection develops, to minimize the possibility of developing infections.

PROCEDURES

Retin-A

Retin-A was originally developed to treat acne and was released for that purpose approximately twenty years ago. People began to observe that those using Retin-A to treat acne did not wrinkle as much as those who were not using Retin-A. This observation led to research that has confirmed that Retin-A does, in fact, reduce wrinkling. Retin-A is beneficial for the skin in many ways. First, it appears to rejuvenate the cells. The cells of a person who has aged skin are very irregular, are often small, and the numbers of cells in each layer of skin are decreased. If this aged skin is treated with Retin-A, the cells appear to be fuller, more uniform, and the skin has more cells in each layer, much like the skin cells of a young person. Retin-A also increases the number of blood vessels that bring nourishment to the skin, which incidentally can increase its youthful pink glow. Further, Retin-A seems to increase the amount of collagen in the skin. All of these changes do help to make the skin appear more youthful. Furthermore, as the cells improve in quality, the older, outer layer of cells are shed more easily. Cells in the skin are constantly changing, with new cells being produced in the deep layers and the older, outer cells being shed. With Retin-A the outer layers of skin are shed more easily, thereby allowing the more youthful-appearing cells underneath to come into view.

In the process of shedding the older, outer layers of cells, some of the damaged cells are also shed. This is beneficial for getting rid of sun-damaged skin cells, and, in fact, some areas of premalignant actinic keratosis can be eliminated over several months with the use of Retin-A. This means Retin-A may be beneficial in actually reducing the possibility of an individual developing skin cancer.

Further, Retin-A seems to help reduce excess pigmentation, and so can help to make liver spots less obvious.

Retin-A Therapy

Retin-A, in most cases, is used every night. An individual is instructed to cleanse the skin thoroughly, and the esthetician can be most helpful in determining which product is going to best cleanse the skin. The individual should then allow the skin to dry completely before applying the Retin-A just before bedtime. Retin-A is most effective if other products are not applied at the same time. However, it is very important that the person using Retin-A also be guided in optimal skin care in order to get the maximum benefit from the Retin-A, and other skin care products can be used during the day. There are several strengths of Retin-A, as well as several preparations. The most commonly used is the cream; however, gel may be more effective in people with oily skin. Most people need to use the Retin-A every night for the first year, and it does take a number of months to see maximum improvement, but some people may see increased improvement up to a year. At about a year, most people have obtained maximum benefit, and often at that point switching to using Retin-A two or three times a week rather than nightly will usually be sufficient to maintain the benefit. If at any time the individual stops using Retin-A altogether, the improvement will disappear, and, within a few months, the skin will return to the same condition that it would have been in had Retin-A never been used. The skin will not be worse after using Retin-A, but it will not be any better. Therefore, Retin-A probably does not actually prevent aging as much as it does decrease the amount of aging present at a given time. For this reason, using Retin-A during the early years when the skin is naturally youthful probably will not help an individual look any better when he or she reaches thirty or forty than waiting until thirty or forty to begin using it.

Some side effects are associated with the use of Retin-A. Most people, when they first begin using Retin-A, will notice some redness and what they may view as dryness. If there is much redness or flakiness, it may be useful to skip a few nights and use the Retin-A only every other night or every third night at first, or to cut down to a lower dose until the skin gets used to it. Most people then, over the months, as the skin gets used to the Retin-A, can go back to using it every night, and/or move up to a higher dose to get a more pronounced improvement. The flakiness really is the physical evidence that the outer layer of skin is shedding more easily; however, this does appear to be dryness, and optimal skin care can help to minimize the amount of flakiness.

Another factor, which is very important, is sun sensitivity. Retin-A does seem to sensitize the skin to the sun, and if an individual gets too much sun while using Retin-A, it can actually increase wrinkling, risk the potential of sun damage, and risk keratosis and skin cancer. Therefore, we recommend to our patients that they not tan the areas where they are using Retin-A, though if they wish to they can tan other areas. The esthetician's advice in helping these patients select proper sun protective products can be very helpful. Some people have literally used Retin-A on almost all areas of the body; however, the face and neck are the most commonly treated areas, with the hands and arms being the second most commonly treated. Certain areas are more sensitive to Retin-A, so smaller amounts need to be used, or need to be used less frequently. The eyelids are a sensitive area, and it is extremely important that Retin-A not be allowed to get into the eye if the eyelid is going to be treated. There have been some reports of Retin-A causing corneal ulceration. The areas around the nose and neck are also sensitive, and Retin-A should be used with caution on these areas. It should not be used on the red vermilion of the lip. Another area that is more sensitive in some people is the crease at the wrist and at the elbow and, in general, areas that sweat more profusely.

Chemical Peel

The chemical peel is designed to treat fine wrinkling. Various types of chemical peels have varying degrees of effectiveness, and some of the newer treatment programs combine chemical peel with other products such as Retin-A to achieve the maximum benefit. Retin-A seems to help the skin heal more quickly at the time of a chemical peel. The most common forms of chemical peel are phenolic and trichloroacetic.

Basically the chemical peel performs three functions. It affects the outer layer of skin in such a way that the older, outer layer of skin peels off. While this peeling is taking place, over about ten days, the body forms a new, fresh, outer layer of skin. This fresh layer of skin has fewer wrinkles, and generally a nicer texture. The chemical peel also penetrates deep into the skin and tightens the collagen. This is why the chemical peel is so effective in treating wrinkling, and why the improvement is very long-lasting for most people. Many people will still notice some improvement from the chemical peel twenty or more years after the initial peel. Although the aging process does continue, some of the improvement is essentially permanent. The third effect of the chemical peel is to decrease skin pigmentation, and so it is most effective for decreasing liver spots. Because it does remove natural pigmentation, the areas treated with chemical peel may become too light to effectively match other areas of skin, and so it is often not appropriate to use in a darker-skinned individual. The chemical peel also will remove natural freckling in many individuals, and so this can be a benefit for those wishing to be rid of freckles, but may mean that it is not appropriate for individuals who wish to retain their freckling. The most common chemical peel, the phenol chemical peel, is applied under general anesthetic in most cases, although small areas can be treated without such anesthetic. It is important to apply the solution slowly because part of the solution is, in fact, absorbed into the blood stream and if it is applied too rapidly can cause changes in the heart rhythm and potentially even death. This is the why an individual who is going to have a chemical peel should have a complete physical examination beforehand and also be observed closely with cardiac monitor during the procedure. With appropriate monitoring, if minor changes in heart rate do occur, these can be easily treated. The phenol solution used in the chemical peel is a combination of ingredients, usually including phenol, croton oil, saline, and a product to decrease surface tension. After the solution is applied to the skin, the physician may elect to apply tapes to the area to deepen the effect of the peel. This would usually not be done; however, in the eyelid areas or in areas with thin or delicate skin it would.

During the peeling process, as the peeling is taking place, crustiness forms on the treated area. This is usually present for approximately ten days, during which very often moisturizing agents are used to keep it more comfortable and to help it separate more easily when it is ready to separate. As the new outer layer of skin develops, the crustiness comes off easily. The newer outer layer of skin, however, is usually somewhat pink for up to three or four months, and while it is pink it is sensitive to the sun. An esthetician can be very helpful during this time, not only in advising patients in camouflage therapy so that they can resume normal activity more quickly, but also in helping the patient select products to provide appropriate sun protection. This can sometimes be accomplished with products that combine cover-up and sunscreen in the same product. Potential complications involve: (1) the possibility of heart rhythm changes during the application if it is done inappropriately or too rapidly; (2) the permanent darkening of certain areas of the skin, especially if the patient gets too much sun during healing phases. This is the reason that sun protection is so important. This risk is minimal, however, with appropriate sun protection and avoidance of sun exposure. Occasionally, a patient will develop some milia, or whiteheads. Good skin care, occasionally with topical antibiotic solution, may be helpful in treating this. But occasionally these will need to be opened using a fine instrument. Scarring and other complications are very unusual following an appropriately-performed chemical peel, but have occasionally been noted in chemical peels performed by individuals who have not had appropriate training in doing this form of treatment.

The trichloroacetic peel generally is a less involved treatment with a shorter recovery period; however, it is also not as deep or as effective, and so it needs to be repeated at regular intervals in order to maintain the same amount of improvement. There also appears to be less potential change in the coloration with the trichloracetic chemical peel.

Overall, the chemical peel appears to be about two to three times as effective as Retin-A in dealing with fine wrinkles, and while the improvement with the Retin-A lasts only as long as the Retin-A is used, the improvement with the chemical peel appears to be essentially permanent. So while the initial treatment and recovery period with chemical peel are more involved, the amount of improvement is greater, the length of time that it lasts is significantly longer, and the improvement in the brown spots is significantly greater.

Dermabrasion

Dermabrasion can have some of the same advantages as a chemical peel. Dermabrasion is a physical sanding process, not a chemical treatment, and is more effective in treating irregularities in the outer layers of skin. Therefore, it is more appropriate and advantageous in treating scars, especially acne scars, which will be discussed later. Dermabrasion can sometimes be used in treating wrinkles, especially around the mouth, and has the advantage of less change in skin coloration to chemical peel. Dermabrasion does not affect the deeper layers of skin as well as a chemical peel, and hence does not improve the collagen, and does not last as long. It should be noted that with certain types of skin, particularly that of people of Asian decent, there is a high risk of pigment changes and darkening following chemical peel, and so chemical peel should seldom, if ever, be used on a person of Oriental extraction, whereas dermabrasion has less risk for this type of skin and may be used cautiously in these individuals.

Collagen Injections

Collagen injections are used to fill indented scars and wrinkles. The collagen used is a highly purified beef collagen. The beef collagen is modified so it is essentially identical to human collagen. Collagen injections are therefore tolerated well by 97–98 percent of individuals. Prior to using collagen treatments on the facial area, skin testing is performed in order to determine whether the patient will have any unusual reactions to it. Most patients who do not react to the skin testing on the arm will tolerate collagen well, although occasionally a patient does have a little firmness and redness in the area where the collagen is injected. Out of the hundreds of thousands of patients who have been treated, there have been a couple of reports of people who have developed some sensitivity to beef products as a result of collagen injections. For most people, collagen injection treatments are an outpatient procedure performed in the physician's office. Most patients are able to go about their normal activity the next day, if not the same evening after the injection, since there is very little black-and-blue bruising. There are many benefits to collagen injections. They can be useful in treating deep lines, smile lines, and frown lines. They can also be helpful sometimes in treating finer lines, especially in the crow's feet area. The skin of the eyelid is too thin to hold collagen well, and the treatment should be avoided there. Collagen can also be used to treat fine lines around the lips and to create more fullness in the lips.

The use of collagen does have many advantages. A note should be made that injectable collagen, which we are discussing, serves a totally different purpose than the collagen that is found in cosmetics. Cosmetics are not able to penetrate down to the deeper layers where the collagen is injected, and so the collagen in cosmetics has its primary effect at the epidermis, or outer layers, of skin, and is beneficial in helping retain moisture in these areas. Injectable collagen is used as a filling material, especially for lines, but can also be used in indented scars, such as acne scars. Collagen is relatively easy to use, with no recovery period for most people. The major disadvantage of collagen is that it is temporary, and most individuals need to have additional treatments two to three times a year in order to maintain the benefit. There is some concern that collagen may cause autoimmune disease, but so far there has not been any proof that this does happen.

Fat Injections A newer method of treating deeper lines is with fat injections. Fat cells have been transplanted or transferred for decades. Newer techniques involve the injection of these fat cells into areas such as the frown lines or smile lines. Fat is removed from an area, such as the abdomen, utilizing suction-assisted lipectomy techniques or aspiration with a needle under local anesthetic. This fat is then prepared for reinjection. Various techniques may be used to prepare it, including rinsing the fat in balanced physiologic solution, sometimes adding insulin to stimulate the fat cells, and possibly reducing the larger masses of fat cells to smaller, more uniform size, so that the injection will be more uniform. An advantage of fat injections is that some of the attachments from the skin to the deep muscles in these areas can be released. Muscle activity in these areas where the skin is more closely attached to the muscle is partially responsible for the formation of deep lines, and so releasing some of these attachments can reduce the effect of the muscle on the deep lines, allowing the skin to be less adherent, and allowing the space between the skin and the muscle to be filled more effectively with the fatty tissue. Fat injection is more complex than collagen injection and it is generally done under sterile conditions. It is usually done under anesthetic, either local or general. The procedure involves more recovery time since there are usually black-and-blue areas and some swelling, which lasts for a week or perhaps two. On the other hand, fat treatment provides more permanent improvement. Some of the transferred fat cells may last for the rest of the life of the individual. On the average, perhaps 50 percent of the volume of a fat injection will be absorbed. Generally, therefore, at the time of treatment, the area is slightly overfilled to allow for some of this absorption. The individual, as the absorption and aging process continues, may require additional fat injections. Fat injections are appropriate for the larger, deeper lines and can be used to fill in contours, for example, to produce fuller lips.

Collagen and Fat Injections

Generally, collagen injection involves essentially no recovery period, so skin care can continue as usual. Following fat injections, it may be useful to the patient to have some instruction in camouflage make-up to cover black-and-blue areas, and massage may help to decrease swelling and help the fat injections blend in more smoothly and quickly.

TREATMENT OF COLOR DEFORMITIES

Certain individuals are born with birth marks, like red hemangiomas or brown nevi, and these are treated in different manners. Raised, red, strawberry hemangioma very often fade naturally during the first few years of life, and so often no specific treatment is needed. If they do persist or enlarge, they may require treatment by laser or by excision, and occasionally residual scarring is treated either with cover-up cosmetics or with scar revision. Flat, or portwine hemangiomas, usually will not fade on their own, but can often be satisfactorily treated with camouflage makeup. However, if they are extensive, or in prominent areas, laser treatment can significantly reduce redness and minimize the difficulties in covering them with makeup.

Laser Treatments of Skin Deformities

The Argon laser, or the tunable dye laser, produces a color in the blue-green spectrum. Since blue-green is absorbed by red more readily than by other colors, when a blue-green Argon laser is aimed at the hemangioma the majority of the energy from the Argon laser is absorbed by the red birthmark. A red birthmark is the result of an increase in newer blood vessels in the birthmark area. The laser energy is literally absorbed by the red blood vessels, and this causes the vessels to shrivel and disappear. A full treatment may involve several sessions, depending on the size and location of the hemangioma. The tunable dye laser is usually more successful in younger children, when the birthmark is often a brighter red color. The Argon laser can be used in adults, where the birthmark tends to be more of a purplish color. Generally it is not possible to totally eliminate the birthmark, but usually the area can be made to appear much more normal and thereafter fairly easily covered with camouflage makeup. After a treatment session, there usually is a fair amount of crustiness in the area treated by laser. It may take several weeks for this to totally clear, often leaving a natural pink color due to new blood vessels which are helping with healing. As the months pass, these vessels will no longer be needed and they will fade, leaving the area a more natural, although not totally normal, color. These treatments can be done often with local anesthetic, although younger children may need a general anesthetic so they don't move. In most cases the procedure can usually be done on an outpatient basis.

Surgical Treatment of Skin Deformities

Brown birthmarks are most commonly excised. Usually the excision is small enough so that the good skin on either side can be brought together, leaving a thin scar. Occasionally, if the birthmark is large, it may be necessary to use a skin expansion technique. This is a technique using a silicone implant positioned under the normal skin next to the birthmark. Each week additional saline or salt water solution is injected into the implant, expanding it and stretching the skin. After the skin has been stretched adequately, the birth-mark is removed and replaced with the expanded skin. If the birthmark is very extensive, grafting may be necessary. The skin grafts are never totally normal in appearance, and there usually is scarring. If there is infection or bleeding under the skin graft, the graft may not survive and then has to be repeated. If the brown birthmark is close to the surface, occasionally it can be treated with dermabrasion or with a carbon dioxide laser.

Moles or skin cancers usually can be excised directly with local anesthetic when they are small, and the good skin is brought together with sutures. Generally planning the incision such that it falls within a natural facial line allows it to heal in an inconspicuous manner. Incisions are red early on because of the new blood vessels that help with the healing. It may take a number of months for this redness to fade; generally, the healing process takes a full year. Early on, camouflage makeup may be helpful in covering the redness.

Medical Treatment of Skin Deformities

Certain aging spots, so called liver spots, can be treated with Retin-A. Aging spots that are darker may benefit more by using a combination of Retin-A and 5 percent hydroquinine, a bleaching agent.

Another area of unsatisfactory color that can be benefited through plastic surgery is dark coloration in the lower eyelids. The skin of the lower eyelid is naturally a different color than the skin of other areas of the face, but in some people there may be a hereditary darkness in the lower eyelids. This darkness can be most effectively treated with a chemical peel. Allergies may also be an important factor in darkening of the lower eyelids. Sometimes treating the allergies will help to lighten the lower eyelids. Darkness in the lower eyelids may be caused by increased shadowing from loose skin, wrinkling, and bags. The lower eyelid lift is most effective in helping people who have this problem. Finally, with age, many people develop small, dilated blood vessels known as spider hemangiomata. These can sometimes be treated with electrocoagulation, a technique of coagulating these blood vessels with a small electrical current. However, better results are obtained by treating these with an Argon or tunable dye laser with less effect on the surrounding overlying skin.

FACE LIFT (RHYDIDECTOMY)

The face-lift (rhydidectomy) reverses sagging in the cheek and neck areas, reduces jowls and fullness of the neck, reduces smile lines, and improves the jaw and neck line. Today, in most cases, this is accomplished by not only tightening the skin in the jaw and neck region, but also tightening the muscles underneath and sculpting the fatty tissue. The incision that is used starts approximately an inch behind the hairline in the temporal region, passes in front of the ear, and then behind the ear lobe and back into the hairline again behind the ear for a couple of inches, and there is often an incision under the chin. See Figure 13-3. The portion of the incision behind the hairline can usually be easily camouflaged by an appropriate hairstyle, even fairly early on. There may always be a small area along the incision where there is decreased hair, and generally this is easily covered by appropriate styles. Most people can, in fact, wear almost any style they wish to wear. The incision in front of the ear can either be placed about a quarter of an inch in front of the ear or be placed into the front part of the ear canal. If the incision has been placed a quarter of an inch in front of the ear, some patients will benefit from use of a camouflage makeup to help blend in this incision area.

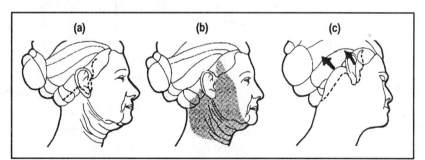

Figure 13-3. A face lift

Occasionally, a mini-lift is performed. Here the skin is only freed up approximately an inch or two around the ear. The mini-lift helps improve the mid-cheek and neck near the ear, but produces virtually no improvement in the mid neck area under the chin. This operation produces some numbness in the cheek and neck. It is important for every professional dealing with someone after a face-lift to be aware of this numbness and minimize the use of heat or cold in these areas.

Generally, sutures in the incisions are removed from the front of the ear and the chin in about five days. The incisions behind the hair are removed at about two weeks. It is important to make certain that the incisions behind the hairline are well healed before using any rinses or stronger hair treatments. Generally, as long as the sutures are still in place behind the hair, we recommend use of baby shampoo as the only hair product. Baby shampoo is pH balanced, so while it is not optimal for hair on an ongoing basis, it is very gentle on the incision and is preferred during early healing.

Potential complications of a face-lift include, along with numbness, a very minimal risk of nerve or muscle weakness in the mouth or forehead area. This is unusual, and normally is only temporary. Infection, bleeding, or anesthetic reactions are very unusual. Occasionally there may be some poor healing and the resulting loss of some of the outer layers of skin behind or just under the ear, where the circulation is the poorest. People who smoke are much more at risk for such healing problems. If there is poor healing, it is important that the esthetician use products that are very gentle on healing tissue. In most cases there is swelling and black-and-blue after the procedure, but in the average patient, by two weeks after surgery almost all of the black-and-blue has faded, and approximately 80 percent of the swelling has decreased so that the individual using a small amount of camouflage makeup can go about his or her normal activities. This is especially true, of course, if the patient has the advantage of a camouflage therapist who is an expert in giving technical instruction in the application of camouflage makeup. Very often, prior to having plastic surgery, an individual may be using excessive amounts of makeup in order to try to cover up some of the signs of aging, and using the same techniques after the procedure can detract from the improvements of the plastic surgery. For that reason, we have all our patients see a clinical cosmetician shortly after the initial healing to receive a full make-over and advice on optimal makeup.

The clinical cosmetician can be very helpful during the preoperative period. The physician and staff will do all they can to prepare the patient and make certain he or she is in the best possible health. During this same preparatory period, the clinical cosmetician can help assure that the patient's skin is in the best possible condition. Cleansing the skin can decrease the bacterial count and decrease the risk of infection. Optimizing the condition of the skin can prepare it so that it will heal as well and as quickly as possible after surgery.

Post-operatively, the clinical cosmetician can be an important part of the professional team in providing emotional support. Many patients do have a letdown after surgery. This is similar to postpartum depression that many women have after childbirth. Before surgery there is a significant amount of anticipation, and, after surgery, the body has to have a way of clearing this anticipation. Suddenly, the event is over, whether it be childbirth or surgery. Often this will be expressed as a letdown; occasionally as more significant depression. Generally this does not last very long, but while patients are experiencing various post-operative emotions, it is very helpful to have caring professionals to empathize with and listen to their concerns, to reassure them that they are healing and physically improving, and to let them know that their emotions will also clear and improve.

Working closely with the plastic surgeon to further understand the procedures and understand what the patient is experiencing will help to make the clinical cosmetician more effective in providing patient support and will also help to assure that the patient is not getting mixed messages.

EYELID LIFT (BLEPHAROPLASTY)

As mentioned above, with time the eyelid skin loses elasticity and becomes loose. Eyelid lift (blepharoplasty) is designed to improve this condition. Excess skin is removed using incisions in the natural furrow in the upper eyelid out into the crow's feet area. After removing excess skin, the eyelid muscles are tightened, and excess fatty tissue resected. See Figure 13-4. The sutures are generally removed in about three days, and the incisions heal into the natural lines. At four or five days the patient is able to begin wearing makeup to cover up the residual black-and-blue.

Side effects and complications include the possibility that patients will have some temporary blurriness of vision immediately after surgery, due to the ointments and swelling. It is unlikely that there will be any permanent change in the vision, though an occasional patient will have minimal change in glasses. According to worldwide statistics, approximately 6 in 10,000 may have some loss of vision. Usually this can be treated successfully. The incisions generally heal very well in the eyelids themselves but are a little pink and firm in the crow's feet area for a longer period of time, requiring more skillful use of cover-up makeup.

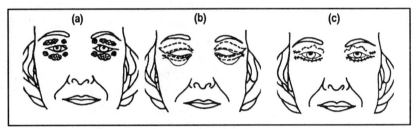

Figure 13-4. An eyelid lift

FOREHEAD LIFT

The forehead lift is designed to restore the eyebrows to a more elevated, pleasant position, and to minimize frown lines. Generally the procedure is done by making an incision approximately one to two inches behind the hairline and then freeing up the skin and reducing some of the forehead muscles by working underneath the skin of the forehead. See Figure 13-5. As with the face-lift, this does produce some numbness in the forehead for several months, and there may be some permanent numbness behind the incision. It is important to be aware of this numbness when doing any type of treatments in the forehead or upper scalp region. The hairline will be moved back approximately half an inch, and for people with a high forehead before surgery this may be a disadvantage. In that situation, an incision in front of the

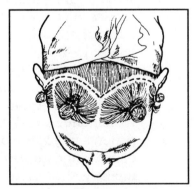

Figure 13-5. A forehead lift

hairline may be used. Covering this incision with camouflage makeup during the early healing process may be helpful.

Complications such as anesthetic reaction, infection, bleeding, and poor healing are unusual, and even black-and-blue and swelling are usually not very marked, although there can be some discoloration and swelling in the upper eyelids.

HAIR RESTORATION AND TRANSPLANTATION

One of the effects of aging is the effect that aging has on the hair. This can be thinning of the hair or receding hairline. Optimal hair care is important in terms of minimizing these problems. Individuals may have diseases which contribute to loss of hair in certain areas, in which case medical treatment by a dermatologist may be very important in minimizing the hair loss. For some, today, a medicine called Rogaine can be useful in minimizing hair loss. This was a medicine originally developed to treat high blood pressure, but it was found that, with topical application to the scalp, as many as 80 percent of individuals with hair loss problems minimized the loss. Often Rogaine caused hair in balding areas to regrow. Rogaine seems to convert nonproductive hair follicles into productive hair follicles to again produce more normal, fuller hair. For this reason Rogaine can be a valuable treatment for a significant number of patients. The effect is temporary, and if the individual stops using Rogaine, the improvement will disappear. Some people do in fact find that the amount of improvement is not enough to justify the expense of continuing to use Rogaine.

Flaps, moving the scalp from areas where there is good hair growth to areas that are bald, are one method of hair replacement. This may include the removal of portions of the bald area and advancement of the hair-bearing scalp, or actually moving a finger of hair-bearing scalp from the side up to the front hairline or to the crown of the head where the hair may be thinning. Hair transplants (or plugs) can also be used, removing small areas of skin from the back of the head most commonly, and transferring them to the frontal hairline or to the crown of the head. The hairs that are transferred in this manner seem to continue to behave and grow in the same manner as would the hairs in the back of the head. Such hair transplants generally are permanent. If you look closely, however, you usually can see small scars around the plugs that have been transferred. Such treatment usually requires several stages, performed usually about three months apart. A series of hair transplant plugs are placed generally around a quarter of an inch apart initially, and then at subsequent stages the areas between the first hair plugs are filled in with additional hair plugs. The hair growth is never quite as full, natural, or youthful hair, but with proper advice in hairstyling it can look quite natural and youthful. The hairline may continue to thin in other non-treated areas.

Complications with this are rare. There may be occasional numbness and infection. It is important to realize that after the hairs are transferred, generally the plugs will not produce for about a month to six weeks. The hairs that were present may drop out, only to re-grow at the end of the four to six weeks and thereafter remain permanently.

CONTOUR TREATMENTS

Rhinoplasty

The nose is the most common area of disproportion, and the most common facial contouring is rhinoplasty, or nose sculpting surgery. The shape of the nose is determined by the framework underneath. The framework is bone in the upper part of the bridge of the nose, and cartilage toward the tip. Incisions on the inside of the nose can be used, and any area of the framework can be sculpted so that it can be modified. See Figure 13-6. The majority of the sculpting can be done through incisions on the inside of the nose, although if the nostrils need to be narrowed or shortened, an incision in the natural fold in the base of the nostril may be utilized. These procedures are usually outpatient procedures and can be done with either local anesthetic and sedation, or with general anesthetic. Following this surgery, usually there will be a splint on the outside of the nose for approximately a week, and the patient may be asked to use the splint part-time for an additional week. There may be packs on the inside of the nose, and very often the packs make it so that the patient cannot breathe through the nose, similar to having a cold. This inability to breathe through the nose is often the only uncomfortable part of the recovery period. At the end of two weeks, the nose bones are pretty well set in place, although it does take approximately three months for the nose to regain its total preoperative strength. Generally, at the end of two weeks the majority of the black-and-blue areas in the eyes and nose have cleared, and approximately 80 percent of the swelling is down. Often it takes six to nine months before all the swelling is down, although usually at two weeks an individual looks good enough to go about normal activities.

The clinical esthetican can be helpful in terms of camouflage makeup during the first week or two to cover black-and-blue areas, and occasionally contouring with makeup is helpful to make the swelling less obvious during the early healing phases.

Complications are unusual but could include an anesthetic reaction, bleeding, or infection.

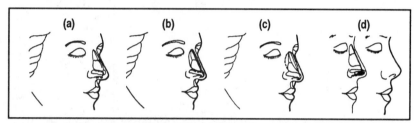

Figure 13-6. Rhinoplasty

Otoplasty

Another relatively common contouring procedure is contouring of the ears, known as otoplasty. Children born with prominent ears often suffer a great deal of teasing from their playmates. This is especially true during the early years in school. Generally children begin teasing each other in the kindergarten or early grade years. Since the ear reaches about 80 percent of its normal adult growth by age four, many of these operations are done at around four-and-a-half or five years of age when the ear is pretty well fully grown but before the child is subjected to a lot of teasing. These procedures, however, can be done in any stage during the individual's life. Basically, the principle involves contouring the cartilage of the ear in order to pin back the ear or place the rim of the ear closer to the head. See Figure 13-7. Other areas of the ear can also be modified. Occasionally the ear lobe is prominent or is too large even from early years, and very commonly as the ear lobe becomes larger with age it is useful to do a small ear lobe tuck at the time of a face-lift, or as an independent procedure in order to erase this telltale sign of aging. These procedures can be done usually on smaller children under general anesthetic, but with adults it can be done with sedation and local anesthetic. Dressings remain on the ears from three to seven days, and often a headband is worn after that, especially at night, to minimize the risk of the hearing being disrupted. There usually is some bruising and swelling, and it may be helpful to use camouflage makeup to minimize this early on.

Complications, such as anesthetic reactions, infection, or recurrence of the prominence are unusual.

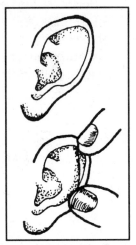

Figure 13-7. Otoplasty

Facial Contouring

Other facial contouring generally involves one of three techniques. The contours can be augmented, usually using implants, or the fatty tissue can be sculpted.

Sculpting the facial skeleton can be helpful in many areas. Occasionally the ridge along the eyebrows, eye socket itself, the cheek bones or the jaw is too prominent. All of these areas can be sculpted to minimize excess prominence in fairly straightforward techniques and can be accomplished usually as an out-patient procedure with local anesthetic and sedation, or with general anesthetic. It is important to remember that no one's face is absolutely regular, either by nature or by plastic surgery.

More extensive deformities such as craniofacial birth defects can leave the eye sockets too far apart, markedly uneven in position, or the skull itself too large or deformed. These also can usually be corrected using moderate craniofacial surgical techniques. These are highly specialized techniques performed by teams of plastic surgeons and neurosurgeons in centers that have had a special interest in this area. These are much more extensive procedures, and usually involve general anesthetic. These procedures can be extremely beneficial to deformed individuals and can allow them to enjoy a much more normal existence without feeling conspicuous.

Implants can be used to enlarge various contours; especially common are the implants that are used in the chin area, the cheekbone area, and now the cheek area. These implants are usually made out of silicone although several other materials can be utilized. The implants are very well tolerated and have never been demonstrated to cause any types of cancers or other illnesses. See Figure 13-8. There is a small risk of infection, and occasionally they do become infected and may have to be removed so that the infection can be cleared up and then replaced. If this were to occur, it generally would occur in the early post-operative period, and seldom is there a risk of problems after the initial healing has progressed. The implants are tolerated very well by the body and there has never been any evidence of rejection as might be seen in kidney or heart transplants.

Silicone injections have been utilized by some researchers, but there have been problems with reaction and movement of the silicone injections, and this technique has never been widely adopted, nor has it been approved by the FDA.

Fat sculpting can also be effectively utilized in a number of circumstances. Fat grafts can be used to fill in smile lines or frown lines, or occasionally in filling in contour defects in the cheek region or in other areas of the face.

Often, cosmetics can be used to help with preoperative contour. They can be used for camouflage makeup immediately after surgery, and contouring makeup can be used to help decrease the appearance of obvious swelling immediately after surgery. After facial plastic surgery, it is important to reconsider how makeup is applied to the face.

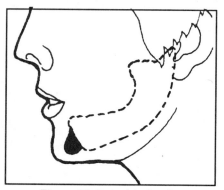

Figure 13-8. A chin implant

Liposuction

Liposuction is the most common plastic surgery procedure performed on the body today. It is primarily designed to help improve proportion or contouring, and to decrease unwanted fat bulges. See Figure 13-9. The human adult has about 30 billion fat cells, and in most cases this number does not change during the adult years. If an individual gains weight, the fat cells enlarge; if weight is lost the fat cells decrease in size but do not change in number. The fat cells that are removed through liposuction, or through any other surgical procedure, are permanently removed and are never replaced, and so the number is permanently decreased. It is important to leave behind a normal layer of fat cells; otherwise the skin would scar down to the muscle and look terrible. The procedure is not a substitute for diet and exercise. If an individual gains weight after having the procedure, the remaining fat cells in the treated areas as well as the fat cells in other areas will enlarge. Generally this would be a more proportionate weight gain, and weight loss would produce a more proportionate weight loss, than would have been true before liposuction treatment. But it is important for an individual to maintain proper weight through diet and exercise after liposuction. Liposuction is not designed to treat general obesity. It is designed primarily to treat localized areas such as the abdomen and "saddle bags" in women, or "love handles" in men. Virtually any area of the body can be treated, but there is a limit to how much can be treated at a single time.

It is important to point out that if there is loose skin before liposuction, there will be loose skin after the treatment, and in fact the skin may even be looser. Liposuction only treats the fat and does not help with the skin. Two areas where this is important is: (1) under the chin; if there is loose skin, and fatty tissue under the chin, after the fatty tissue is removed

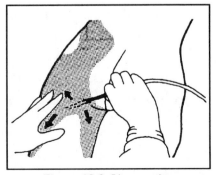

Figure 13-9. Liposuction

with liposuction the loose skin may hang even further; and (2) in the abdomen; if fatty tissue in the abdomen is removed from under loose skin, the loose skin may hang even further. The only effective way of treating this is with a tummy tuck. The swelling from liposuction is usually significant enough that at the end of the first week the dressings are taken off and the sutures removed, most people notice no real difference in the contouring. Even though there is less fat, it takes usually four to six weeks to begin to see a nice improvement, and often even more improvement will be noticed as much as six to nine months later, as the swelling continues to decrease. When this procedure is performed by individuals who are adequately trained and who have had general training in the aesthetic factors of contouring, such as board-certified plastic surgeons, there are few complications.

There have been a few cases reported of some darkening of the skin in the area especially after marked sun exposure, and so it is important to not get excessive sun exposure during the early postoperative period. There have been a very small number of deaths reported with liposuction. These were primarily because too much was removed at a single time by people who were inexperienced in the procedure. Of hundreds of thousands of cases of liposuction that have been performed by experienced plastic surgeons, there have been very few complications.

Post-operatively, patients are able to resume light activity generally the next day, and by three weeks are usually back to almost full normal activity.

BREAST ENLARGEMENT

The second most common area of the body for plastic surgery is the breast. Breasts can either be enlarged or reduced, made more symmetrical, uplifted, or reconstructed.

Over two million women in the United States have had breast enlargement procedures utilizing silicone implants. The silicone implant can be placed immediately under the breast tissue, or, more commonly now, immediately under the chest muscle. The implant helps the woman's own breast tissue project upward and forward, and produces better proportions. Various sized implants can be used, depending on how much enlargement is desired. The procedure is generally done on an outpatient basis under either local anesthetic along with sedation, or under general anesthetic.

The incision for the breast enlargement is generally small, and is placed in an inconspicuous location, either under the breast, around the nipple, or under the arm. The exact selection of the incision depends upon the desires of the patient and surgeon, and the surgical requirements, but needs to be individualized for each patient. See Figure 13-10.

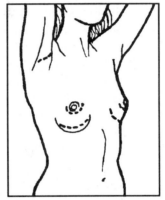

Figure 13-10. Breast enlargement

A space is then created under the breast or under the pectoralis muscle where an implant can be placed. See Figure 13-11. The implants are mostly silicone and are designed to be the same weight and consistency as normal breast tissue. See Figure 13-12 and 13-13.

Questions have been raised about whether breast implants could cause autoimmune disease or cancer. These are ques-

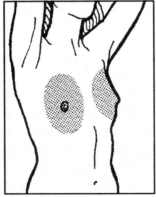

Figure 13-11.
Breast implant site

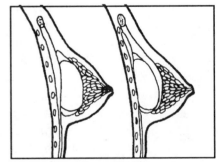

Figure 13-12.
Breast implant

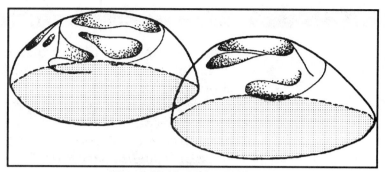

Figure 13-13. Breast implants

in the medical profession for many years. The FDA (Food and Drug Administration) undertook extensive review of the safety of breast implants in 1991. As of this writing in 1992, the FDA, after reviewing the hundreds of research studies published in the medical literature and also having had access to manufacturer's files, found that there was "no concrete evidence" that the implant caused any disease and that "we don't see any cause-and-effect relationship" between silicone breast implants and autoimmune disease, cancer, or any other illness. The FDA did call for additional research concerning the safety of the breast implants and did place restrictions on the use of gel-filled implants for breast reconstruction while additional research is being pursued. Silicone implants are being made available for breast reconstruction patients. At the same time, the FDA was very explicit that there is no need to remove or replace implants unless a specific problem has developed with the implants, such as rupture (and even then there is no evidence that ruptured implants would cause any of these illnesses or be dangerous). They further recommended that women who have implants should have mammograms and exams at the same frequency as women of similar age who do not have implants in place. Virtually all medical organizations, including the American Medical Association, the American College of Surgeons, and the American Cancer Society, felt that the safety of implants was well enough established that women should have free access to the use of silicone implants and choice as to whether they wish to use them. Virtually nothing in life is totally risk-free, but the benefit-to-risk ratio of implants appears to be extremely high. As of 1992, the FDA is also reviewing the safety of saline-filled implants, and they remain available for all patients who wish to utilize them.

BREAST REDUCTION, UPLIFT, RECONSTRUCTION

Women with large breasts may have significant symptoms, including neck pain, back pain, bra straps cutting into the shoulders, and shoulder pain. See Figure 13-14. In order to reduce the breasts to a more proportionate size, it is necessary to remove part of the breast tissue, rearrange the residual breast tissue into a more desirable shape, remove excess skin since the skin has been stretched, and elevate the nipple. All of this rearrangement generally does require significantly more incisions than breast enlargement requires, often an incision around the nipple, from the nipple to the fold underneath the breast, and another incision in the fold under the breast, though for smaller reduction patients it may be possible to use an incision just around the nipple itself. See Figure 13-15. Most patients, however, are very pleased with the results, even though they do have larger incisions, because they feel better physically as well as feeling better about their looks.

Generally, breast reduction is done with a one- or two-night stay in the hospital with a general anesthetic, and there is the possibility of infection, bleeding, or anesthetic reaction.

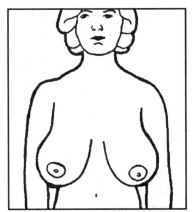

Figure 13-14. Breast reduction
– before

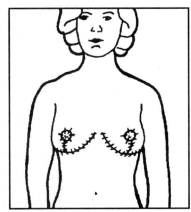

Figure 13-15. Breast reduction
– after

Breasts are never exactly the same on both sides, either by nature or by plastic surgery, and it is important that patients be aware of this.

The same basic principles apply for breast uplift. Again, this usually involves a fair amount of rearrangement, and can involve the same type of incisions as used in the breast reduction, and the same potential complications, though the operation usually is not as extensive, and can more commonly be done on an outpatient basis.

Breast reconstruction has become much more common in recent years. Breast reconstruction can be done in the form of subcutaneous mastectomy and reconstruction, which is designed to help women who are at high risk for developing breast cancer reduce the risk before they develop actual cancer. In this procedure, the nipple is preserved, and after the breast tissue is removed the shape is reconstructed utilizing the silicone breast implant and generally placing it under the chest muscle.

Breast reconstruction after cancer and mastectomy can be performed as a delayed procedure, three to six or more months after the original mastectomy, or in more and more cases, at the time of the initial surgery. Again, after the mastectomy is performed, the implant is positioned under the muscle in order to re-establish the shape, and then three to six months later the nipple can be reconstructed if the patient so desires (see chapter on cancer.)

Alternative methods involve moving some of the skin and muscle from the back to provide more skin and better coverage for an implant, or doing what is called a TRAM (transverse rectus abdomens muscle) flap, moving skin, muscle, and fatty tissue from the tummy up to the breast area to totally reconstruct the breast without using an implant.

Over the last twenty years, it has been demonstrated that breast reconstruction is a safe procedure. It does not interfere in any way with the treatment of the original breast cancer. Techniques have improved to the point that today a woman with a breast reconstruction will generally look quite natural, especially if she is wearing clothing, even a bathing suit.

There are some differences between the reconstructed breast and the natural breast, especially the mature breast. The reconstructed breast is more like a youthful breast in that it does not sag, has more fullness, usually in the upper areas, and produces more cleavage. The reconstructed breast generally does not have normal sensation because some of the nerves that go to the nipple area especially pass through the breast tissue, and when the breast tissue is removed, these nerves also are removed, leaving some areas of numbness in or around the nipple. Occasionally there may be problems which lead to the breast having less than optimal shape, and this may have to be revised. Other potential complications include the usual possible anesthetic reaction, infection, bleeding, and possible loss of part of the nipple or skin if the circulation is not adequate in these areas.

The procedures for the breast deal with the problems of aging and sagging, secondary to aging or pregnancy, and also deal with the quality of proportion and contouring. The breast is a very important psychological aspect of the female figure; the absence of a breast can have a devastating effect on the self-image of some women. For that reason, breast reconstruction can be critically important for a woman.

TUMMY TUCK AND OTHER BODY LIFTS

The tummy tuck is designed to reverse some of the effects of pregnancy on the belly, namely reduce the loose skin, remove many if not all of the stretch marks, remove some of the extra fatty tissue that may be left, and tighten the muscles to trim the waist and abdomen. See Figure 13-16. The tummy tuck can also be used for men and women who have had weight fluctuations and who have excess skin because of weight gains and subsequent losses.

The incision is designed in the lower abdomen, in what is called the bikini line because it is covered by most bikinis, although some French-cut bikinis do not cover it. See Figure 13-17. There usually is also an incision around the belly button. Excess skin is removed near the incision. The belly button is maintained in its original position, and the incision is closed after tightening the muscle and then the skin. See Figures 13-17 and 13-18. This procedure has commonly been done as an in-patient procedure, although it is now possible to do it under general anesthetic as an outpatient procedure. Recovery time is generally three to four weeks.

A modification of this is the mini tummy tuck, which is designed primarily to help only the lower part of the abdomen. This procedure involves less surgery and a shorter recovery period. The full tummy tuck is designed to help both upper and lower abdomen. The same potential complications exist including the possibility of anesthetic reaction, infection, or bleeding. There often is some numbness in the lower part of the belly afterwards; much of the feeling may return but some numbness may remain permanently. If there is any poor healing, it is usually in the lower abdominal

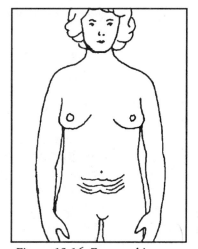

Figure 13-16. Excess skin

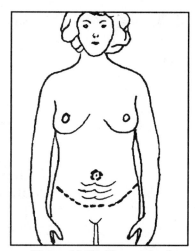

Figure 13-17. Tummy tuck — before

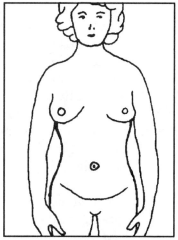

Figure 13-18. Tummy tuck — after

incision. Generally this will heal without further surgery. It is important for patients to walk after surgery in order to minimize the risk of blood clots in the legs.

The same basic principles can be applied to removing excess, loose skin on almost any area of the body. More common lifts include arm lifts, thigh lifts, and buttocks lifts, although lifts can be done in almost any area. These lifts do involve removal of skin and, hence, generally moderately long incisions, and it is important that the patient be aware of the trade-offs involved in terms of improved appearance and tighter skin in exchange for the incisions.

SPECIAL RECONSTRUCTIVE PLASTIC SURGERY AREAS

One area where the clinical esthetican-plastic surgeon team can be very helpful to patients is in reconstructive plastic surgery.

Reconstructive surgery follows many of the same principles involved in cosmetic surgery. The difference is that in cosmetic surgery, the goal is to enhance the existing beauty; in reconstructive surgery, the goal is to re-establish the beauty that was present before accident or disease. The principles are much the same in terms of trying to re-establish an appearance that is as youthful as possible, while re-establishing the optimal proportions and contours, and attempting to re-establish the natural color, ultimately attempting to re-establish the individual's radiance.

Space does not allow an extensive discussion of the multiple types of reconstructive procedures available, but we would like to share a few basic principles.

The first preference would be to reconstruct using skin, fatty, tissue, muscle, and bone, which is already in the area. Therefore, if someone has a simple laceration, the principle is to attempt to close the laceration in such a way that leaves minimal scarring. All healing takes approximately a year to full maturity, and so incisions and cuts generally are a bit red at first. This is due to the new blood vessels that grow into the area to help with the healing, and as the healing progresses, the red usually fades and the color blends in better. Likewise, there is usually swelling and some firmness, and with time, often with some massage, this firmness and swelling will decrease.

If the injury is deeper, for example, a person is in an automobile accident and has a laceration as well as a fracture of the nose, the principle is to replace the bones to their normal position, close the laceration, and protect the bones with a splint to allow healing, and then treat the laceration in much the same way as you would treat a simple laceration.

Very often a secondary dermabrasion or sanding procedure may be helpful for scarring. This is basically a sanding procedure utilizing a special diamond frase instrument, which can help to smooth the outer surface of skin, and help to blend in the scar. This usually would not be done for six to twelve months after the initial injury to allow the early healing to be completed prior to the dermabrasion.

Another procedure that may be helpful is a scar revision, usually removing the old, unattractive scar, and often rearranging the tissue, perhaps with some special procedures, so that the incision can be closed in a more natural line or in a less conspicuous location. Healing after this procedure goes through the normal maturation, and does take time.

If there is skin missing, the tissue expansion procedure can be used to stretch some of the skin in a nearby area so that the missing skin can be replaced by skin that has the same texture and color as that which is missing. If a significant amount of skin is missing, it may be necessary to bring in skin from a distant area, utilizing a flap or a skin graft. With a flap, the skin is left attached to the original donor area for approximately three weeks while it picks up a new blood supply from the recipient area, and then it is detached from the original area and moved fully into recipient area after it has picked up the new blood supply from the recipient area. With the skin graft, literally the outer layers of skin are removed from a donor area, leaving the inner layers of skin to heal in that area. The outer layers are removed as a thin sheet and are totally separated from the patient, and then placed in the new position.

The skin graft is very commonly used in treating burns, and the outer layers of skin will heal in the burned area where new skin is needed. Unfortunately, the skin graft, while it does become tougher over the months, is never quite as tough as the original skin; it never has quite the same color or the same texture as the original skin, the color very often being a little darker than the surrounding skin, and sometimes a little more yellow. Even though the shape and contour is often reconstructed with a skin graft, the color leaves something to be desired, and this, of course, is an area where an expert in camouflage makeup can be very helpful to burn patients.

If some of the deeper structures are needed, cartilage grafts can be taken from the ear, or bone grafts can be taken from a rib or even from the hip bone and used to reconstruct contour. In an ear, cartilage or bone can be used to establish the framework, a flap of skin to re-establish the cover. Often these reconstructed structures will be as nice as the original, but if the patient has the benefit of expert plastic surgery, as well as expert makeup advice, a better result is obtained than otherwise would be possible.

In overall summary, there are four hallmarks to beauty, the first youth, the second proportion, the third optimal color, and the fourth radiance. Together, the esthetician and the plastic surgeon as a team can help individuals optimize beauty in all of these areas. Together the esthetician and the plastic surgeon can be a winning team.

REVIEW

You should now be familiar with:

- what is plastic surgery and who performs it.
- how an operating room is set up.
- equipment used for plastic surgery.
- procedures used in plastic surgery.

Esthetic Therapy for Cancer Patients

Almost everyone knows someone who has had cancer. Studies indicate that as many as one third of all Americans will at some point in their lives develop cancer. The clinical esthetician/cosmetologist should be prepared to address not just the cosmetic aspects of aesthetic therapy but to attend to any concerns the patient with cancer may have about his or her overall appearance.

There is a very strong correlation between how attractive we feel physically and our overall self-image. The enhancing effects of appearance counseling, then, can be extremely therapeutic to cancer patients even if there is no outward evidence of side effects. Studies have proven that when patients feel positive about the way they look, they are more confident and in general approach life with a more assured attitude.

Understanding the special needs of the cancer patient is an important part of clinical cosmetology. The information contained in this chapter will offer the clinical esthetician/cosmetologist some insight into what cancer is, how it is treated, and what aesthetic options are available to patients who are either about to undergo cancer therapy, are in the process of being treated, or who are in the recovery stage.

Cosmetics can improve the overall appearance of the cancer patient's skin by camouflaging skin discolorations and visible scarring; hair alternatives can minimize the effects of temporary hair loss; recommendations on nail care can counteract nail damage and improve the presentation of the patient's hands. In addition, professional skin-care treatments can promote relaxation and ease the surface dryness and dehydration that can occur from chemotherapy or radiation treatments, while suggestions on special clothing to assist the patient in concealing evidence of surgical cancer therapy or the existence of special appliances (catheters, ostomy bags, and chemo-pumps) can ease some of the stress associated with illness.

UNDERSTANDING CANCER

Cancer is defined as a group of diseases that are caused by the uncontrolled growth of cells in one or more of the body's organs or tissues. Cancer may affect any body tissue. The cell is the fundamental unit of the body. See Figure 14-1. The human body is made up of cells organized into various organs or tissues: skin, muscle, bone, blood, glands, etc. These tissues are composed of special cells that conduct specific functions. Inside every cell is a nucleus that contains chromosomes. In the body there are twenty-two sets of what is referred to as "regular chromosomes" and one set of "sex chromosomes." Each chromosome contains several thousand genes. The chromosomes and genes are comprised of deoxyribonucleic acid (DNA). The DNA contains the information required for the cell to perform its function.

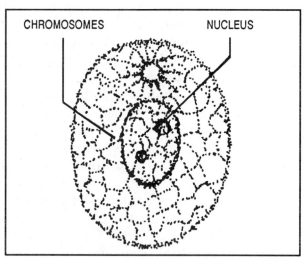

Figure 14-1. The cell

Cells reproduce by splitting in half to create new cells. As this process occurs the DNA makes a copy of itself to form a nucleus for each of the two cells. See Figure 14-2. Healthy cells reproduce in an ordered way, coordinated with the cells around them, and perform their specialized tasks. Cancer cells function independently; they do not contribute to the function of the affected organ. They often reproduce at a faster rate, preventing the affected organ from functioning normally. Cancer cells may also spread from the original organ to other organs. This spread is called metastasis. These abnormal cells are referred to as malignant. The malignant cells are extremely harmful because they invade and injure vital organs.

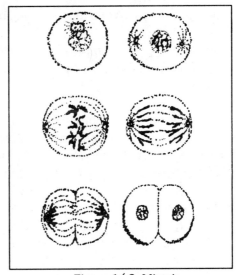

Figure 14-2. Mitosis

DIAGNOSIS

Hundreds of thousands of people in this country will be diagnosed with some form of cancer this year. The probability of cancer developing increases with age. Those in their 20s have less than half the chance of developing cancer as those in their 30s, while those in their 40s are twice as susceptible. This pattern continues each decade, doubling the risk.

It is important to diagnose cancer as soon as possible, because early detection insures a better chance of survival. If a cancer is suspected, tests are performed. These may include microscopic examination of tissues obtained by biopsy, cytology test (a microscopic examination of the cells obtained from superficial or internal lesions, like a pap smear), imaging techniques (like x-rays), chemical testing (chemicals are used to reveal the presence of substances indicative of cancer; i.e., blood in feces, high levels of a certain enzyme in the blood), or by directly looking in an organ (endoscopy: a tube with a viewing lens is passed into the organ to examine it).

CANCER THERAPY

Joanna M. Cain, M.D.

Cancer therapy, at present, can be divided into the disciplines of surgery, chemotherapy, and radiation therapy. While most people are familiar with some of the effects of chemotherapy — hair loss, for example — we may be less familiar with the effects of the other arms of therapy.

SURGERY

Cancer surgery includes many procedures that alter body function and feeling. It is important to recognize these alterations when planning cosmetics and clothing for these areas. The major types of operations and their side effects include:

Skin and Muscle Grafts

These grafts are employed to attempt to restore more normal anatomy and bring in a better blood supply than would otherwise exist when an area has had a radical removal of tissue. When these grafts are moved, they continue to have the same sensation that they originally had. For example, a graft from the back to the neck will "feel" like the neck when touched; a graft from the inside of the thigh to the groin will "feel" like the inside of the thigh. For some patients this "abnormal" sensation can be quite distressing. In addition, the nerve supply to the area can be damaged and the grafted muscle and skin will not sweat or change its blood supply appropriately for the environmental circumstances. In addition, damage to the nerve

supply may increase a feeling of numbness in the area, increasing the likelihood of injuries such as cuts and burns. These grafts are used for reconstruction in virtually all parts of the body.

A particularly common area of surgery for reconstruction is the breast. It is rare now to find patients for whom a true radical mastectomy with removal of all the muscle groups under the breast is required. In fact, even the modified radical mastectomy that preserves a portion of the pectoralis muscle that sits under the breast is less common. However, for those procedures and for simple mastectomies, reconstruction of the breast shape either immediately or at a later time is quite common. These reconstructions can cover a variety of types including the movement of muscle tissue without the overlying skin or movement of skin only (as in reconstruction of a nipple). The use of breast implants of various types is also common.

RADICAL SURGERY AND OSTOMIES

Many of the body functions impacted by cancer and affected by cancer surgery can be resorted by providing new openings (ostomies) for those functions. Tracheostomies (opening of the airway through the neck); gastrostomies (opening of the stomach to the front of the abdomen); colostomies (opening the colon or bowel to the front of the abdomen); and the various

Joanna M. Cain, M.D., is an associate professor at the University of Washington Medical Center. She teaches in the department of obstetrics and gynecology, a division of gynecologic oncology.

forms of urostomies (opening the urine tract either by placing ureters or a loop of bowel with the ureters attached to the front of the abdomen) are the more common examples. Because the body fluids these ostomies handle were never meant to drain off the skin, elaborate systems of skin care must be followed in the ostomy area, and often plastic bags are placed to handle the body fluids as they exit the openings. Any product used in the area must therefore not add to the increased moisture around the ostomy, must not add to the potential for infections, and must be unlikely to incite a local skin allergy.

VENOUS ACCESS CATHETERS

These catheters are an important part of cancer management as they allow rapid access to the blood system. These catheters come in two main types — those that are buried under the skin in the upper chest wall or elsewhere and those that exit through the skin with a closed end. Clearly, the need for prevention of infection in these areas is paramount. Of the two types the subcutaneous catheters (implanted) are less susceptible to infection, but anything used in the area must be able to be completely removed from the skin when that catheter must be used.

EDEMA WITH CANCER SURGERY

Swelling, or edema, of any area of the body can occur with alteration in the blood or the lymphatic flow in the area, but for cancer therapy more often is associated with surgically removed lymphatic channels. The dissection of the lymph nodes in the axilla for breast cancer, for example, can cause permanent swelling in the arm. The dissection of the lymph nodes in the groin or pelvis for gynecologic cancers may cause permanent swelling of the leg. This lymphedema creates particular problems as it decreases the body's ability to fight infection in the region. For this reason, extra care must be taken to prevent cuts, burns, and other destruction to the integrity of the skin in the area.

RADIATION THERAPY

Advances in radiation therapy have significantly improved the effects on the skin. Areas that previously were severely affected are no longer so. However, it is still necessary to treat certain areas that are close to the skin — for example head and neck cancers, some breast cancers, and lymph nodes areas, like those over the clavicle or in the groin. The short-term effects of this are much like severe skin burns, and are treated the same way that local burns would be treated. The more profound effects of radiation doses on or near the skin are in the long term. Radiation changes the texture and the blood supply of the skin, and the effect can be progressive so that skin integrity may be at more risk ten years from radiation than it is initially. Specifically, radiation will cause some measure of local skin tanning and fibrosis or thickening. The local blood vessels — primarily the smaller vessels — decrease in number and have difficulty repairing damage to their walls. This poor repair can lead to the formation of tiny collections of small vessels called telangiectasia that appear like little red stars on the skin. These are very fragile and likely to bleed with abrasion. This loss of adequate blood supply thins the skin and increases the likelihood of infection in the area because oxygen, nutrients, and white blood cells are unable to reach the area. Over time, rare patients may even develop skin ulcerations because of this effect.

CHEMOTHERAPY

Chemotherapy and immunotherapy refer to those drugs or immunologically active agents that are given to stop the growth of cancer cells. There are now a large number of such drugs available, and each one has a different set of side effects with implications for skin care. Chemotherapy, in general, does its work by preventing growth of cancer cells because of damage done to the DNA or the metabolic factories of the cell. Normal cells with rapid growth are also affected by these agents but are more able to overcome and repair the damage these drugs cause. Therefore, the damage is greater to the cancer cells, and the balance between the potential damage to the cancer cells versus the rate of repair of damage to normal cells is the basis for the doses of these drugs that are given. Also, the particular side effects of the drugs on normal cells are matched so that in two or three drug treatments, the side effects of the drugs used will be heaviest in different areas. The normal body cells that are the most affected by chemotherapy are those whose rate of growth are the highest. Therefore, hair growth anywhere on the body, the lining of the gastrointestinal tract, the skin in general, and especially the cells of the bone marrow that make the red cells, white cells, and platelets, are affected by chemotherapy. The effect on the bone marrow is exceptionally important as the risk for infection with low white cell counts can be extremely high. It can be so high that tooth brushing or washing the skin with a rough cloth are temporarily forbidden. It is always important to know what a patient's counts are, as white blood cell counts below 2000/mm3 or platelet counts below 50,000/mm3 can be associated with infection or bleeding from otherwise seemingly innocuous skin care. Patients should check with their physicians for guidelines about the level of "counts" for which they should exercise caution.

The particular effects of any one drug on any one patient can vary widely, but the side effects can be classified as follows:

Skin

Some drugs are particularly associated with skin rashes, hyperpigmentation, and changes in the nails. Bleomycin, for example, is a drug that will leave patients with permanent stripes of hyperpigmentation in scratch marks and can cause nails to thicken. Other types of drugs and skin effects include:

- "Hormone" type drugs (Prednisone, Decadron, etc.) can cause an acne-type rash and the development of thin skin and stretch marks on the skin.

- Darkening can occur with bleomycin, cytoxan, adriamycin FUDR, and 5-FU.

- Rashes and/or skin scaling can be caused by most agents.

- Recall phenomena is an unusual effect of some drugs (such as adriamycin) where the acute effects of radiation therapy are "recalled" in the area of the former radiation when the drug is given.

- Burning of the skin with exposure to the sun is more common simply because of thinning of the epidermis, but some drugs heighten the sensitivity to the sun even more producing severe sun burns with limited exposure.

The protective mechanisms of the skin can be affected by thinning of the epidermis, leading to moisture loss and dryness. The need for good skin integrity with the low white counts is even more accentuated in this setting where cracking of the skin can lead to infection. It is quite possible with cracks in the skin and low white cell counts to introduce a serious infection not only into the skin but also into the blood stream. For this reason, constant skin care to prevent dryness and special efforts to keep any product used free of contamination is important.

Other side-effects of chemotherapy and immunotherapy can include nerve damage to the fingers, making it difficult for a patient to use small instruments or to sense the temperature of an object. In addition, temperature regulation can be poor and protection of the area from extremes of temperature is very important.

COMBINATIONS OF THERAPEUTIC ARMS

Most of cancer therapy is given with combinations of more than one arm of therapy. For example, a patient with breast cancer may have local surgery, radiation, and then chemotherapy; or a patient with uterine cancer may have surgery and radiation. Sometimes these are given at the same time, and sometimes one following the other. When we combine these different therapies we also combine the toxicity of each especially for the therapies that are given at the same time. This presents particular problems for patients who have radiation therapy and chemotherapy at the same time as the local reaction might be significantly more brisk than without the chemotherapy. An appreciation of the escalation of side effects by combining more than one modality of therapy is important.

WORKING WITH THE CANCER PATIENT

Three to four months after being diagnosed with cancer, most patients are in the process of redefining their lives, striving to cope with the medical treatments they must endure, and trying to manage a host of emotions that accompany a serious diagnosis.

Most patients will probably not be prepared for any really drastic physical changes during this period. A patient whose appearance has been altered because of cancer will not want unrealistic promises or cosmetic gimmicks from a beauty professional. What the patient will need however, is a few simple suggestions on how to normalize his or her appearance.

The patient should be carefully evaluated by the clinical esthetician/cosmetologist, and his or her concerns should be repeated back for clarification. The therapist should never do more than the patient wants to do, or the clinical esthetician/ cosmetologist could sabotage an otherwise admirable effort, which ultimately could result in the patient feeling even more defeated about his or her appearance than before the session started. The treatment should work for and not against the patient.

Not all cancer patients will require or even want cosmetic makeovers. A patient may just wish to lift his or her spirits by having a consultation with a clinical esthetician/cosmetologist. Such a patient may only be seeking the services of the beauty professional to elevate his or her mood by learning new techniques to enhance his or her appearance with medical cosmetics, skin-care advice, wardrobe suggestions, or with a new hairstyle. Whether or not you are a fully licensed hair stylist you should have enough of a background in appearance counseling to make some interesting recommendations that will appeal to the patient. The following information will target specific areas that may concern a patient who has cancer.

HAIR LOSS

In our culture we have an overwhelming preoccupation with hair. Hair is frequently referred to as a person's "crowning glory." In addition to hair being a symbol of beauty and sensuality, hair also provides protective covering for the body that protects the scalp and skin from friction, scratches, and abrasions, and insulates it from extreme environmental temperature changes.

Patients maintain that one of the most devastating side effects of cancer therapy is hair loss. *Hair loss* can be anything from loss of hair in patches, to diffuse hair-fall, to baldness, or even complete hair loss over the whole body. See Figure 14-3. Unfortunately, the patient's physician cannot accurately predict exactly how much hair a patient will lose or when exactly he or she will lose it, but hair loss on the average usually occurs within two to six weeks after chemotherapy begins. The amount of loss generally depends on the side effects of the cancer therapy and how well the patient's body tolerates treatment. The medications that destroys cancer cells travels through the bloodstream. Hair follicles are tiny organs buried in the dermis layer of the skin. They are nourished by the substances in the bloodstream carried through a network of capillaries. The medications patients are administered in chemotherapy are so powerful that they paralyze the follicle, resulting in hair loss. The hair falls out at the root. Fortunately, even though the hair stops growing, the follicle remains intact, and eventually the hair will grow back once the cancer treatments have ceased but it takes time. Regrowth generally does not occur until three to five weeks after the last cancer treatment.

There are basically four different types of hair loss, mild (hair loss less than 25 percent), severe (50 percent or more), baldness (loss of all scalp hair), and complete hair loss (scalp and all other areas of the body including eyelashes and eyebrows).

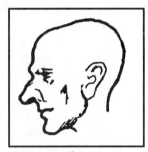

Figure 14-3. Hair loss

HAIR REPLACEMENT

There are several ways in which the cancer patient can cope with hair loss, depending on its severity. False eyelashes, eyebrows, hair extensions, hairpieces, wigs, and headwraps can all provide excellent alternatives to patients suffering from the effects of temporary or permanent hair loss.

Facial Hairpieces Ready-made facial hairpieces such as artificial mustaches, beards, sideburns, and eyebrows can all be used by the clinical esthetician/cosmetologist to camouflage the loss of facial hair. See Figure 14-4. All facial prostheses are made in much the same way; hairs are tied by hand onto a delicate lace net. A surgical adhesive is applied to the net, and the gauze net is attached to the patient's facial area, securing the facial hairpiece. False eyelashes are made by hand and tied to a nylon thread, cut, shaped, and curled. Artificial eyebrows can be constructed by hand or by machine with individual strands of hair tied to a lace foundation.

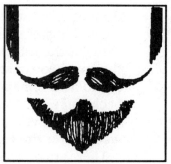

Figure 14-4. Facial hairpieces

Artificial Eyelashes

False eyelashes may be needed if the patient temporarily loses his or her eyelashes due to radiation or chemotherapy treatments. See Figure 14-5. Properly applying eyelashes requires time and practice. Your patient will need a supervised lesson. You will also have to trim the lashes for the patient, fit them on his or her eyelids and instruct the patient on the appropriate technique with which to apply them. Recommend that the patient select an inexpensive pair of feathered (ends of the lashes vary in length) false eyelashes (see cosmetic therapy chapter on how to apply). If the loss is permanent, the patient may have eyelashes from another part of his or her eye transplanted surgically.

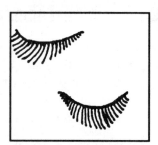

Figure 14-5. False eyelashes

Camouflaging with Eyewear

Eyewear — eyeglasses with wide, distinctive frames and tinted lenses will conceal missing eyebrows and eyelashes (see chapter on adaptive techniques for the visually impaired, the section on eyewear). See Figure 14-6. The frames should be wide enough to cover the area where the eyebrows should be.

Eyebrow Alternatives

To temporarily replace eyebrows patients can draw them on with pencil, use theatrical eyebrows, or apply artificial brows (for more information see cosmetic therapy section of this chapter). See Figure 14-7. If part of the patient's eyebrow is unlikely to grow back an eyebrow transplant is possible or micropigmentation may provide be a suitable camouflage alternative.

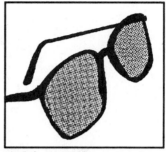

Figure 14-6. Camouflaging with eyewear

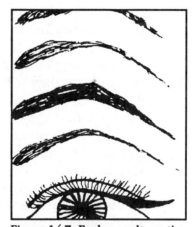

Figure 14-7. Eyebrow alternatives

Wigs Not every patient will want to wear a wig; however, patients should be presented with enough information to make that decision for themselves. See Figure 14-8. The camouflage therapist, although he or she may not be a cosmetologist, should know enough about hair replacement to advise the cancer patient of his or her options. Selecting the wrong wig or hairpiece could end up causing the patient unnecessary anxiety and also prove to be quite costly.

A wig could never replace the real hair the patient lost, but it can help to temporally camouflage his or her hair loss until hair grows back in. Several different types of wigs are available today. Some are hand-made using human hair or synthetic fibers. Many wigs look and feel so much like real hair that it is difficult to detect the difference, while others, like fashion wigs, will look extremely artificial.

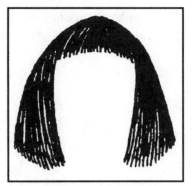

Figure 14-8. Wigs

Helping the Patient Select the Right Wig

Not every patient will have the same expectations or requirements, nor will all be able to afford the same type of hair replacement. The following information is provided to assist the clinical esthetician/cosmetologist in helping patients choose a wig or a hairpiece that will best serve their needs and one that they will feel good about wearing. See Figure 14-9. But, before the clinical esthetician/cosmetologist can help a patient find the right form of hair replacement, he or she must conduct some research beforehand. First, it is important for the clinical esthetician/cosmetologist to identify the various types of wigs and hairpieces available today, how they are made, and how much they cost. If at all possible the following considerations should be brought to the patient's attention by the clinical esthetician/cosmetologist before the patient decides on any one of the following hair replacement solutions.

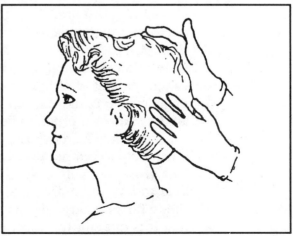

Figure 14-9. Choosing a wig

Quality and Construction

Type of wig or hairpiece

- Is the hairpiece or wig that the patient is considering purchasing made from human hair or synthetic fiber?

Workmanship

- How well is it made? Suggest that the patient turn the wig or hairpiece inside out and examine it.

Color

- Does the color look natural, and does it work well with the patient's own natural coloring? (The wig or hairpiece must complement the patient's coloring.)

Fit

- Comfort — is the wig the right size, not too loose or too tight? (Remind the patient that a wig will not stretch after wearing it the way shoes will!).

Life expectancy of the hairpiece or wig

- How long will the patient need the hairpiece or wig?, and will the patient be wearing the hairpiece on a daily basis?

Financial considerations

- How much can the patient reasonably afford to spend on a wig or partial hair piece? Is the patient financially restricted?

Hairpieces

Not all cancer patients will lose all of their hair. A hairpiece can be worn to supplement partial hair loss. There are three types of hairpieces: hair extensions, add-ons, and hair replacements.

Hair Extensions

- A hair extension is an addition of hair or fiber to pre-existing hair. This entails attachment of the hair extension, which allows the patient to wear the extension four to eight weeks. It becomes a part of the patient's own hair until it is time to remove it for cleansing, service, and re-attachment.
- The materials are made from either human hair, synthetic fiber, or a combination of both, usually in the form of a weft or a cluster or strands of the hair or fiber.

Add-ons

- Add-ons are hair items that are designed to be added and removed by the patient. These may include postiches, banana clips, wiglets, and falls. These materials are made from human hair, synthetic fiber, or a combination of the two.

Hair Replacements

- Hair replacements are "pieces" that are attached to the patient's hair or scalp. These pieces will replace or augment missing hair or may cover the patient's own hair. Hair replacements may be made from human hair, synthetic fiber, or both. They may be hairpieces or full wigs.

Ready-made Synthetic Wigs

A synthetic wig is the least expensive form of hair replacement on the market. See Figure 14-10. The price range of a synthetic wig can vary from as low as $50 to as high as $2,500 for a good synthetic wig, with the average cost ranging between $100 and $150. One of the nice things about a synthetic wig is that it requires very little maintenance; it is easy to obtain and affordable to purchase, which makes it the most convenient form of hair replacement available.

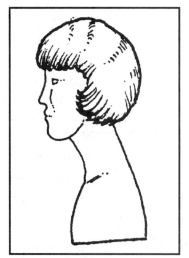

Figure 14-10. A synthetic wig

Wig Construction

Synthetic hair is actually a plastic fiber that is manufactured in Japan. It is formed from hot, molten plastic that is poured through a device that resembles a shower head. While the plastic is still wet it is placed in cold water until it solidifies. After it hardens it looks like long spaghetti strands. Once it has cooled the plastic is thrown into a large vat that contains dyes. After the plastic has been dyed it is cut. It is then sewn into wefts. Wefts are fringes of hair generally six to twelve inches long. See Figure 14-11. The synthetic fibers are then shaped into different curl patterns and sewn onto a mesh base. Starting on one side of the ear, a very long weft is sewn around the head, and this process is repeated until the weft reaches the top of the head, at which point it is secured onto a mesh base. This process continues until the wig resembles a full head of hair.

Hairpieces are better designed for persons with only partial hair loss because gaps in the mesh base will appear if the wig becomes disheveled. Furthermore, because of the way in which it is made, this type of wig can be very uncomfortable for a patient who has complete hair loss; the way in which the wefts are sewn to the mesh foundation can cause the underside of the wig to scratch the patient's scalp by constantly rubbing against the skin.

A cotton scarf in the same color as the wig can be worn underneath the hairpiece to prevent the scalp from being exposed in the event that the artificial hair becomes parted and the scalp becomes exposed. This will ease the discomfort caused from the hairpiece coming in contact with the scalp and also absorb perspiration. Changing scarves frequently will prevent the hairpiece from absorbing perspiration, and this will help to preserve the wig because it will not have to be shampooed as frequently, thereby increasing its longevity. Most wigs should last for six months to two years with weekly washings.

Wig longevity is another dilemma a patient may have to face when purchasing a synthetic wig. This type of wig only

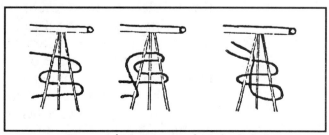

Figure 14-11. Fringes of synthetic hair

lasts from two to four months when worn on a daily basis, because inexpensive wigs are constructed from plastic fibers that cannot tolerate heat. If the hairpiece comes in contact with heat it frizzes. Even though a synthetic wig is less expensive initially, in the long run it may end up costing the patient more because it will have to be replaced with another wig within a few months.

Color plays a major role in how natural the wig will look. This can pose a problem for female patients because most synthetic wigs are dyed in ash color tones. When a woman wears a synthetic hairpiece in natural light it tends to look artificial due to the absence of highlights. The color of synthetic hair can be altered, however, by an experienced wig stylist. Highlighted hair strands can be discreetly woven into the synthetic hair that will give the wig a natural looking sheen in daylight.

Synthetic wigs are stock made (one size is presumed to fit all) as opposed to custom made (individually sized). Since everyone has a different head size, the synthetic wig will more than likely have to be adjusted to fit the patient's head. The original fit may be too loose or too tight for the patient (generally, synthetic wigs tend to fit loosely).

Achieving the Right Fit

There are several ways in which the hairpiece can be adjusted to fit the patient's head. Little darts can be taken in at the center, or an elastic band can be placed on the underside of the piece. Most patients find that they do have to make some sort of adjustment to secure the fit. The elastic band does prevent the hairpiece from shifting, but it must be attached with double sided tape, and unfortunately most synthetic wigs do not have an area where the tape can adhere. Double sided tape will stick to the head but it will not adhere to the inside of the hairpiece. A security patch or a piece of toupee patch material can be placed on the inside of the hairpiece to provide a base in which to attach the double sided tape. This material can be purchased at most wig salons. It is a polyester material impregnated with plastic. The patient will need a piece of material about one inch by one inch sewn onto the underside of the hairpiece on the area where the wig will be covering each temple and also at the back of the wig where it fits over the nape of the neck. The double sided tape should be attached to the inside of the hairpiece and pressed firmly down so that it adheres the hairpiece to the patient's head. This will keep the wig from shifting without the addition of an elastic band to secure the wig, which over a long period of time can become extremely uncomfortable.

Re-styling the Synthetic Wig

Because of the weft construction method that is used to make synthetic hairpieces, most synthetic wigs are too full to look natural. Even though the wig is conveniently pre-styled for the consumer, a patient considering purchasing a synthetic wig should never plan on wearing it out of the shop. Have the patient investigate whether styling is included in the purchase price of the wig. An experienced stylist can take a bushy, synthetic wig, thin it by trimming it, and custom style it to complement the facial features of the patient. The proper hairstyle and the right amount of hair thickness can make all the difference in how convincing the artificial hair will look.

Handmade Wigs

Natural hairpieces are hand made from Chinese hair. They are individually constructed by attaching hairs to a netting, which is cut and sewn to conform to the shape of the head. How well a wig is constructed can be determined by the type of material that was used to make the hairpiece, the type of base to which the hairs were tied, and the method that was used to attach the hair to it. These factors will play a major role in the direction in which the hairs will lie.

A wig base may be made from one or a combination of the following: hair lace, silk gauze, imitation-silk net, nylon, or elastic net. If nylon or elastic net is used it will stretch to fit any head size and will hug the scalp. Silk gauze or imitation silk is used to create a part in the hair to imitate a natural looking hairline. The quality of a handmade hairpiece also depends on how fine the mesh and how many hairs per knot are tied to it. The smaller and the finer the lace the more delicate and the more expensive the hairpiece.

The following information has been included in this chapter because many cancer patients who are in need of a hair prosthesis will inquire as to the construction of a hairpiece. It is therefore important for the clinical esthetician/cosmetologist to have an overall understanding of the methods used.

The hair is attached onto the base by a method called ventilating. It is then tied onto the mesh cap in small sections by hand, a process similar to the method used to make a rug. An instrument called a latchet hook, which looks like a large ventilating needle, is used to perform this procedure. The wig maker uses the latchet hook to pull out one or several hairs at a time from a large bundle of hair. The hair is then hooked onto the needle, and the needle is drawn through the mesh foundation, a knot is tied, and the needle is removed. Knotting the hair into gauze is a very slow and tedious process. It requires a delicate technique in which hairs are drawn individually through another piece of gauze to prevent the knots from being visible. This painstaking method ensures that the ultimate result will be a wig or a hairpiece that looks completely natural. Men's and women's wigs differ in that a man's hairpiece or wig must have ventilation around the front and side edges to appear natural. This is not as important in the construction of a woman's wig because these areas are usually concealed by hair. However, women's wigs can be custom made by a professional wig maker to expose the hairline by incorporating a lace front or a lace insert into the wig. Most hand-tied hairpieces are not made in the United States, but come from Korea and China. Their prices range from $300 to $700 or more.

Handmade Human Wigs
The outside layer of hair is made of a cuticle layer that resembles shingles under a microscope. Before a wig can be made from human hair three procedures must be performed: the cuticles must be removed with an acid wash and scrub, the color must be stripped from the hair, and the hair must be dyed a color that is desirable.

Removing the Cuticle
The process of removing the cuticle involves dipping the hair into muriatic acid, which softens the outside coating of the hair (cuticle). The hair is then gathered into small bundles and brushed by hand to remove layers of the cuticle. The hair is then rinsed in an acid-neutralizing solution. Because Chinese hair is black, the hair must be bleached (decolorized) so that it can be re-colored to a desired shade. After this process has been completed the hair has been weakened because of the chemicals that were used, which generally makes the life expectancy for a human hairpiece worn on a daily basis approximately one year.

The hair is ready to be made into a prosthesis. This is done by dividing it in half, putting it into the mesh, tying it into a knot, and pulling it out into two strands.

This is the process that is used to construct most hand-tied pieces. Occasionally, a hairpiece is made with hair that still has its cuticle. Instead of dividing the hair down the center (in half), it is divided 90 percent verses 10 percent. The wig maker goes into the end of the hairpiece, at the root end, ties the hair, and clips off the tail. This leaves a "beard effect." If you were to run your hands gently over the top of the wig you would experience a stubby feeling. This type of construction is still not as effective as completely removing the cuticle because if you were to wash this type of hairpiece it would matte and tangle at the base.

The Vacuum Fit Wig

Recently a new type of wig has come onto the market. Instead of the traditional mesh base, it has a suction skull cap formed from a soft, pliable, plastic that is molded to fit the wearer's head. The wig is held on the head by a vacuum, which is created by the molded shape. The wig stays secure regardless of weather or activity without pins or tape. Because of the suction cup, patients can brush their hair without the fear of the wig falling off, and can even wear their hair up if they so desire.

This form of hair replacement is an excellent solution for active children; because of the suction cap a secure fit is always guaranteed. The cap can also be replaced for a larger one if a child outgrows it.

It generally takes four months to construct this type of wig, and the cost is approximately $2,500. It can last up to two years, depending on how often it is worn and how well it is cared for.

To custom fit the vacuum cup wig, a plaster mold is taken of the patient's head. The outside perimeter line of the hairpiece is drawn directly onto the patient's scalp using a water transferable pen. A plaster of paris mold is placed directly on the scalp, until it is completely dry. It is then popped off the patient's head, and an exact mold in the shape of the head has been created. From this mold a flexible, pliable, plastic base is made. This is placed on the patient's head, pushing down and back until the air has all escaped, creating a vacuum and forming a suction cup. Once a fit has been established a piece of "skin" is made out of silicone. This skin fits the base exactly and is then tinted to match the patient's scalp.

Hair that is used to make wigs is obtained from hair merchants or hair brokers. Most of the hair is imported through England. The hair must not have been treated. Usually Chinese and Rumanian women grow their hair until it reaches a certain length, at which time they cut it off, or they gather it up over a prolonged period of time from their brushes and save it, until they have collected enough of it to sell to the hair merchants. This is the reason why it is so expensive to have non-processed human hair in a hairpiece or wig.

Once the hair has been sold it is transported to a collection center, where it is cleaned and sorted according to color, length, and cuticle direction. When a wig is going to be made a wig maker specifies a certain hair color and orders it. To make one wig, anywhere from 6 to 8 ounces of hair may be required. Many wigs are eight, ten, and twelve inches in length. The patient who is being fitted for the hairpiece is sent the hair first to examine it and to determine if it is the correct hair color they specified (natural highlights are used for women, and a combination of highlighting and ash tones for men). If the color of the hair and the silicone flesh-colored base is acceptable, then both the base and the hair are sent to Korea where they will made into a custom designed wig.

Once the hair and the silicone scalp arrive in Korea, a wig maker sews in a few hairs at a time to the base, using the ventilating method; this process usually takes about two weeks. Instead of tying the hair to a mesh net and knotting it (the standard method), the hair is poked through the silicone skin and glued underneath. When this process is completed it is glued again to the pliable plastic base, which fits the patient's head. Because of the way in which it is constructed this hairpiece can be easily permed and styled.

Measuring the Wig

Before the right wig can be selected for the patient, his or her head must be measured to insure that the wig will fit properly without being too tight or too loose. See Figure 14-12. The following four measurements will guarantee a good fit.

1. Temple to temple — A cloth tape measure is used to measure the area extending from temple to temple around the back of the neck.

2. Ear to ear — The end of the tape measure is placed by the top of the ear and brought over the top of the head across to the other ear.

3. Hairline to nape of neck — This measurement is taken from the base of the hairline in the front across the top of the head and down to the nape of the neck.

4. Around the head — The distance around the base of the head is measured, starting at the nape of the neck and wrapping the cloth measuring tape in such a way that it completely wraps around the head and the temples, stopping at the top of the hairline.

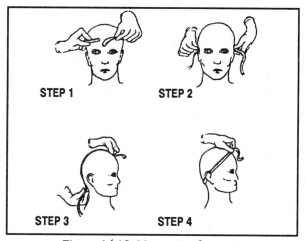

STEP 1   STEP 2

STEP 3   STEP 4

Figure 14-12. Measuring for a wig

Styling

Regardless of the type of wig or hairpiece the patient selects, he or she should have it styled appropriately to complement his or her facial features. It should also balance the proportions of his or her body. This would include thinning it and trimming it and in some instances, if the hair is natural, coloring it. If you are not familiar with styling or coloring wigs, locate an experienced stylist in your area for your patients. This person should have a lot of experience styling both synthetic and real hairpieces — falls, hairpieces, and wigs.

The wig or hairpiece should be styled so it resembles the patient's previous hairstyle. Depending on how the patient feels, changing the patient's image or individual style may not be appropriate. If possible, before the patient begins cancer therapy advise him or her to take a photograph of himself or herself wearing a favorite hairstyle. When and if the patient should need to purchase a wig this picture can communicate the style preferred. The patient should select a wig in a realistic hair length and style. This decision should be based on the amount of time and money required to maintain the wig.

Hair Extensions

Patients who only experience mild hair loss may want to consider wearing hair extensions. Hair extensions can be attached to the natural hair in one of four ways: bonding, braid and sew, individual braids, and weaving. See Figure 14-13. In all techniques hair is added to the patient's own hair. The added hair will have to be re-attached as the patient's own hair grows out (four to eight weeks). However, because hair extensions must be attached to existing hair, they may not be appropriate for patients experiencing a great deal of hair loss. Hair extensions would only be appropriate for filling in thinning areas or small patches of hair loss. Consult an experienced hair extension expert to see if this service would be an appropriate solution for the patient.

(For more information on this subject read *Hair Additions — The Fourth Dimension*, by Charlotte Jayne, Milady Publishing Company, Albany, N.Y.).

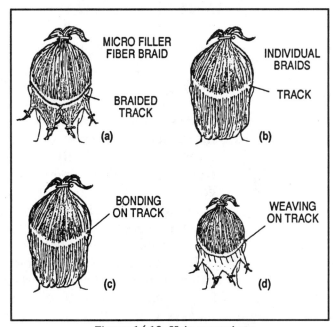

Figure 14-13. Hair extensions

Head Wraps If the patient does not feel comfortable wearing a wig she can wear the following hair replacement alternatives: turbans, scarfs, or hats in a variety of different styles. One company called Designs For Comfort (see directory below for their address and telephone number) manufactures a very special product called a "Headliner."

The company's creative consultant, Kitty Costikyan, designed a hair replacement alternative with her friend Peggy Childs that was originally for cancer patients. The concept for the Headliner was developed when Costikyan lost all her hair during a bout with cancer. She needed something to cover her head during her hospitalization. At the time there were no head coverings available. Recognizing they could fill an unmet need the two women set about to design a special head wrap, a prototype cap with a small hairpiece inserted in the front, which they appropriately called a Headliner, that could be worn as a cover-up for social activities or during hospital stays or even while sleeping. The Headliner is a combination cap and hairpiece (not a substitute for a wig) that is light and comfortable to wear. The Headliner Plus creates an even greater illusion of natural, healthy hair by inserting a second hairpiece in back. The caps are made from soft, washable fabrics and are available in over thirty colors and patterns. The hairpiece is made from a high-grade synthetic fiber that can easily be styled and washed and is available to patients in fourteen common hair shades.

Other hair replacement options are also available to patients. The following section was taken from the book *Beauty and Cancer*, by Diane Doan Noyes and Peggy Mellody, R. N. Published by AC Press, Los Angeles, 1988.

Headwraps

The headwrap is a stylish alternative to a wig, as well as a sensational way to accessorize any ensemble. A headwrap can complement your looks, enhance your style, and add versatility to your wardrobe. See Figure 14-14.

Making headwraps out of scarfs is easy, but takes a little practice. The emphasis should be on color and texture rather than complicated tying techniques. For beginners, it is helpful to purchase a mirror that you can hook around your neck, in order to free both of your hands. This type of mirror can be purchased at most drug stores, variety stores, or beauty supply stores.

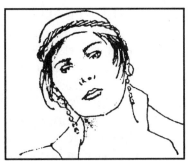

Figure 14-14. A headwrap
*Courtesy Diane Doan Noyes and
Peggy Mellody*

Department stores are filled with a variety of beautiful scarfs, but many are unsuitable for use as a headwrap, especially for women experiencing total hair loss. The following tips should make your selection easier.

- Choose cotton or cotton-blend scarfs. Unlike silk or polyester, these materials will not slip off your head.
- For basic headwraps, choose 26-inch or 28-inch square scarfs. You can use larger squares, up to 32 inches for fancier wraps, and oblongs for headwrap trims.
- Fabric stores' remnant counters are a great source of inexpensive material. To make your own scarf, ask the sales clerk to cut the material into the desired size. Finish edges by turning in fabric to make a 1/4- to 1/2-inch border on all edges; stitch.
- Mix and match contrasting prints and colors by accessorizing with more than one scarf.
- Dress up a headwrap with ribbons, braids, twisted scarfs, hats, berets, or jewelry.
- Wash scarfs according to the manufacturer's directions.

Presented here are the step-by-step directions for a basic headwrap, plus several stylish variations. Once you have mastered these techniques, use your imagination and build on the basics.

Basic Headwrap 1

Step 1   Lay scarf flat; wrong side facing you. Fold scarf into a triangle, leaving one point slightly longer than the other (a & b). See Figure 14-15.

Step 2   Drape scarf over your head with the shorter side on top and points in the back. Pull scarf

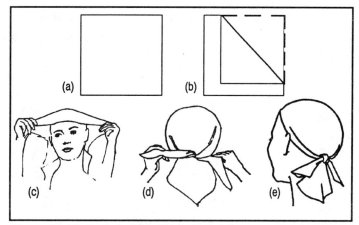

Figure 14-15. Basic headwrap 1. *Courtesy Diane Doan Noyes and Peggy Mellody*

down until about two to three inches above your eyebrows (c).

Step 3   Tie scarf ends in a half-knot behind your head. The flap should be anchored beneath the knot (d).

Step 4   Tie scarf ends into a square knot (e).

Basic Headwrap 2

Step 1   Perform steps 1–3 of Basic Headwrap 1.

Step 2   Using both hands spread lower flap out under half-knot. Try to spread the scarf as close to the back of your ears as possible. If you are experiencing hair loss, this will help conceal that fact (f). See Figure 14-16.

Step 3   Carefully bring flap up over knot and tuck flap and loose ends in behind knot securely (g & h).

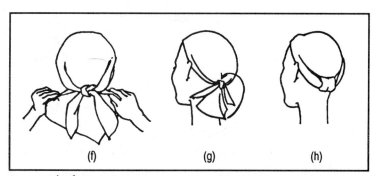

Figure 14-16. Basic headwrap 2. *Courtesy Diane Doan Noyes and Peggy Mellody*

Contrasting Twist Headwrap

Step 1   Follow steps 1–3 outlined in Basic Headwrap 1.

Step 2   See Figure 14-17. Select a second scarf in a contrasting print or color. Lay fabric flat; wrong side towards you. Fold fabric into a triangle (i). Fold top point down to bottom fold (i).

Step 3   Fold top fold to bottom fold (j).

Step 4   Take ends, one in each hand, and twist (k). (For added interest, fold two scarfs separately and twist together.)

Step 5   Place twisted scarf over basic headwrap; tie in a half- knot at back of head (l).

Step 6   Bring ends of headwrap up over both knots; tuck all ends in securely (m).

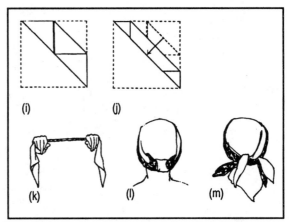

Figure14-17. Contrasting twist headwrap. *Courtesy Diane Doan Noyes and Peggy Mellody*

Basic Side Twist

Step 1   Tie Basic Headwrap 1 as described in steps 1-4, but place the knot over one ear instead of at back of head. See Figure 14-18. Let the ends hang down loose (n). For an interesting touch, add an earring to the opposite ear.

Contrasting Side Twist

Step 1   Tie scarf as described in Basic Side Twist.

Step 2   Twist a second scarf as described in Contrasting Twist steps 1-4.

Step 3   Knot; twist over headwrap above the same ear. Allow ends to hang loose (o). See Figure 14-19.

Basic Headwrap with Hat

Step 1   Tie Basic Headwrap 2 as described in steps 1–3.

Step 2   See Figure 14-20. Add hat of your choice (p).

Side Twist with Hat

Step 1   Tie Basic Side Twist headwrap according to directions.

Step 2   See Figure 14-21. Add hat of your choice, leaving scarf ends dangling at side (q).

Headwrap with Beret

Step 1   Tie Basic Headwrap as described in steps 1-4, but place square knot over one ear instead of a back of head.

Step 2   Add beret, covering knot.

Step 3   See Figure 14-22. Tuck loose scarf ends up into beret (r).

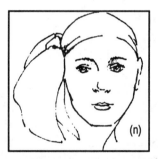
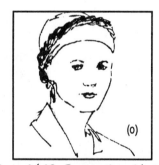

Figure14-18. Basic side twist   Figure14-19. Contrasting side twist
Courtesy Diane Doan Noyes and Peggy Mellody

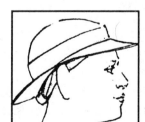
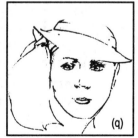
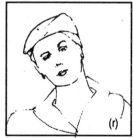

Figure 14-20. Basic   Figure 14-21. Side twist   Figure 14-22.
headwrap with hat   with hat   Headwrap with beret

Courtesy Diane Doan Noyes and Peggy Mellody

The following directory will provide the clinical esthetician/cosmetologist with a list of names and addresses of wig manufacturers and retailers. Write to or call any of the companies listed below for a catalog and a complete price list. Be sure to investigate how long it takes to order a wig and what the refund policy is, should the patient be dissatisfied. Keep this information in your files to share with your patients. You should also contact wig shops and hair replacement centers in your immediate area (the names and telephone numbers of hair replacement centers are listed in your local telephone directory). Find out what they can offer your patients by contacting the center in advance and then paying them a personal visit.

Alkin Hair Co.
264 West 40th St.
New York, NY 10018
(212) 719-3070

> Alkin Hair Company sells hair to cosmetologists and salons for weaving, braiding, hair extensions, and complete wig construction.

American Hairlines
1808 Jerome Ave
Brooklyn, NY 11235
(800) 221-8082
(718) 332-0020

> American Hairlines specializes in medical hair prostheses for men, women, and children. Both the Alopecia Foundation and the Hairloss Council refer patients to this company. They manufacturer wigs in a variety of lengths and styles.

Anna-Mae Products
9251 Orco Parkway, Suite D
Rieverside, CA 92509
(714) 681-8395
(800) 343-9477

> Anna-Mae Products has designed a wig adapter for women with partial or complete hair loss. The adapter creates a natural-looking hairline while cushioning sensitive areas, helping the wig to stay in place without tape or bobby pins. It works with any wig and comes with a 30 day money back guarantee.

Designs For Comfort, Inc.
P.O. Box 8229
2156 New Willow Road
Northfield, IL 60093
(800) 443-9226
(708) 446-9190 in Illinois and Canada
FAX# (708) 446-9224
> Wig alternatives are their specialty (refer to the section in this chapter on head wraps).

Edith Imre
8 West 56th Street
New York, NY 10024
(212) 758-0233
> This company specializes in supplying hair prostheses for patients who suffer from hair loss, chemotherapy, radiation, surgery, disease, or genetic causes.

Eva Gabor International
55 W. 39th St
New York, NY 10018
(800) 223-9812
> Eva Gabor is one of the largest manufacturers of ready made synthetic wigs in the country. The telephone number listed is their national sales office. When you call, tell the operator your patient's zip code and they will immediately refer you to the nearest retail outlet in the area.

Louis Feder/Joseph Fleisher
14 East 38th Street
New York, NY 10016
(212) 686-7701
> Custom-made from design to completion, all wigs for men and women are made from Italian hair. Their innovative designs have been acclaimed by *Vogue, Town & Country,* the fashion world, and Hollywood.

Jacques Darcel
50 West 57th Street
New York, NY 10019
(212) 753-7576
> This company offers a complete selection of wigs, which includes synthetic and human hair hand-tied wigs, hair pieces, and semi- custom (pre-made wigs custom styled for the patient), toupees for men, as well

as wig-care products such as special shampoos and conditioners. The patient can contact the company directly to order a brochure. They will also color match the patient's real hair to their new wig or hairpiece by mail.

Knight & Day Hair Products, Inc.
P.O. Box 849
Corte Madera, CA 94925
(800) 333-8018

Knight & Day Hair Products manufactures an undetectable, custom-made, vacuum fit hair replacement for patients with alopecia areata, chemotherapy, burns, and pattern baldness. "More Hair" creates the illusion of natural hair growth and scalp. Wigs are made from 100 percent human hair.

Lugo Hair Center, Ltd.
20 Synder Ave
Brooklyn, NY 11226
(718) 284-0370
(800) 348-2379

Lugo Hair Center supplies different textures of hair for weaving and braiding to beauticians and to the general public that require hair for weaving. They specialize in both Afro and European hair.

Nisus Concepts, Inc. or *Girouard Hairgoods*
2315 Fairplay Drive 9401 W. Beloit Rd. 305
Loveland, CO 80538 Milwaukee, WI 53227
(303) 667-9465 (414) 327-6050

The company produces Headliner and Kairfree (identical products), a state-of-the-art cranial prostheses custom made for the wearer's head. A specialized mold of the patient's scalp is made, creating a vacuum base which fits his or her head like a second skin and is comfortably held in place by suction, thus eliminating tape completely. Human, synthetic, hand tied, or wefted wigs can be interchanged at will.

Rene of Paris
15551 Cabrito Road
Van Nuys, CA 91406
(818) 376-1300
(800) 528-5678

patient can write or call their toll free number directly for a brochure.

Top Priority
174 Fifth Ave.
New York, NY 10011
(212) 206-6785

Top Priority specializes in wigs for chemotherapy, head trauma, and alopecia patients. In fact, they received so many referrals from physicians that they were able to obtain their own major medical provider number, which makes it easier for patients to file a medical claim with their insurance carrier to reimburse the purchase of their hair prosthesis. They custom design full and partial wigs for men, women, and children who experience hair loss due to medical problems. They use a special type of synthetic hair, which they developed in France, called "Ultra Hair," to construct their full wigs and hair pieces. They also copy the patient's previous hairstyle before their hair loss. Their wigs are lightweight and comfortable.

Mail Order Wig Companies

Wigs by Paula
21 Bristol
South Easton, MA 02375
(800) 343-9695 for ordering a brochure or a wig by mail
(800) 472-4017 for any additional information

The Wig Company
P.O. Box 12950
Pittsburgh, PA 15241
(800) 245-6288
(412) 221-4790

This convenient mail order company offers a complete selection of synthetic wigs and hair replacement accessories. Call or write for a free catalogue. Personal shopping advisers are on hand to answer any questions your patient may have and to help patients select the right wig and style. The Wig Company offers an unconditional guarantee, which means that a patient can return a wig for a different style or color.

Wilshire Wigs
13213 Saticyo St.

N. Hollywood, CA 91605
(800) 927-0814
FAX # (818) 982-2416

Wilshire Wigs has been supplying wigs to the entertainment industry and the general public for over twenty-five years. They have a wide selection of ready-made wigs for women, men, and children. They have over 6,000 sq ft of hair goods with over 800 different styles and 40 different hair colors of each of their 800 styles on display. In addition to both their ready-made synthetic and human hair wigs they also custom make wigs to order. Facial prostheses (eyelashes, eyebrows, mustaches, beards, and sideburns) are also available or can be custom made, and Wilshire Wigs repairs hairpieces as well.

SKIN CARE

Any number of the following skin disorders can result from cancer therapies: severe dryness, edema (swelling), erythema (redness), hyperpigmentation, hypopigmentation, radiation burns, possible skin cancer from radiation treatments, and increased photosensitivity. The patient's reaction will vary depending on the types of medication and therapies he or she is being treated with. Most of these side effects disappear within four to six weeks after the patient's last cancer treatment. Appointments, regardless of the aesthetic service that is to be performed, should not be scheduled for patients for a week to two weeks after the patient's last chemotherapy treatment, and not until the patient's white blood cell count recovers.

Helping the Patient Care for His or Her Skin

Statistics show that two-thirds of all patients diagnosed with cancer want to participate in their own recovery process by actively involving themselves in their rehabilitation. Although patients with cancer lose some control, washing and grooming are important everyday activities that the patient still will have control over. Most patients will be eager to learn new ways with which to maintain appearance.

The clinical esthetician/cosmetologist can advise the patient on the proper use of cosmetics and the right skin-care routine. A healthy complexion is an important part of the patient's appearance. The following recommendations may be made to patients to help them care for their skin on a daily basis.

Suggest mild, non-greasy, fragrance-free, sensitive, skin-care products. The patient should be advised not to re-dip into cosmetic containers. If at all possible the patient should use skin-care preparations that are packaged in tubes to prevent cross contamination.

Keep the patient's skin-care regimen simple — the fewer products the patient has to use the less likely he or she is to have a negative skin response. A cleanser, a gentle toner, and a moisturizer, along with a sunscreen or sunblock with an SPF of 15 or more, is all the patient really needs.

Caution the patient to avoid using harsh cleansing agents, or any skin-care product with alcohol, as that may dry out the skin.

Washcloths or complexion brushes are too rough for the skin and therefore should not be used by the patient because they will cause irritation.

Many patients after undergoing radiation or chemotherapy treatments, regardless of their skin type, experience some level of surface skin dryness. Some patients even develop open sores. If you encounter a patient with dryness that is this severe, recommend immediately seeking medical assistance because an open sore could easily become infected.

Chemotherapy patients will sometimes experience mild skin flaking caused by the rapid turnover of skin cells. The result is a thinner skin surface, which is more prone to dryness. Certain anticancer drugs (Adriamycin, Busulfan, Chlorambucil, Methotrexate) also contribute to dry, itchy, flaky skin. Daily use of emollient creams and lotions is recommended for dryness. A variety of effective products are available, both cosmetic and dermatologic, to help soothe and alleviate the discomfort caused by dryness. Suggest skin-care products that are fragrance free with simple, basic, ingredients because they will cause less irritation.

At-Home Skin Care

Cleansing Instructions

Urge the patient to replace his or her regular cleansing soap with a creamy, gentle cleanser. Recommend that patients wash their hands before cleansing their face. Instruct patients to use only tepid water. Overscrubbing the skin will cause irritation; be sure to tell the patient to use a gentle massaging action. The cleanser should never remain on the skin for very long. Tell the patient to be sure to rinse thoroughly; residue left behind on the surface of the skin can cause redness, stinging, and may lead to dryness. After the patient's skin has been rinsed clean, suggest that he or she pat it dry. Patting is easier on the skin than vigorous rubbing.

Advise the patient to use cleansing lotion not just on the face, but all over the body. Excessive bathing and harsh detergent soaps can exacerbate dryness; caution the patient against their use. In addition advise patients to reduce the number of baths and showers they take. Extreme water temperatures (hot or cold) should also be avoided. Recommend that the patient only use lukewarm water for bathing or rinsing.

Restoring the pH to the Skin

A toner is the final step in the cleansing routine; it makes the skin feel fresher and cleaner, and it also helps to remove more of the stratum corneum cells. A toner without alcohol can be applied to the face and neck immediately after cleansing. Aloe juice has been shown to relieve irritation and reduce inflammation, and the citric acid in lemon when mixed with water (1 part lemon juice to 7 parts water) has excellent astringent properties and yet will not overdry the skin.

Moisturizing

Lubricating the skin with a moisturizing cream or lotion will seal in precious moisture. If the patient is experiencing some dryness, a cream will provide a better barrier of protection than will a light lubricating lotion. Suggest that the patient moisturize the skin immediately after cleansing and toning. To trap surface moisture into the skin recommend that the patient hydrate his or her skin first by lightly splashing water on it or by spritzing it with a spray mist of mineral or rose water before applying cream. Before the patient retires at night he or she should apply a nourishing night cream to his or her skin by massaging it in gently. A patient can also place a humidifier in the bedroom at night, which will help increase moisture in the air, preventing surface dryness.

Daily Sun Protection Is Required

The use of sunscreens and sunblocks (with a SPF of at least 15) should be applied daily by the patient to prevent sunburn. Be careful about recommending moisturizers with sunscreens; they usually do not provide enough protection. Patients will require a full strength sun shield (a sunscreen with an SPF of 15 or higher or a total sunblock). Also remind the patient to wear protective clothing when outdoors.

Weekly Skin Treatment Recommendations
The patient should be advised not to use grainy scrubs because they cause too much friction and can irritate sensitive skin. If the patient's skin is acne-prone, he or she can use a mud masque up to two times a week. If the patient's skin is sensitive and tends to be dry, recommend a mild cream or gel masque, and advise him or her to use it no more than twice a month.

Skin Care for Patients Undergoing Radiotherapy

When a patient is undergoing radiation treatments, he or she is advised to use only tepid water to cleanse the area being treated. The patient is instructed to allow the water to run over the area and told to pat, not rub, the skin dry. The patient must not scrub or scratch the site. Brushes and washcloths should not be used for cleansing the skin because of the coarse texture. All cleansing creams, toners, moisturizers, sunscreens, cosmetics, and powders (particularly talcum powder because it contains an abrasive) must be approved by the patient's physician first. In most instances patients are instructed not to apply any cosmetics or skin-care products on or around the treated area for up to three weeks after their last treatment.

How to Respond to the Patient's Skin-Care Questions

If a patient should ask you a question about skin care that you do not know the answer to, admit to the patient that you are not certain and offer to check into it. Assure the patient that you will respond as soon as possible. When in doubt about any aspect of a patient's treatment always confer with his or her physician.

EDEMA

Certain medications (such as steroids) will cause swelling and puffiness in facial tissues, creating puffiness under the eyes. The following suggestions can be offered to patients to help control edema. To reduce puffiness around the eye area, suggest that the patient elevate his or her head slightly at night while sleeping with pillows. This will prevent fluid from accumulating under the eyes and will allow it to drain through the sinuses. A plastic eye mask or a five- to ten-minute application of cold, moistened, cotton compresses (soaked in ice water or milk) will help reduce swelling temporarily. Cosmetics can also be skillfully applied to camouflage facial puffiness (see chapter on cosmetic therapy — contouring). Makeup techniques such as highlighting and shading will temporarily minimize the appearance of swollen facial features.

ERYTHEMA

Erythema (redness) and rashes are common side effects of radiation treatments and chemotherapy. Medications such as Actinomycin D, Bleomycin, and Mithramycin sometimes perpetrate allergies that result in skin irritations. If the patient is undergoing radiotherapy neither heat or cold should be used on or near the irritated area, including warm or cold compresses, electric heading pads, or infrared light therapy on treated areas.

RADIATION BURNS

Every patient who is treated with radiotherapy will experience different levels of sensitivity, depending on the type of tissue treated and the amount of radiation administered. Since the radiation dose must be strong enough to destroy cancer cells, it can also damage surrounding healthy tissue. This treatment may end in permanent injury to the surrounding areas, causing painful skin burns. Some patients, usually three weeks after the first treatment, may appear sunburned or their skin reddened. The skin may blister or crack in the treated area. Many of these skin reactions are temporary and will reverse after the patient's treatments have ceased. The skin may appear rough and may peel, leaving some residual redness. Cosmetic therapy can conceal long-lasting erythema but should not be considered until the patient's cell count has recovered. For more severe scarring caused by radiation burns, the use of collagen can in some instances make a substantial cosmetic improvement in the appearance of scar tissue (see chapters on dermatology and plastic surgery).

CHANGES IN SKIN TONE

The side effects from cancer therapies, such as radiation and chemotherapy, can cause changes in the patient's skin tone. A patient may lose skin pigment because of the body's reaction to certain medications, or he or she may develop light pink or brown patches on areas of skin exposed to radiation, similar to sunburn, age spots, or melasma. Other forms of discoloration can also appear on the skin as bands or stripes. Most of the pigmentary problems patients experience will resolve once cancer treatments have stopped. Discoloration that is caused by changes in melanin will fade over a period of six to twelve months after the patient's last treatment. Pigment can sometimes be lightened with a bleaching solution prescribed by a dermatologist; however, if the pigmentary changes were caused by the patient's reaction to large dosages of chemotherapy, it is unlikely that these areas will diminish. Fortunately, both hyperpigmentation and hypopigmentation can be easily camouflaged cosmetically with special opaque cover creams (see chapters on dermatology and cosmetic therapy).

PHOTOSENSITIVITY

Radiation and medication increases the patient's chances of photosensitivity. Patients who have had radiation treatments or those who are taking chemotherapeutic drugs (especially Methotrexate, Dacarbazine, 5-Fluorouracil, or Vinblastine) must be extra careful to protect their skin from phototoxicity (exaggerated sunburn reaction). Even after their cancer treatments have ceased patients are cautioned by their physicians to continue to protect their skin. Pigmentation is also intensified by exposure to the sun. Be sure to remind the patient to use a sunscreen with an SPF of 15 or higher as well as a lip protector with a sunscreen in it, to keep lips from drying out, cracking, and bleeding.

SKIN CANCER

Cancer patients who have undergone radiation treatments must be particularly alert to skin irregularities since they are extremely vulnerable to skin cancer. Always be attentive to any notable signs of skin cancer such as moles that have changed color, that have irregular borders, that crust or bleed, or that itch or are tender. If you encounter any irregularities, recommend that the patient have the area in question examined by a physician immediately.

SKIN-CARE TREATMENTS AND FACIAL PREPARATIONS

As long as the patient's physician does not object, there is no reason why the patient cannot have a professional skin-care treatment. A professional facial that includes a massage can help soothe surface dryness, improve circulation, and restore color tone to the patient's complexion. Facials can also relax patients and help to relieve some of their stress.

Because cancer patients are so susceptible to bacteria, all products used in skin-care treatments must be as bacteria-free as possible. The best way to ensure that the patient will not be at risk is to use skin-care preparations that are packaged in tubes.

You can also prevent the patient from coming in contact with bacteria by preparing natural skin-care treatments specifically for his or her facial treatment. There are definite advantages to doing this; the patient will not have to worry about cosmetic contamination, harsh preservatives, or fragrances that could cause skin allergies. These are all very serious considerations since after undergoing chemo- or radiation therapy cancer patients tend to have very sensitive skin. Sensitivity can lead to skin irritation, resulting in a rash. A rash will make the skin tender, raw, and vulnerable to scratches or surface cracks (fissures), which can easily become infected. When performing any type of skin-care treatment on a patient, use a gentle touch, and avoid using any type of cosmetic that might produce friction. Irritation to the skin is potentially harmful because of the patient's increased infection susceptibility.

Extreme caution should be taken to avoid any area that is broken open (such as a scratch, abrasion, or blisters on or around the mouth area). The patient's immune system is not functioning properly and cannot fight off infection; therefore the patient is extremely vulnerable to surface bacteria; the slightest scratch could easily become infected. Be especially cautious of blisters around the patient's mouth. Many patients who have undergone cancer treatments are susceptible to mouth sores. Herpes virus is often present at the site of infection, and you could very easily become infected yourself.

FACIAL TREATMENTS

The following are suggestions for natural skin-care preparations. There is no guarantee, however, that fruits and vegetables are any less allergenic than cosmetic preparations, especially if the patient is sensitive to a specific ingredient in a homemade preparation. Always make sure that you question the patient about any allergies he or she may have before you begin the facial treatment.

All the supplies you will need for your facial preparations can be obtained at a health food store or a pharmacy. Skin-care preparations should be made in advance, the same day as the appointment, and safely stored in the refrigerator to preserve freshness.

Make sure that all your utensils are cleaned and sterilized before using them for preparations. Discard the remainder of any treatment products that are left over from the patient's facial; they cannot be salvaged because there is nothing in them to preserve their freshness.

Preparing Natural Cosmetics

The following preparations are suggested to relieve surface dryness; their action is always gentle and soothing.

GENTLE YOGURT AND ALOE CLEANSER
Ingredients:
>An ounce to two ounces fresh plain yogurt
>or fresh liquid yogurt (keifer)
>1 T. or more Aloe gel

To apply:
>Thoroughly incorporate the gel with the yogurt by mixing. Apply to the patient's skin in the same manner as you would any creamy cleansing solution, warming it up in your hands first and then massaging it gently onto the skin. After a few minutes remove it with disposable warm moistened cotton wool squares.

PH BALANCING FACIAL TONER
Ingredients:
>2 T. apple cider vinegar in 6 oz. glass of mineral water.

To apply:
>Put mixture in a container with a spray nozzle and place in the refrigerator; when you are ready to use shake well, spray onto the patient's skin, and gently blot off excess moisture with a clean, dry, cotton square.

LEMON FACIAL TONER
Ingredients:
>1/8 cup fresh squeezed lemon juice
>7/8 cup mineral water
>Put mixture in a spray bottle and shake before spraying on to the patient's skin.

PAPAYA ENZYME FACE PEEL

Papaya contains the enzyme papain, and pineapple contains the enzyme bromelin. Both dissolve keratin, which is why they are used frequently as ingredients in peeling lotions and facial masks. For years cosmetic surgeons have been recommending that their patients rub fresh papaya onto their skin after facial rejuvenation surgery, because papaya acts as a natural exfoliant.

Ingredients:

2 ounces mashed, fresh papaya or pineapple
1 tsp. honey
1/2 tsp. fresh lemon juice

To apply:

Mix all the ingredients together in a bowl. Cover the eyes with cool, moistened cotton pads soaked in water or camomile tea. Brush the peel onto the face and neck. Turn on facial vaporizer and direct the warm, humid mist toward the patient's face at a distance of 16 to 18 inches. The honey in the peel will bind moisture to the surface of the skin and hydrate it, while the papaya or pineapple dissolves away the dead skin cells. After 5 to 8 minutes turn off vaporizer and wipe off the peel with disposable moistened cotton wool pads and apply a mask.

MILK MASK FOR DRY SKIN

1/4 cup powdered milk
1 tsp. wheat germ oil
2 T. plain yogurt
1 tsp. aloe gel

Mix all the ingredients together in a bowl until they turn into a paste. Brush the mask onto the patient's face, taking care to avoid the eye area. Leave on for 10 to 15 minutes and remove with cotton squares saturated with warm water. Follow up the mask treatment with a light spray of the pH face conditioner and complete the treatment by applying a cream moisturizer.

The following books will supply the clinical esthetician/cosmetologist with additional recipes for natural skin-care treatments.

Jeanne Rose's Kitchen Cosmetics, Panjandrum Aris Books, San Francisco.

Cosmetics from the Earth, by Roy Genders. Alfred van der Marck Editions, New York.

The Medically Based No-Nonsense Beauty Book, by Deborah Chase. Alfred A. Knopf, New York.

Draping the Patient for the Facial

If the patient is wearing a wig, he or she may wish to remove it before the facial treatment begins, and may not want to be seen without it. To prevent patients who are suffering from temporary hair loss from feeling self-conscious or uncomfortable, place a head drape right next to the facial gown so that the patient can put it on without your assistance.

The Facial

The following information is designed to guide you through the the facial.

1. Place wet, warm face towels over the patient's face.

2. Remove the towels and brush on the yogurt cleanser or pour a milky cleanser into the palm of your hand. Gently apply the creamy cleanser by spreading it onto the patient's face, neck, and shoulder areas.

3. Steaming hydrates the skin by adding moisture and cleanses the skin naturally. Use a misting device that dispenses warm (not hot) steam vapor at the face. Adjust the facial steamer at a comfortable distance from the patient's face (at least 12 to 18 inches).

4. Turn the steamer on. Using light, circular, outward movements, massage the cleaning lotion in around the shoulders, up and around the throat, over the chin, around the mouth, over both sides of the jaw, up and across the bridge of the nose, over the sides of the cheeks, around the eye area, between the eyes, onto the forehead, and outward toward the temples .

5. Gently remove the cleanser with warm cotton-wool pads soaked in warm water.

6. Cover the patient's eyes with cotton compresses, and apply the papaya peel or a gentle enzyme peel by brushing or spreading it onto the face and throat with your hands.

7. With the peel on, allow the patient to relax under the warm steam for three to five minutes.

8. Completely remove the peel with warm cotton wool pads moistened with water.

9. Wrap the patient's face in warm towels again to prepare it for massage.

10. A brief facial massage is good at this point, but use a light touch. A non-greasy lubricant should be used if the patient has oily skin. This step should be omitted from the facial treatment completely if the patient has acne-prone skin. For extremely dry and scaly skin, you can massage oil onto the face, neck, and shoulder areas, but make sure it is not fragranced (refer to the chapter on burns — skin-care section). Massage the patient's shoulders, clavicle, throat, chin area, cheeks, bridge of the nose, around the eyes, and forehead.

11. Wrap the patient's face and shoulders in the warm towels again, then gently remove the oil from the skin with moistened cotton squares.

12. Cover the patient's eyes with cotton compresses, apply the milk mask to the patient's face and throat, and leave on for fifteen minutes. The mask will form a barrier between the skin and the environment and will lock in moisture.

13. Remove the mask with warm cotton wool pads.

14. Spray a gentle toner onto the patient's face, neck, and shoulders.

15. Gently massage in a light lubricating lotion.

COSMETIC CAMOUFLAGE

Cosmetics can be used by the patient to conceal uneven pigmentation, broken capillaries, or to disguise surgical scaring. Remember, the area along or around the suture line must be completely healed before it can be camouflaged with cosmetics.

To prevent the possibility of infection, all cosmetic applicators used on the patient during treatment must be disposable. Cotton swab cosmetic applicators can be used to apply eye shadows, powder blusher can be applied with cotton squares or cotton balls, and cream rouge with a disposable cosmetic sponge.

You should refrain from using mascara on a patient with cancer, and you should discourage the patient from using it. Water-proof mascara can be irritating to the eyes, and even water-based mascaras (which are considered the least sensitizing) can easily become contaminated with bacteria, posing a threat to the cancer patient. Recommend instead that the patient curl her eyelashes and wear a soft shade of pencil-type eyeliner to define and draw attention to her eyes. A pencil liner can be easily disinfected by sharpening it. Once it has been sharpened, exposed eyeliner is removed, diminishing the risk of contamination.

COSMETIC THERAPY AFTER RADIOTHERAPY

If the patient's skin is about to blister or crack, advise him or her to seek medical care at once. Under no circumstances should the clinical esthetician/cosmetologist attempt to apply cosmetics to an open area of skin or to an area that is obviously red and inflamed. Instead, the patient should be advised to report all skin irritations to his or her physician since a rash could be an indication of an adverse reaction to medication. If the patient's skin irritation persists or becomes more severe, his or her physician will most likely want to substitute his or her medication. Generally, most redness and skin rashes disappear anywhere from four to six weeks after the last cancer treatment.

CORRECTING DISCOLORATION

Skin discoloration is one of the most common side effects of cancer therapy. Some of the medications patients must take have been known to cause photosensitivity, especially if the patient is exposed to the sun. Sun overexposure while on cancer drugs can trigger or worsen changes in skin color. The areas most frequently affected are the face, the backs of the hands, nails and the nail beds, elbows, and the creases in the body. Much of this uneven pigmentation can easily be camouflaged with cosmetics.

A patient's skin may become pale, sallow, ruddy, or may turn what many physicians refer to as bronzy color. Color correctors can be applied under a sheer makeup base as a makeup primer to correct skin discoloration. Red undertones can be concealed by a green color corrector, and yellow undertones can be camouflaged by a lavender or mauve color corrector.

A creamy, whipped (light textured), water-in-oil-base foundation can be applied over a rich moisturizer and a color primer to minimize the appearance of surface dryness. Eliminating the appearance of dryness will make the foundation appear less obvious. When applying foundation over the color corrector make sure that you first wait for the makeup primer to completely dry. To speed up the setting process apply a light coating of translucent powder over the primer before covering it with foundation. To apply, use a clean sponge, gently pressing the foundation into the skin by dabbing it over the color primer. Start by applying it sparingly, make sure to blend out the edges; if necessary you can always repeat the process and add more coverage.

If your patient is a young child, an adolescent, or a man, correct skin discoloration by applying a translucent bronze powder directly over the facial area. Translucent bronze powder is easy to use and more acceptable to these patients. The powder will camouflage the unevenness of the skin tone and at the same time will add a hint of healthy color to the patient's complexion. Began by scraping a small amount of the powder off the powder cake with a spatula. Place the loose powder in your hand, and dip a clean powder brush into it. Test the strength of the application by dabbing the brush first on the back of your hand. Dust any remaining powder lightly onto the patient's forehead and out toward the temples, working your way down the nose and across the cheeks, and distributing it evenly over both ears, on the chin, onto the jaw area, and onto the neck. Be sure to instruct the patient to repeat the application exercise until he or she can confidently apply the powder without it being detectable.

A very sheer skin stain such as a bronzing gel could also be used to discreetly correct uneven skin tone. This form of cosmetic complexion color is excellent for patients who are plagued with problematic skin conditions such as acne.

Powder blushers and creme rouges can also be used to restore complexion color, but the application of any cosmetic coloring agent used on the facial area must produce a natural appearance and not look artificial. The most effective way to prevent an unnatural result is to make an assessment of the patient's skin type beforehand in order to determine what consistency of coloring agent (powder blusher or creme rouge) should be used. If the patient has dry, mature skin, apply a creamy rouge or light mousse over the foundation and use a light application of loose face powder to set. If the patient's skin is oily or acne-prone use a powder blusher by applying it over the final application of setting powder. Choose a setting powder that has a high concentration of talc in it to help reduce surface shine.

Peach, terracotta, or brick shades will warm up ashy, gray undertones in the skin; soft pinks or corals will help to correct sallow, yellow undertones. If you are working on a patient with a dark complexion be sure to use a color with a lot of depth to it. It is important to evenly match the value of the patient's skin tone, or the colored blusher you select will make the patient's complexion look washed out. Choosing too dark a shade will create too much of a contrast and will end up making the complexion look even paler. Patients with fair skin, for example, should use either soft peach or light pink blush shades, whereas dark complexioned patients should apply deeper shades such as brick, terracotta, or coral. Face color should be applied to cheekbones, forehead, and chin.

For patients with acne, or for extremely active children, gel stains provide a nice alternative to a powdered coloring agent because the gel stains the skin temporarily and is not rubbed off as easily, so it will remain on the skin longer.

TRAUMATIC SCARRING

Sometimes it may have been necessary for surgery to be performed to remove the cancer, leaving the patient with some highly visible scars. Several techniques can be used to cosmetically conceal incision marks or to draw attention away from scarring. For additional information on the therapeutic cosmetic approach to any of these problems see the chapter on cosmetic therapy.

COSMETIC THERAPY FOR MASTECTOMY PATIENTS WITH BREAST RECONSTRUCTION

Eighty percent of female cancer patients who have mastectomies are excellent candidates for breast reconstruction. Although surgery restores the shape of the breast so that the patient does not have to wear a prosthesis, it does not make the breast look as it did before the patient's cancer surgery. The breast is usually left scarred with incision lines, and the nipple looks as if it has been reconstructed.

Two operations are performed to reconstruct the breast. In the first operation an incision is made by a surgeon between the skin and the muscles, and an implant is inserted. The nipple of the breast, however, is not immediately replaced. It is reconstructed several months later in a second operation. The surgeon attaches grafted skin, generally taken from a donor site behind the ear or from the labia, to the reconstructed breast (see plastic surgery chapter).

Cosmetic therapy can be used to normalize the appearance of the nipple graft. An artist's flat brush (a # 6 or a # 8) can be used to outline the areola with a light brown or tan cover cream, and the areola can be shaded with a rose or mauve shade cover cream to match the color of the other nipple.

Incision scars can be easily camouflaged with a thick, opaque application of a cover cream that matches the skin tone of the breast. To camouflage a scar, apply cover cream directly into the hair-line scar, feathering out the edges with a cosmetic sponge. If the scar is hypertrophic (red and raised) apply a slightly deeper shade of cover cream over the raised area and a paler shade of cover cream to the flat area around it. You can lighten up the original cover cream shade by tinting it until it is lighter in value.

Remember that the patient must view the scar from the same angle in which you are concealing it, or the color will appear incorrect. Ask the patient to view her breast in a full-length mirror, or have her hold a hand mirror to evaluate the result of the cosmetic therapy. The corrective cover should provide coverage for several days, especially if the patient's skin tends to be dry. Although the cover cream is waterproof, it can still rub off, so advise the patient to check the area periodically and touch it up if necessary.

Micropigmentation is also an excellent solution for restoring permanent color to the nipple graft. The areola (the round, pigmented area that surrounds the nipple) can be outlined and filled in to match the nipple on the other breast by permanently tattooing the areola. This tattooing is micropigmentation (see chapter on micropigmentation).

CARING FOR THE NAILS

You will need to take into account several clinical factors that can affect cancer patients when you are thinking about nail care: slow re-growth cycle, malformation of the nails, the possibility of bacterial infection, pigmentary problems, and nail fragility.

Slow Re-growth Cycle

Because the growth of the nail is influenced by nutrition and the healthy condition of the body, cancer, chemotherapy, and radiation treatments can greatly affect the growth of the cancer patient's nails. Blood vessels supply nourishment to this area for the continued growth of the nail. If a person is in poor health or suffering from the side effects of medical treatments or medication, it can retard the growth of the nails.

Malformation of the Nails

If the nail does not receive the proper nourishment, it may become poorly shaped, with wavy ridges or furrows due to uneven nail development. To minimize the ridges and furrows, recommend buffing the nails slightly with pumice powder to smooth out these nail depressions.

Infection

The most important consideration of the clinical esthetician/cosmetologist should be the possibility of infection in or around the nail area. If you are performing a manicure or pedicure on a patient make sure that all your implements are thoroughly disinfected. Disinfect your work space and wash and sanitize your hands before you begin the treatment. ISAGel lotion hand gel by Sween Corporation, North Mankato, Minnesota 56001, (800) 533-0464, or Instant Hand Sanitizer by Cinema Secrets, Inc., Burbank, California 91505, (818) 846-0579, is a gel solution that can be used prior to manicuring treatments to disinfect your hands.

Appointments for professional manicures or pedicures should only be scheduled when the patient has the ability to fight off infection, and not immediately after radiation or chemotherapy treatments. Generally two to three weeks is required for the patient to restore his or her white blood count. If any area of the skin is punctured during the manicure or pedicure procedure an infection is likely to result; for this reason removal of the cuticle is not recommended. If hangnails are present, advise the patient to abstain from peeling off the loose skin around the nail. Picking could result in a tear in the skin, which could become an open wound that may result in infection.

Pigmentary Problems

The side effects of cancer therapies and the influence of strong medications, although rare, can cause nail discoloration, making the nails appear darker. A colored nail polish will camouflage nail plate discoloration, and a special nail treatment referred to as a french manicure will help to normalize nail pigmentation on children and men.

Nail Fragility

Chemotherapy can cause the nails to become brittle. When the free edge of the nail becomes weak the nail can crack, tear, flake, and in some instances may break off painfully. To prevent this from occurring recommend professional hot oil manicures or paraffin hand treatments (gauze strips dipped in warm, herbal wax; see chapter on burns, the skin-care section) to soothe and moisturize the nails. Nightly nail soaks in warm water and applications of either cuticle cream or cuticle oil massaged onto the nails and around the cuticle afterward will help correct brittle nails and dry cuticles. Recommend that the patient wear protective rubber gloves when performing housework.

Caution patients to avoid using alcohol-based polish removers. They are too harsh and can cause nails to split. Instead recommend that patients use a creamy nail polish remover that contains lanolin to remove old nail polish.

To strengthen the nails, suggest that patients file their nails slightly round at the tips but leave the corners square. This will prevent the nails from breaking quite so easily. Special nail polishes and nail hardeners will provide a protective coating over the patient's nails to help strengthen them. Nail polishes that contain nylon fibers will support and protect nails. The patient should apply as many coats as necessary to build up a protective shield on the nail. They can be purchased at a pharmacy or a beauty supply store.

Artificial Nails

Artificial plastic nails are not an appropriate camouflage solution for cancer patients because they further damage the nail bed by causing severe dryness, because of the strong possibility that the patient could contract a fungal or a bacterial infection from the use of unsterilized implements, and because of the adhesive (acrylic glue), which is used to adhere the artificial nail to the nail bed, and is a known allergen. If the liquid should come in contact with the patient's skin it could cause an allergic reaction such as contact dermatitis.

CLOTHING ALTERNATIVES

A person's outward presentation is a testament to his or her inner feeling and emotions. With the assistance of a clinical esthetician/cosmetologist the cancer patient can select clothing that will express his or her positive traits and will create in the minds of outside observers moods and emotions in harmony with what he or she intends.

COLOR

Color is an important tool that patients can skillfully incorporate into their look to normalize their appearance. Studies have proven that color has a powerful effect on the human psyche. A careful selection of the right wardrobe colors (bright, vibrant, pure colors) will help the patient appear healthier, whereas dull or dark colors will make the patient's features look drawn and his or her complexion pale. Suggest that the patient refrain from wearing dark colors or neutrals such as gray, dark brown, navy blue, or black next to the skin; these shades can drain the skin of its natural color and will make the patient look pale. Instead, recommend that the patient wear bright touches of color next to his or her face to counterbalance the severity of darker shades. The influence of cheerful colors around the patient will also lift his or her spirits.

WEIGHT FLUCTUATION

As with any serious illness severe weight loss can result. Cancer therapies could influence the patient's body weight in either direction, causing weight loss or weight gain. Radiation treatments, for example, can cause nausea, which can result in the patient experiencing a temporary loss in appetite, promoting weight loss, while chemotherapy treatments may cause a patient to gain weight, anywhere from eight to ten pounds. After a mastectomy, weight gain is considered part of the recovery process. The clinical esthetician/cosmetologist can help the patient conceal weight gain or loss and visibly correct body proportions with the illusion of color, fabric texture, and style design. Horizontal prints will make the patient's body frame appear wider and will create the illusion of weight gain, while vertical prints will create the illusion of length.

RE-IMAGE COUNSELING FOR POST-MASTECTOMY PATIENTS

The type of cancer surgery the patient will undergo will depend on the extent of cancer found. One or both breasts may be affected. If the cancer is localized, the surgeon may try to save the breast by performing a lumpectomy (removal of the cancerous lump and the adjacent underarm lymph nodes through excision), but if the cancer has spread a complete mastectomy (removal of breast tissue) may be required. There are three types of mastectomies: simple, modified, and radical. A simple mastectomy removes only the breast, leaving the axillary lymph nodes and the breast muscles. A modified mastectomy is a surgical procedure that requires the removal of the entire breast and the axillary lymph nodes, and a radical mastectomy involves the excision of not only breast tissue but the underlying breast muscles as well.

The purpose of wearing a breast prosthesis is to create symmetry by correcting figure problems. It is used to fill out the line of a garment. If cancer was removed from only one breast the term unilateral (affecting only one side) is used to describe involvement; bilateral pertains to both breasts, and reconstruction refers to the reassembly of a breast such as the replacement of lost tissue or the use of a graft or an implant.

Breast reconstruction is not usually performed until months after a mastectomy. It is delayed to allow tissues to soften and heal. In the interim a patient selects a temporary breast form to balance her figure and to reduce discomfort on her back, neck, and shoulders. Patients with small- to average-size breasts may wear padded bras or lightly molded brassieres. Women with larger breasts need to balance their body proportions by wearing a weighted prosthetic device. A patient can purchase a prostheses from a hospital, medical supply, or specialty store. A variety of styles are available; they can range in price from $5 to $500 or more. In most instances the patient's health insurance pays for the device.

There are several breast forms available, but the three most common are:

Contour light — a form with a cavity in back. This type of breast prosthesis was specifically designed for patients with sensitive tissue who cannot tolerate or are uncomfortable with anything coming in contact with sensitive nerve endings. The contour light breast form is favored by women who have had modified or radical mastectomies.

The teardrop — it has sides that are tapered so they can be adjusted to supplement areas where tissue has been removed. This is generally the type of breast form selected by patients who have had modified or radical mastectomies.

The heart shape — its rounded form adds to the crest of the patient's brassiere, creating the illusion of symmetry. This breast form is an excellent choice for a patient who has had a lumpectomy.

Along with the breast forms, other mastectomy accessories are available, which include bras, bra extenders, pockets that can be sewn into bathing suits, and brassieres that will support the breast form. Artificial nipples are made from silicone and can be attached directly onto the device or onto the skin.

One of the complications that may occur after a mastectomy is lymphedema, a chronic swelling due to the accumulation of interstitial fluid. The edema may just be confined to under the arm or shoulder, or it can affect the entire arm.

CLOTHING SUGGESTIONS

Patients who experience cancer have special clothing requirements that the clinical esthetician/cosmetologist should be aware of. The following suggestions should prove helpful to cancer patients.

Patients must select non-constricting clothing styles.

Clothing should be made from natural, soft fabrics that, if necessary, will easily drape over chest appliances.

Clothing styles with padded shoulders or shoulder pads sewn into garments will keep material from resting against the patient's chest and will help create the illusion of body symmetry.

Pants and skirts with elastic waistbands and pleats in the front will camouflage weight gain and will be more comfortable for the patient to wear.

Bright, cheerful colors will make the patient not only look healthier but may make the patient feel better as well.

Accessories such as scarves, earrings, or pins can be used to divert attention away from the area. Suggest that the patient select a piece of interesting costume jewelry that can be worn on her clothing as a conversation piece.

The *Beauty and Cancer* video from Beauty and Cancer/ Appearance Concepts Foundation (1-800-227-7730) will provide you with tips on hair-loss alternatives, suggestions on clothing for above and below the waist surgeries, camouflage makeup techniques, skin care and hair care for the cancer patient.

The American Cancer Society, in conjunction with the Cosmetic, Toiletries, and Fragrance Association has established a nationwide public service program: "Look Good, Feel Better." It is designed to assist the cancer patient in improving the quality of his or her life through personal appearance and body image. For more information contact:

American Cancer Society
90 Park Ave
New York, NY 10016
(800) 4-CANCER

C.T.F.A. Foundation
The Cosmetic, Toiletries, and Fragrance Association
1110 Vermont Ave., NW
Suite 800
Washington, DC 20005
(202) 331-1770

REVIEW

You should now be familiar with:

- cancer therapies.
- issues in working with cancer patients.
- effects of cancer on outward appearance.
- camouflage techniques effective with cancer patients.
- sources for wigs and hairpieces.
- special skin-care issues for cancer patients.

CHAPTER

15 AIDS

Acquired immune deficiency syndrome (AIDS) is caused by a virus called HIV that damages the human immune system. AIDS is an acronym for *Acquired* — meaning that this disease is not inherited, *Immune* — the immune system is the part of the body affected by the disease, *Deficiency* — it is the lack of immune function that characterizes this disease, leading to a series of clinical features that define this syndrome. Most doctors now refer to the spectrum of disease caused by HIV as "HIV disease." It is divided into two phases: asymptomatic and symptomatic. Symptomatic disease is divided into two phases: pre-AIDS, or ARC, and AIDS, the end stage of HIV disease. See Figure 15-1.

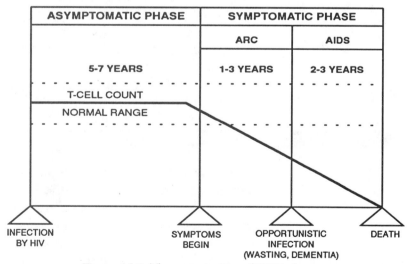

Figure 15-1. The progression of HIV infection

AIDS is defined by the progressive failure of the immune system, allowing the development of certain infections, tumors, or neurologic disease. At least 75 percent of infected persons will develop symptomatic HIV disease (ARC). Every-one developing ARC will probably develop AIDS and die from the disease. AIDS occurs on average about ten years after HIV infection, and death occurs on average about two years after developing AIDS. See Figure 15-2.

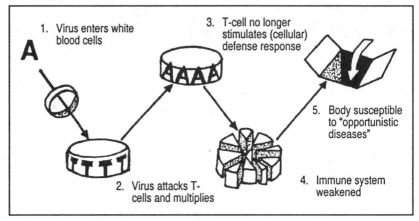

Figure 15-2. How the HIV virus affects the body

TRANSMISSION

This year it is estimated that 750,000–1.5 million people are infected with the AIDS virus, HIV. Of this total number 171,846 had full-blown AIDS as of March 31, 1991.

The only way in which the AIDS virus can be acquired is through exchange of bodily fluids, usually (semen or blood). This is during homosexual or heterosexual sexual contact, blood transfusion, intravenous drug use, or at birth from mother to child.

HIGH-RISK GROUPS

Those at risk of being HIV infected are homosexual men, bi-sexual men, heterosexuals who have had sexual contact with infected persons, intravenous drug users, hemophiliacs, people who received blood transfusions before blood was searched for HIV (1981-1985), and babies born to infected women.

Although once thought of as "a disease of homosexuals," AIDS can no longer be defined as a "gay disease." Fifteen percent of HIV infected persons in the United States are women. The AIDS epidemic has now spread to every popu-lated continent. However, virtually all infected persons can be identified as having one of the risks of acquiring HIV discussed above. The AIDS virus cannot be transmitted through casual contact.

When exposed to the HIV virus by the risk behaviors stated above, infection may occur. Usually for the first several years the infected person has no symptoms. Yet during this time the infected person's blood and secretions may be capable of transmitting the disease. Most persons infected with HIV in the United States now are in this asymptomatic phase. After an average of about five to seven years the person begins to develop symptoms of infection. This symptomatic phase is called AIDS Related Complex, or ARC. Fever, weight loss, diarrhea, thrush, coral yeast infection, and shingles are common forms of ARC. As of this writing, no one has developed an immunity to the virus.

DIAGNOSIS

Testing for HIV involves taking a sample of the patient's blood and examining it for the presence of antibodies (white blood cells) to HIV. If a patient tests positive it is an indication that he or she has been exposed to the virus. All patients who test positive are infected with HIV and can transmit it. Positive test results are possible from six weeks to three months after exposure. All persons in the risk groups defined above or who have symptoms suggesting HIV infection should be tested. Testing should be done after counseling. The results of HIV tests must be kept confidential. See Figure 15-3.

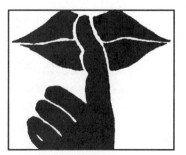

Figure 15-3. Confidential HIV test results

OPPORTUNISTIC INFECTIONS AND AIDS

Certain agents cause human infection only when immune failure gives them the opportunity to do so. They are called opportunistic infections. In AIDS certain opportunistic infections are characteristic.

Pneumocystis Carinii Pneumonia

Pneumocystis Carinii Pneumonia (PCP), is the most common opportunistic infection occurring in AIDS patients. It is also the leading cause of death in AIDS patients, although many patients have been treated for and have recovered from PCP. It is caused by a micro-organism called pneumocystis carinii. Symptoms can develop rapidly or slowly and last from a few weeks to a few months; they include fever, chest discomfort from coughing, and shortness of breath.

Treatment for PCP is generally administered in a hospital because patients may require oxygen and are given potent antibiotics.

Toxoplasmosis

Toxoplasmosis (or TE) is another type of opportunistic infection associated with AIDS. It is usually found in animals, but humans can become infected from the undercooked meat of infected animals. It is very serious and usually results in brain inflammation and seizures. The initial symptoms of the disease are seizures, confusion, dizziness, headaches, visual disturbances, fever, and fatigue. Another major clinical manifestation of TE is dementia (loss of intellectual function resulting in altered consciousness or a defect in cognition). Diagnosis is made through blood tests and highly developed x-ray techniques (WMR or CAT scan) to locate and identify brain lesions.

The treatment for toxoplasmosis is antibiotic therapy, but there is no complete cure. AIDS patients generally relapse within a few months if therapy is discontinued. Because of this, AIDS patients with toxoplasmosis are kept on these drugs indefinitely.

Cytomegalovirus

Cytomegalovirus (CMV) is a blindness-causing virus and is more common than toxoplasmosis. It is one of the family of Herpes viruses. It causes the cells it infects to take on a characteristic enlarged appearance. It is very common and has been associated with a syndrome resembling infectious mononucleosis. According to the *American Medical Association Encyclopedia of Medicine*, approximately 80 percent of adults have antibodies to it in their blood (an indication of previous infection). In most cases, it produces no symptoms. More serious CMV infections can occur in people with impaired immunity, such as the elderly and those with AIDS.

Many AIDS patients excrete cytomegalovirus. Since this virus can cause birth defects, it may be advisable for pregnant women to be excused from the direct care of any known CMV excretor.

MEDICAL TREATMENT

While not curable at this time, HIV disease and AIDS are treatable. Treatment depends on the stage of infection and whether or not an opportunistic infection or cancer has occurred. A patient may be administered any of the following therapies: antibiotics, antiviral drugs, chemotherapy, radiation therapy, and, frequently, new experimental treatments and medications. Patients also often take underground or non-prescription medications such as mega-vitamins, organic extracts, and non-licensed drugs. There is no way to correct the underlying immune deficiency, and even though opportunistic infections can be controlled through medical therapy, the patient always remains vulnerable to new cancers and/or many other opportunistic infections.

AZT

AZT (also called zidovudine) is an antiviral drug approved in 1987 for use in treatment of HIV infection. AZT has been shown to decrease the occurrence of opportunistic infections caused by AIDS, such as pneumocystis pneumonia and infections of the brain and nervous system, and therefore extends the life of patients with both ARC and AIDS. For these reasons many patients with HIV infection are taking AZT.

The most common side effect of AZT use is anemia. Blood tests are routinely performed on patients to monitor the red blood cell count, and blood transfusions may be required for such patients. AZT can also cause fever, muscle aches, nausea, restlessness, and insomnia.

NEOPLASMS AND AIDS

Two particular forms of cancer are prevalent among AIDS patients.

Kaposi's Sarcoma

Kaposi's Sarcoma (KS) is an uncontrolled growth of the cells that line certain blood vessels. Before the outbreak of the AIDS epidemic KS was rare and was seen almost exclusively in elderly Italian or Jewish men. In these cases the cells usually grow slowly. KS can cause lesions on the skin, internally, or both. In patients with AIDS, KS may be more aggressive and can create widespread tumors. The lesions can be raised or flat, and are usually blue, purple, or red. KS lesions generally appear first on the feet and ankles but can spread to the face and the rest of the body. KS causes severe body image problems for patients. It is the visible stigma of a fatal, infectious disease that interferes with their personal interactions.

KS lesions can also often be found in the mouth, lungs, lymph nodes, stomach, intestines, rectum, or other organs. Because the lesions' appearance may resemble other skin conditions, they must be examined by a pathologist, who performs a biopsy, where a small piece of lesion tissue is removed and analyzed. Other tests such as lab work (blood, urine, stool tests), x-rays, or pulmonary function tests (breathing) may be given to search for other opportunistic infections. The KS lesions may or may not be accompanied by other HIV related symptoms such as fever, night sweats, chills, enlarged lymph glands, weight loss, and diarrhea.

Treatment of KS is determined by how far the disease has advanced and how quickly the cancer is progressing. If other opportunistic infections are present, treatment for these infections takes first priority. The goal of KS therapy is to stabilize the disease. Since most AIDS patients with KS have limited disease, and since treatment does not prolong survival, most receive no local treatment. In severe cases chemotherapy is the most common form of treatment for KS (see chapter on cancer), but low-dose radiation therapy is also effective for local small or larger lesions. Both chemotherapy and radiation therapy may reduce swelling and discomfort by partially shrinking the KS lesions. The side effects of radiotherapy may cause surface skin burns, partial hair loss in localized areas, loss of appetite due to nausea or stomach upset, weight loss, and fatigue. How many of these side effects the patient will experience and how long the effects will last depends on the amount of radiation given and the part of the body treated. Aside from chemotherapy and radiation therapy, local treatments such as injections or freezing may also cause resolution of small KS lesions and are frequently performed by a dermatologist. Most patients try to conceal these lesions. In most instances they can be easily camouflaged.

Camouflaging KS Lesions

To a certain extent you can alter or conceal the appearance of KS lesions with the use of cosmetic preparations; however, special clinical considerations must be assessed when working with patients with AIDS. The following should be taken under consideration prior to beginning the treatment.

Clinical Considerations

The cosmetic solution must be sensible and financially feasible for the patient. If the patient only requires a small amount of cover cream, he or she should be advised accordingly. The patient should never be supplied with unnecessary items that he or she will not really need in order to perform the camouflage procedure. Properly equip the patient with only the pertinent cosmetic items he or she will actually use.

The patient's lifestyle must be taken into consideration, and the question of what type of lighting the patient will be in must be addressed. See Figure 15-4. The shade of the cover cream must be matched in the same lighting conditions under which the patient will be seen. Indoor and outdoor lighting varies drastically and will dramatically alter the color of the cover cream. The patient may need two separate cosmetic solutions. Another possibility is a color corrector, which can be added to the cover cream shade to compensate for changes in lighting (see chapter on cosmetic therapy).

Because most KS lesions are elevated and not flat on the skin, there will be some contour distortion. Be sure to advise the patient accordingly and recommend that the cover cream is well blended into the surrounding skin at the base of the lesion to prevent demarcation.

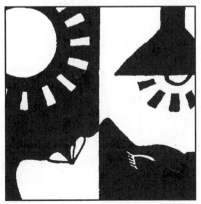

Figure 15-4. Clinical considerations

Cosmetic camouflage is not always the appropriate solution. If, for example, a patient has a KS lesion on a certain area of the face and he or she wears glasses, the frames may rub against the makeup, removing it from the skin. In such a case constant re-application, a second application of setting powder, or different eyeglass frames may be required to correct the problem. If the lesion is located on an area of the body that is exposed to constant friction (such as on the sides or nape of the patient's neck or on the hands), it is more than likely that some of the cover cream will end up on the patient's clothing. Be sure that your camouflage suggestions are sensible, and above all be realistic with the patient about what he or she can and cannot expect from the cosmetic camouflage solution. If necessary consider other camouflage options, such as color, to draw attention away from the area, the use of facial hair for covering, or clothing alternatives.

Evaluate the patient's physical and intellectual capabilities to determine how well he or she can perform the necessary camouflage techniques. Patients who are on heavy medication may be disoriented or lack the dexterity to perform even the simplest of cosmetic techniques and may need the assistance of a health care aide, friend, or family member. Some patients with CMV (cytomegalovirus) may have severely impaired vision or may be completely blind (see chapter on adaptive techniques for the blind) and will have great difficulty performing precision cosmetic techniques. Be sure to consider all these factors in your final assessment.

The Camouflage Session

1. Prepare the patient's work station prior to the treatment. Place all items the patient will need to perform the camouflage process in front of him or her in the order he or she will be using them. Be sure that all objects are appropriately labeled. Place a waste receptacle within the patient's reach so he or she can dispose of waste as you go along.

2. Most patients have lesions on different parts of their bodies. From the feedback the patient gives you determine which lesions take first priority; it is on these lesions that you will begin teaching the patient the camouflage process. If time permits you will be able to work on more than one area during the first session. If not, you will have to reschedule the patient

for a second session. The number of camouflage therapy appointments the patient will require will depend on how many locations on the patient's body are affected and how many of those areas the patient chooses to conceal with cosmetics.

3. Put on a pair of disposable examination gloves. Drape the patient with a makeup cape, or, if necessary (if the KS lesions are on an area of the patient's body covered with clothes), ask the patient to change into a gown for the treatment. Disposable gowns are available at a medical supply store but are more convenient than they are necessary.

4. Prepare the patient's skin first by massaging in circular motion a light cleansing solution into the area where the camouflage cosmetic is to be applied. Remove the lotion with warm, moistened cotton wool squares and discard. Apply either a toner (for dry skin) or an astringent (for oily skin) with a clean, dry cotton square or cotton ball. Dot onto the area a light moisturizer, and blot off any excess with a clean tissue. The moisturizer needs to be completely absorbed (ten to twenty minutes) before cover creams are applied.

5. Because the patient will be performing the camouflage process under your supervision, you will need to spend a few minutes acquainting him or her with the color matching technique. You can use poster boards to illustrate skin undertones (golden or rose). These visual aids will enable you to involve your patient in the selection of the appropriate cover cream shade or shades that will match his or her skin tone. It is important that the patient participate in this process because he or she must be able to alter the shade of the camouflage cosmetic if his or her skin tone changes because of medication or illness.

6. Once you and the patient have decided on three different color matches, proceed to remove the cover creams from their containers. Use the wooden end of a disposable cotton-tipped swab, or cut a cotton swab in half and use the end you cut to remove the cover cream from the container. Place the cover cream on the back of the patient's hand. Dispose of

the swabs immediately so as not to re-dip. Be sure you use a clean swab each time. See Figure 15-5.

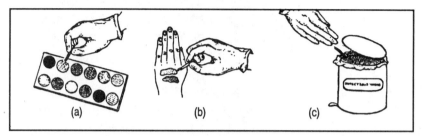

Figure 15-5. Matching cover cream color

7. Instruct the patient to mix the cover creams together on the back of his or her hand, experimenting with the correct proportions while performing this process. This helps the patient determine how a certain amount of cover cream can alter the color, making it more or less compatible with his or her skin tone.

8. Do not allow the patient to become discouraged if he or she was unsuccessful in achieving the appropriate shade the first time; instead encourage the patient to evaluate what he or she should have done and suggest he or she begin again. The second application is often easier than the first, and the patient's confidence is restored.

9. When both you and the patient are satisfied with the color match, instruct him or her to apply the cover cream to the lesion by pressing it directly into the skin. Depending on the size of the area involved and the patient's preference, any one of the following application tools can be used: disposable sponge (for large areas), sponge tip applicator or a cotton tipped swab (to apply the cover cream directly onto the lesion), or the fingertip application method. See Figure 15-6. This involves pressing the pad of the finger into the cover cream and applying it directly to the lesion, pressing and carefully blending the edges at the base to avoid a line of demarcation.

10. Once the cover cream has been applied and blended, the patient is ready to apply powder. A colorless translucent powder should be used to set and waterproof the application; a tinted powder can be used to slightly alter the original color match.

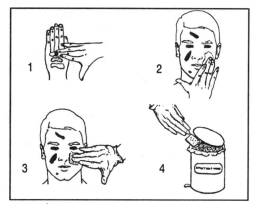

Figure 15-6. Applying cover cream to a facial lesion

11. Shake the powder into the palm of the patient's right hand. Ask the patient to press a clean cotton ball (instead of a powder puff) into the powder, and apply the powder directly over the cover cream. If the patient is only covering a few lesions he or she can use the tip of a cotton swab to directly apply the powder.

12. Advise the patient to wait three to five minutes for the oils in the cover cream to be absorbed by the powder, and then lightly brush off the excess with a clean cotton ball.

13. If the discoloration from the lesions still bleeds through, a second application of cover cream may be applied directly to the lesions with a clean cotton-tip swab. Instruct the patient to re-set the second application with setting powder again, and wait three to five minutes before lightly dusting off the setting powder with a clean cotton ball.

Lymphoma

Lymphoma is a cancer of the lymph system. Patients with AIDS are more likely to develop lymphoma. It affects the lymph nodes, lymph drainage system, and lymph tissue throughout the body. When functioning properly, the lymphatic system drains all the tissues of the body and filters fluid through the nodes. This part of the immune system identifies, attacks, and destroys cancer cells and infectious agents. Lymphoma occurs when an uncontrolled number of abnormal cells develop in the immune system. There are many different types of lymphomas. In some instances lymphoma may be the first indication of AIDS in an HIV-positive patient. According to where the abnormal growth develops, the following symptoms may occur: rapidly growing lymph nodes, fever, night sweats, and weight loss. If lymphoma occurs in the brain, confusion, memory loss, localized weakness, paralysis, aphasia (speech impairment or difficulty understanding speech), headaches, or seizures can result.

Chemotherapy is the most common form of treatment for AIDS-related lymphoma. It may or may not be combined with radiotherapy or surgery. Although this form of treatment may control lymphoma it will not cure AIDS. AIDS patients usually die soon after the development of lymphoma.

THE PSYCHOLOGICAL ASPECTS OF AIDS

The majority of people with AIDS are young or middle-aged. AIDS can, however, affect people at any time of life. A positive HIV test result will usually have a major impact on a patient's life. The shock and the fear is unimaginable for most of us. Patients diagnosed when they are young feel cheated out of the rest of their lives.

Patients are sometimes less afraid of dying than they are of the ravages of this deadly disease. Many AIDS patients have had friends or lovers who have suffered and died of AIDS. AIDS can transform a strong, independent, healthy person into a weak, helpless, emaciated, vulnerable person in great pain. A fundamental aspect of any serious illness is loss of control. No matter how self-disciplined an HIV-infected person is, he or she cannot physically remain in control of the body. Eventually, AIDS may rob the patient of every right to govern even the simplest of bodily functions. Often patients with AIDS suffer from paralysis, mental confusion, loss of coordination, speech disorders, partial or complete vision loss, and incontinence (inability to control bodily discharge).

Slowly many patients learn to surrender, realizing that their fight will be in vain and that they must yield to the inevitable. The new hope for the patient then becomes the assurance that all the discomfort will soon end and that he or she will at last be at peace. The patient resigns himself or herself to the actuality that he or she must passively wait for death, growing weaker and more powerless every day. At this point the only choice the patient is given is to tolerate the pain and the indignity of the disease.

The fight against HIV is exhausting. There are very few positive directions in which an AIDS patient can channel growing anxiety. It is no wonder that some patients who test positive for the virus or develop AIDS contemplate suicide.

INTIMATE RELATIONSHIPS

The AIDS patient's past and present relationships face serious challenges. If the patient is in a long-term relationship, an HIV positive test result can compromise if not destroy any emotional feelings the couple have for one another. A loved one may abandon an AIDS patient.

THE FAMILY

Depending on the patient's relationship with his or her family, their actions can greatly affect the patient's state of well-being. Family response can contribute greatly to the patient's attitude about testing positive for the virus. For patients who already have a strained relationship with their families because of their lifestyle, a positive diagnosis can completely sever all family ties, leaving the patient alone or in the care of strangers, facing the debilitating aspects of this disease.

FRIENDS

There is no way of foreseeing or predicting who will stand by the patient after he or she has been diagnosed. Friends who were previously a part of the patient's social life may avoid socializing with the patient for fear of what might be in store for them. They may not be able to handle the patient's anger or depression after being diagnosed. Many AIDS patients also lose friends to the epidemic. Some claim they can hardly make it through a week without hearing about a friend, casual acquaintance, or close business associate who has died from AIDS.

MEDICAL INSURANCE

Testing positive for HIV may make it difficult for the patient to sustain insurance coverage. Those who test positive for HIV may have their health-care program canceled, have their insurance carrier deny them certain benefits, or even refuse to insure them at all. Some patients have lost everything they owned trying to pay their hospital bills.

For uninsured AIDS patients, being without coverage means spending endless hours waiting in public clinics. Before state and federal agencies will help, patients must prove that they are indigent. A person who has always been independent, after becoming infected with the virus, may be forced to depend on others for not only emotional support but financial support as well.

PHYSICAL ASPECTS OF THE DISEASE

Patients also must struggle to accept the physical aspects of AIDS. Since AIDS is a disease in which the patient's condition is constantly changing, the patient never knows from one day to the next how he or she will feel. On a good day the patient may feel only slightly fatigued and mildly nauseated, only to find the following day that every physical movement requires tremendous exertion. Often too weak to walk, too nauseated to eat, too fatigued to dress, the patient remains house-bound and isolated.

AIDS IN THE WORKPLACE

A patient may have his or her salary docked or may be demoted because he or she is taking too much time off to see doctors or because of the effects of the illness. Some AIDS patients are even fired because they are too slow or too weak to perform their duties on the job. Losing one's job may mean losing insurance.

SOCIAL INTERACTION

Social situations can also become uncomfortable for patients who feel self-conscious about the appearance of KS lesions. Many patients are embarrassed or humiliated because they are infected with the virus and are often afraid others will shun them. Unfortunately, some people still believe that they can catch the disease through some form of casual contact such as shaking hands or breathing the same air. In an attempt to camouflage the purplish lesions KS patients try, often unsuccessfully, to cover them with inexpensive, dime-store cosmetics. Unfortunately such attempts usually makes their appearance even more obvious.

KEEPING UP APPEARANCES

Each patient will handle the news of the infection differently. Patients may either interpret the illness as a fight they must win by challenging themselves, or see themselves as martyrs to a useless cause. Regardless of how the patient really feels, for one reason or another he or she has made a decision to maintain his or her personal appearance and has sought you for your knowledge of aesthetic services.

THE IMPORTANCE OF TOUCH

Our efforts will never make the patient well, but we can help the patient feel better, if not physically, then mentally. The laying on of hands can make a world of difference to a patient who may be sensory deprived because others fear to touch him or her. Touch is a language that goes beyond words. To an AIDS patient the gentle touch of a hand can provide a healing warmth that offers reassurance. Our touch can lift the patient's spirit and demonstrate that we care. See Figure 15-7.

WORKING WITH PATIENTS WITH AIDS

The following information will provide the camouflage therapist with some general information and some basic guidelines to observe when working with AIDS patients.

Figure 15-7. National Task Force on AIDS Prevention

The AIDS virus cannot be transmitted through the air, by shaking hands, hugging, or by shared contact with objects (doorknobs, light switches, telephones, etc.). Only semen and blood have been proven to transmit infection.

KS lesions are not contagious because they are not open lesions. Therefore, you cannot contract the disease from applying cosmetics over the discoloration. You should never work on an open wound or any open area on the skin, because it may be infectious. A safety rule that should always be observed is to *always wear disposable examination gloves* when performing camouflage procedures.

An AIDS patient who has recently been diagnosed with KS may not know about the services of a camouflage therapist. Make sure that you contact physicians who treat HIV positive patients or patients with AIDS about the services you can provide for their patients suffering from the side-effects of chemotherapy, radiotherapy, or KS.

Remind patients that they can always come back for more sessions if they discover a new lesion or lesions, or if they have a flare-up and the appearance of their lesions suddenly worsens (getting darker or growing in number).

Never work on a patient when you have any type of infectious condition (a cold or a flu). His or her immune system is already compromised, and his or her body may not be physically strong enough to resist exposure to another virus.

Examination gloves should be worn when you anticipate any type of contact with blood or bodily fluids, or as a precautionary measure when you perform skin-care treatments. Avoid all procedures that involve sharp instruments. Facial procedures that might draw blood (comedo extractions) should not be performed on AIDS patients (see the chapter on cancer — the section on skin-care treatments).

You should know what to do if you are stuck with a sharp instrument during a procedure. Cosmetologists and cosmeticians should know the telephone number of their local AIDS clinic or the contact number of a physician who treats AIDS patients in their area. These doctors will know what to do and will advise you of the necessary steps to take. These contact numbers should be clearly posted by the telephone in every salon and clinic as a precautionary measure. The Centers for Disease Control recommends that employers provide the necessary equipment, supplies, and ongoing AIDS education to all public service workers in order to minimize the risk of infection with HIV and other blood-borne diseases.

For additional information on AIDS or AIDS educational materials, contact your local AIDS agencies, public health department, or similar organizations. Information for workers can also be obtained through the SEIU (Service Employees International Union) or through Impact AIDS, Inc., 3692 18th St., San Francisco, California 94110, (415) 861- 3397.

Use only disposable materials for facial and cosmetic treatments. Waste materials should be handled and disposed of in accordance with hospital procedures for controlling the spread of all infectious diseases. Check with your local hospital or your local health department for applicable regulations.

Some patients are chronically fatigued, while others will have good and bad days. Always contact the patient the day of your appointment to confirm. Try to be understanding if the patient with AIDS has to reschedule his or her appointment at the last minute because of being too tired to participate in the cosmetic session.

Many patients with AIDS are extremely weak, so keep that in mind when scheduling their camouflage sessions. The lesson may take longer than you had originally anticipated, and because of the illness the patient's response time may be slower. Be patient when giving instruction.

Keep the cosmetic therapy procedures as simple for the patient to perform as possible. Remember, some days the smallest task can prove exhausting. Patients with AIDS can easily become fatigued. To prevent the patient from becoming overly tired during the session, allow scheduled intervals for the patient to rest. When you are working on a patient do not be surprised if the patient becomes nauseated, as this is not unusual. It can be caused by gastrointestinal infection or can be the side-effects of medication. If the patient should vomit, the appropriate way to clean up any type of infectious waste is to first put gloves on, then clean up the bulk of the material with paper towels or something else you can dispose of, putting the contaminated waste in an infectious waste container, and then clean the area with a bleach solution. Bleach kills HIV. You can use either a full strength bleach solution or dilute the bleach 10 parts water to 1 part bleach. Clean the area twice and dispose of your gloves.

Chemotherapy and radiotherapy often cause changes in the skin and hair (see chapter on cancer for suggestions on hair replacement and skin-care therapy), although each patient will react differently to these treatments. Anticipate some of the more common side effects of these cancer therapies, which are: dry skin, surface burns (from radiation), hyperpigmentation, rashes, and hair loss (see cancer and cosmetic therapy chapters for camouflage and skin-care recommendations).

Some patients will have insurance that covers the cost of the camouflage session and all supplies, while others may not have the financial means with which to pay for their treatment. It may be necessary on occasion for you to offer your services free, at a reduced rate, or to set up a special payment schedule if needed.

Do not patronize the patient. He or she already is being made to feel helpless by the effects of the disease. Be empathetic and compassionate toward him or her.

The friends or family of a patient are sometimes not prepared for the sacrifices that must be made on the patient's behalf. They may be incapable of dealing with the sorrow. To avoid burdening those closest to him or her a patient may seek the company of an impartial listener, such as you. Allow the patient to take advantage of the opportunity to honestly reveal his or her feelings by lending your support (see chapter on patient management — working with the terminally ill).

Information regarding every patient's diagnosis, sexual orientation, and general medical condition is strictly confidential. Because people with AIDS face discrimination in housing, employment, and provision of services, maintaining confidentiality is vitally important.

To help ensure confidentiality, infection control precautions should be indicated only by general labels; for example, "Blood/Secretion Precautions" should be posted on charts, on doors, and in treatment areas.

The patient alone must determine who will have specific information about his or her condition (this is the law !).

Since AIDS is not spread through normal casual contact that occurs in the workplace, you are not at risk by working with a person with AIDS/ARC. Cosmeticians or cosmetologists with HIV or AIDS, however, should always wear gloves when working.

Workers with AIDS have a lot to offer both professionally and personally. Co-workers, in turn, can be an important source of support for them.

Below are the guidelines for the state of California regarding AIDS and the cosmetology workplace. Check with your individual state board requirements.

BOARD OF COSMETOLOGY
Sacramento, California

ACQUIRED IMMUNE DEFICIENCY SYNDROME (AIDS) AND THE COSMETOLOGY WORKPLACE

There have been no documented cases of the transmission of the human immunodeficiency virus (HIV, or the "AIDS virus") in a cosmetology establishment (personal-service setting) as of this writing.

The U.S. Centers for Disease Control (CDC) has indicated that there is a risk of transmission of the AIDS virus "when instruments contaminated with blood are not sterilized or disinfected between clients" and when the blood from one person enters the bloodstream of another person. However, CDC has suggested that the risk of transmission in personal-service settings is "extremely low."

The Centers for Disease Control recommends that all instruments that are not intended to penetrate the skin but which may become contaminated with blood be used for only one client or cleaned and disinfected after use.

Board of Cosmetology regulations require that all instruments and equipment used by cosmetologists* be disinfected after each use. These regulations were recently reviewed and amended to ensure the highest practical level of disinfection possible in order to protect the consumers of California. The amendments were developed by working with the California Department of Health Services, in conjunction with the CDC.

The regulations now include a specific requirement to ensure the disinfection of instruments that may be contaminated with blood in order to prevent the spread of blood-borne diseases such as AIDS and Hepatitis B. The regulation requires that all instruments with a sharp point or edge that may on occasion pierce the skin and draw blood (scissors, razors, tweezers, cuticle nippers, etc.) be cleaned with soap (or detergent) and water and then totally immersed in 70 percent Isopropyl Alcohol for at least ten minutes.

The Centers for Disease Control points out that personal-service workers (this would include cosmetologists) infected with the AIDS virus should not be restricted from work unless they have other infections or illnesses for which any person should be restricted from work, and points out that workers should exercise care to avoid injury to hands when performing services. To enhance protection of both patron and operator, non-sterile, disposable gloves may be used, if appropriate.

If cosmetologists disinfect all instruments and equipment according to Board of Cosmetology regulations, and take simple precautions (such as avoiding injury to the hands and being aware of any bleeding cuts), they and their clients should not be at risk of transmitting or contracting AIDS virus infection.

*"Cosmetologist" refers to all persons licensed to practice cosmetology or any of its branches, except the branch of electrology.

Note: All references to information from the CDC were obtained from "Morbidity and Mortality Weekly Report," Centers for Disease Control, November 15, 1985. The Board of Cosmetology confirmed with the CDC that all information is current. (November, 1988.)

REVIEW

You should now be familiar with:

- facts about AIDS and its transmission.
- opportunistic infections that attack AIDS patients.
- medical treatments available to AIDS patients.
- camouflage issues that are particular to AIDS patients.
- psychological effects on the AIDS patient and those people he or she is close to.

The Use of Glycolic Acid

Melvin L. Elson, M.D.

Alpha hydroxy acids, also known as fruit acids, are naturally occurring substances present in foods and have actually been used to treat skin problems for centuries. Lactic acid occurs in sour milk and has been used for a long time as a moisturizer and a balm for burns. It is even reported that Cleopatra bathed in sour milk to soften and hydrate her skin. Moisturizers containing various strengths of lactic acid have been available for years in both over-the-counter preparations and by prescription. Malic acid is formed as apples begin to rot, citric acid is contained in fruits such as lemons and has been used to bleach the skin, and tartaric acid is contained in grapes and was used in ancient Greece as women applied the sludge from the bottom of the vats in which wine was being made to smooth the facial skin.

Glycolic acid is made up of the smallest molecules of all the alpha hydroxy acids, making it capable of penetrating the skin barrier, which is usually so effective in keeping substances from entering the protective covering of the body. Glycolic acid is derived from sugar cane and has the ability to affect the skin in a number of ways.

Melvin L. Elson, M.D., is medical director of the Dermatology Center, Inc., in Nashville, Tennessee, and is concurrently director of the Cosmeceutical Research Institute, Inc. in New York City. He has conducted scientific research for a number of pharmaceutical and cosmetic companies and serves as a consultant for the American Board of Dermatology and other pharmaceutical companies. In 1991 Dr. Elson served as co-chair for the Chemical Peel Workshop, which included a presentation on "Glycolic Acid Peels," at the International Congress for Dermatologic Surgery.

Its use in the skin is not new, again having been used to treat the skin, especially for hydrating the skin, in ancient Egypt. In the modern era research began a number of years ago with the use of glycolic acid as a moisturizer and to treat conditions in which the skin cells build up in an abnormal fashion — ichthyosis or fish skin conditions of various types. Products have been available for many years to treat these conditions with glycolic acid.

More recently Van Scott and Yu have conducted a great deal of research regarding other uses of glycolic acid. Originally, evidence began to accumulate using glycolic acid as a peeling agent for seborrheic and actinic keratoses and other benign overgrowths of the skin, such as warts, etc. From this original work with high concentrations of the acid, milder forms of the acid were used to treat acne and other conditions of the face. A good deal of the work in light chemical peeling, especially for acne, was done by Stagnone and his colleagues of the University of New Mexico Medical Center.

From the work of these investigators anecdotal data indicated a possible benefit from glycolic acid in the treatment of photoaging. Clinical studies were then instituted to determine the validity of the treatment for both photoaging and related conditions such as melasma (mask of pregnancy), true sun damage, and early cancerous changes and to determine the mechanism of action of the acid in the treatment of both sun damage and acne.

CURRENT USES OF GLYCOLIC ACID

The purpose of this section is to review the current understanding of glycolic acid and to discuss the products that have been developed over the last couple of years for use by estheticians and physicians.

Anatomy of the Skin

A basic review of the anatomy of the skin is necessary to understand the mechanism of action of glycolic acid in the treatment of acne and photoaging. The skin is an active organ of the body consisting of three compartments — the epidermis, which is constantly turning over and replicates itself every twenty-eight days; the dermis, made up of the elastic fibers and collagen network embedded in the ground substance; and the subcutaneous tissue, which consists of the fat and the fascia supporting the skin and providing the cushion between the skin and the underlying structures.

The epidermis is a five-layered structure formed in the basal layer of the skin, which produces the cells of the epidermis, which then move up through the layers of the skin, flatten, and lose the nucleus to become the outermost layer of the skin, the stratum corneum or horny layer of the outer skin. Skin cells in the epidermis are held together by a number of different mechanisms — a number of different types of fibers anchoring the cells together and some intercellular cement or glue helping to hold these cells in a manner to allow orderly progression from the bottom to the surface.

The pilosebaceous unit, which is composed of the hair follicle and the sebaceous gland, is a continuation of the epidermis to form the hair shaft to which is connected the sebaceous gland. The development of acne begins when this unit begins to malfunction. In the upper portion of the follicular canal, which does contain a stratum corneum, cells are shed in scales or sheets. In the lower portion of this unit the stratum corneum is thin, and cells are shed singularly into the space to be carried to the surface with sebum produced by the associated gland. When sebum production undergoes changes secondary to androgen production or other factors that increase or change the nature of the production of sebum, the cells begin to clump together, beginning the process of microcomedone formation, which is the earliest stage of acne. The follicle becomes irritated, and this leads to an overproduction of skin cells inside the follicle, eventually building up in the top of the follicular canal, and the skin cells accumulate. This obstruction is the first step leading to the formation of acne lesions.

Effects of Glycolic Acid

One of the primary effects of glycolic acid is on this ability of skin cells to stick together either in the skin layers on the surface of the skin or in the pilosebaceous unit that is participating in the formation of acne lesions. It is not yet well understood at which point glycolic acid exerts its effect on this intercellular space — it could be on the fibers that are linking the cells together or it could affect the glue that is holding the cells in the loose network. At any rate, the effect is the same: glycolic acid loosens the skin cells, they cannot remain attached, and they come off the skin. When one is considering how glycolic acid works in acne it is obvious that if the cells cannot stick together to produce a plug it would be difficult for acne lesions to occur.

The Aging Process

When considering the use of glycolic acid in the overall treatment of the aging face, it is important to have an understanding of not only the anatomy of the skin, but the dynamics of the aging face, before implementing therapy with this substance.

The aging face is affected by five factors — intrinsic aging, sleep lines, gravity, expression lines, and photoaging. Photoaging is manifested as fine lines over the entire surface of the face, a great deal of play on color (both increased and decreased), enlarged pores, broken blood vessels, dryness of the surface, a yellowish caste that the skin takes on over a period of time, as well as the inability of the skin to hold water. All of these manifestations are due to the chronic action of the sun on the skin over a period of time and can be treated in a number of different ways.

The daily use of appropriate sunscreens will actually begin to reverse these manifestations of the aging face. In addition this is the area in which Retin-A is most effective and is also where chemical peels as a surgical method of treatment have been performed by dermatologists and plastic surgeons. This is also where glycolic acid is appropriate.

The mechanism of action of glycolic acid in the treatment of photoaging is not yet completely established but if one returns to the concept that glycolic acid decreases the ability of the skin cells to remain attached to one another, then a theory can be built as to a possible mode of action. In lower concentrations (i.e., dilute solutions), glycolic acid's primary effect will be on the outermost layers of the epidermis — the stratum corneum. As the concentration of the acid is increased, its penetrating ability increases and the viable epidermis begins to dehisce, or lose its ability for the epidermal cells to remain attached in the viable epidermis. This will simply lead to deeper removal of skin cell layers.

A body of evidence is accumulating that indicates that there may be an effect by glycolic acid on the dermis as well. The dermis is the layer of tissue just under the epidermis. It contains the collagen and elastic fibers, which are manufactured by the fibroblast, and these fibers rest in a bed of material known as the ground substance, which contains glycosaminoglycans, proteoglycans, and other complex molecules, primarily mucopolysaccharides. It is this ground substance that may be affected by glycolic acid in the treatment of photoaging.

The clinical effect of these actions is to have smoother skin with less debris (layers and trapped material removed from the surface of the skin), so that the effect is much the same as wiping the mirror clean to be able to see the skin. In addition, there is a response of the skin to slightly increase the turnover of the epidermis to keep viable tissue coming to the surface, which is fresher and smoother in appearance. The integrity of the skin is increased, and this increases the ability of the skin to retain moisture. The effect on the dermis may allow a milieu for better production by the fibroblast as well as possibly increasing the vascular support in the area. This will be manifested as smoother and pinker skin on the surface.

PRODUCTS CONTAINING GLYCOLIC ACID

A number of products containing glycolic acid from a variety of companies have recently become available for use. While it is possible to buy manufactured glycolic acid topical agents, it is imperative to purchase these products from licensed, reputable companies. At the moment only four companies are licensed by the holder of the patents to manufacture and distribute glycolic acid products — Neostrata to physicians, Murad to estheticians, Avon to the consumer, and Herald Pharmacal through its MD Formulations line to the esthetician and physician. In addition to products from these sources, skin exfoliation kits are available for the physician and the esthetician in differing strengths from Herald Pharmacal in Richmond, Virginia.

It is imperative for the client to understand that glycolic acid is not used for a period of time until the skin condition being treated is brought under control, but is a skin-care program to be used for life. Proper skin care is not a treatment; it is a life-style. The at-home products that are available through physician's offices and salons contain anywhere from 8 to 12 percent glycolic acid and take a variety of forms — cleansers, lotions, night creams, toners, and astringents, as well as products for specific areas, such as a smoothing complex available in the MD Formulations line, containing glycolic acid in liposomes, for use around the eyes and lips.

At the moment one product is licensed and available to the physician for in-office use, and two dry-skin exfoliators are available for estheticians — Murad's 30 percent partially neutralized system and Herald's 40 percent partially neutralized system. The concept of partial neutralization of glycolic acid is important. Glycolic acid is manufactured as a 70 percent aqueous solution with a pH of 0.5. If this substance is placed on the skin a significant burn can result. The addition of an alkaline substance such as ammonium hydroxide has the effect of partially neutralizing the solution by producing the ammonium glycolate salt and adjusting the pH upward towards neutral. These resulting preparations will contain certain concentrations of free glycolic acid and certain concentrations of glycolate salt at an adjusted pH. The solution maintains its ability to act on epidermal cells and to affect the dermis, but with a great deal less discomfort to the client and fewer possible side effects. The final product available to the salon from Murad is known as Murad's AHA Rapid Exfoliator, and the one from Herald contains 28 percent glycolic acid adjusted to pH 3.65.

Before going into greater detail regarding the use of these products at home and in salons it is necessary to discuss the one other substance used widely in the treatment of both acne and photoaging — Retin-A (tretinoin or retinoic acid).

Retin-A This derivative of vitamin A, manufactured by Ortho Derm in Raritan, New Jersey, has been on the market since the early 1970s, approved by the F.D.A. for the treatment of acne, and is available in the United States only by prescription. Although its use is primarily in the treatment of acne, many patients use Retin-A as part of their regimen in the treatment of photoaging.

Tretinoin works primarily intracellularly; that is, it changes the way the skin cell manufactures itself so that there is less tendency for skin cells to adhere to one another, which leads to a sloughing of the cells in the microcomedone, the early stage of acne formation. This is one of the primary methods by which tretinoin is effective in the treatment of acne. It also increases the response of white blood cells to the area to help in the healing process and increases the blood vessels in the area, again facilitating healing.

As far as photoaging is concerned, tretinoin has actually been used for this purpose by dermatologists for almost a decade, but a significant increase in its use occurred after an article by Weiss et al, from the University of Michigan, was printed in the *Journal of the American Medical Association* in 1988. Tretinoin normalizes the production of epidermal cells so that there is a normal progression of skin cells from the basal layer to the surface with less disarray and more organization. In addition, studies have shown that tretinoin increases the formation of blood vessels in the skin as well as repairing damaged vessels. Tretinoin also has an affinity for the fibroblast, increasing fibroblast activity in the area of application and thereby increasing the synthesis of collagen. All of these effects combine to produce the clinical results seen with the use of tretinoin — decrease in fine lines, increased ability to retain water, increased blood flow, and an apparent increase in the turgor of the skin.

Although tretinoin is not currently approved for photoaging by the F.D.A. in the United States, Ortho Derm is currently awaiting final approval by the F.D.A. to release Renova® (tretinoin in an emollient cream base) for the treatment of photoaging.

PROGRAMS FOR USING GLYCOLIC ACID

With a basic understanding of the normal anatomy of the skin, the pathogenesis of acne and photoaging, as well as what is available in glycolic acid, programs can be developed to treat clients seen by estheticians. It is also important to understand the role of tretinoin, since many patients are already using this drug or are being seen by a dermatologist or cosmetic surgeon.

The typical program for the treatment of acne utilizing glycolic acid follows.

At-home Care

Morning

1. Cleanse with glycolic acid facial cleanser.
2. Apply 12 percent facial lotion (four drops on moist skin).
3. Apply sunscreen with SPF 15.

During the Day

Apply 5 or 10 percent toner as needed for oiliness.

At Bedtime

1. Cleanse with glycolic acid facial cleanser.
2. Apply tretinoin as directed by the physician on moist skin.

   Other treatment during the day may consist of appropriate antibiotic therapy prescribed by the physician in either topical or systemic form.

In the Salon

After the patient has been on therapy for two weeks, the patient returns for the first application of the esthetician's dry skin exfoliation, and this is repeated every two weeks for a total of six sessions. As home therapy is continued a session can be repeated as needed on a single basis.

The typical program for the treatment of photoaging follows.

At-home Care

Morning

1. Cleanse with glycolic acid facial cleanser.
2. Apply four drops 12 percent facial lotion.
3. Apply moisturizing sunscreen with SPF 15.
4. Apply under-makeup moisturizer and foundation.

At Bedtime

1. Cleanse with glycolic acid facial cleanser.
2. Apply tretinoin as prescribed by the physician on moist skin.
3. Apply glycolic acid night cream.
4. Can apply smoothing complex to the eyelids and lips at this time on moist skin.

In the Salon

Return in two weeks for the first application of the esthetician's dry skin exfoliation. This is repeated every two weeks for six applications and is repeated every three months on a single basis as the client continues the skin care program.

The following is the method used for dry skin exfoliation using the esthetician's dry skin exfoliation kit containing 40 percent glycolic acid (MD Formulations, Herald Pharmacal, Richmond, Virginia).

1. All makeup should be removed.
2. The face should be cleansed with a mild cleanser such as Johnson's Baby Shampoo, Cetaphil, or CAM.
3. Prepare the skin with the prepping solution contained in the kit, using cotton balls or gauze.

4. Pour 5 cc Accelerated Dry Skin Exfoliation into a container.

5. Set the timer for six minutes.

6. Apply the material to the face with cotton swabs or balls (be sure to wear gloves to protect your nails), beginning with the outside of the face and proceeding to the center, leaving the eyelids and upper lip skin for last. This should take two minutes.

7. Allow the solution to remain on for two minutes.

8. Apply fresh gauze saturated with cool water to remove the material, beginning at five minutes and continuing until time is up.

9. Apply moisturizing sunscreen, and allow makeup to be applied.

Helpful Hints

- During the procedure some stinging is not unusual. If undue redness occurs or the client complains of much discomfort apply the cold water early.

- If any material gets into the eyes flush the eyes out with cool distilled water immediately.

- This method of application is appropriate for both acne and photoaging.

- An effective moisturizing sunscreen that can be used at home and in the salon is Catrix Correction Cream (Donnell Dermedex, New York, New York).

Although the programs outlined above will provide a general background on how to implement glycolic acid into your practice, every person's skin is different and only experience and appropriate training will allow you to become adept in the use of this innovative product. All companies who provide salons with glycolic acid products provide training sessions and manuals for your use.

B The Patient Diagram

Since patients will ultimately be performing the camouflage process alone, they are more likely to benefit if they can emerge from the cosmetic treatment with a practice tool. The patient's diagram/form is represented here to stress the importance of giving patients a reference guide that they can later use at their own discretion. The form will enable them to visually recall all the details of the step-by-step cosmetic procedure. Camouflage therapists will find that it will be more helpful to their patients if they permit them to record their own version of the cosmetic process on the form. This will insure that the patient clearly understood the instructions given. It will also make it easier for patients to recall what they learned if they draw from a record of their own experience.

The reference form should always provide for the date of the patient's appointment, the name of the camouflage therapist, a telephone number where the patient can call to request additional information, and where the cover cream products can be purchased.

The forms shown here also provide a special section for listing the cover creams that will be used in treatment and in what percentages they will be combined. The base color (which is the dominant cover cream shade of all the cover creams blended together) should be recorded on line 1. Line 2 is for a second cover cream shade, which may be needed to accurately match the color of the patient's skin. Line 3 provides for any additional tints or color correctors that may be necessary to achieve the best cosmetic result.

The section below is for checking off any applicators, setting powders, cream rouges, or powder blushers that the therapist may recommend. The skin care portion of the form is to provide the patient with additional information on proper skin care and the cover cream removal process.

PATIENT'S NAME _____

DATE_____
CLINICAL COSMETICIAN_____
ADDRESS_____
PHONE_____

_____
_____
_____

Camouflage Application:
Cover Creams Used

#1 _____

#2 _____

#3 _____

Applicators

Flat Brush	☐	Powder Brush	☐
Liner Brush	☐	Powder Puff	☐
Wedge Sponge	☐	Cotton Ball	☐
Stipple Sponge	☐	Cotton Square	☐
Cotton Swabs	☐		

Setting Powders
Translucent ☐ Tinted ☐ Noncolored ☐

Cream Rouge _____

Powder Blusher _____

Blusher Brush _____

Skin Care Recommended:

_____

_____

Sunscreen _____ SPF_____

Moisturizer

Cream_____

Lotion _____

Removal Method:
To loosen up and soften cover cream use a cleanser with an oil base to break down the waxes. Massage gently in circular motion. Wipe off with warm cloth or moistened cotton square, follow with an oil free cleanser to remove residue. Follow with a non-alcoholic based toner or astringent. Then moisturize.

Sample form for the camouflage therapist, which can be copied to give to patients before the camouflage therapy session begins.

PATIENT'S NAME _____

DATE_____
CLINICAL COSMETICIAN_____
ADDRESS_____
PHONE_____

_____

_____

_____

Camouflage Application:
Cover Creams Used

#1 _____

#2 _____

#3 _____

Applicators

Flat Brush	☐	Powder Brush	☐
Liner Brush	☐	Powder Puff	☐
Wedge Sponge	☐	Cotton Ball	☐
Stipple Sponge	☐	Cotton Square	☐
Cotton Swabs	☐		

Setting Powders

Translucent ☐ Tinted ☐ Noncolored ☐

Cream Rouge _____

Powder Blusher _____

Blusher Brush _____

Skin Care Recommended:

_____

_____

Sunscreen _____ SPF_____

Moisturizer

Cream_____

Lotion _____

Removal Method:
To loosen up and soften cover cream use a cleanser with an oil base to break down the waxes. Massage gently in circular motion. Wipe off with warm cloth or moistened cotton square, follow with an oil free cleanser to remove residue. Follow with a non-alcoholic based toner or astringent. Then moisturize.

Sample form for the camouflage therapist, which can be copied to give to patients before the camouflage therapy session begins.

APPENDIX

C

Selected Readings

Chapter 2

Thunberg, Ursula. "The Dying Adult: Clinical Perspectives." *Understanding Human Behavior in Health and Illness*. Third Edition. Ed. Richard C. Simons. (1985): 513-521.

Chapter 3

Adams, G.R. "Attractiveness Through the Ages." *The Psychology of Cosmetic Treatment*. Ed. J.A. Graham. New York: Prager Press, 1985.

Adriaenssens, P., W. Boeckx, B. Gilles, S. Mertens, P. Nijs, and K. Pyck. "Impact of Facial Burns on the Family." *Scand. J. Plast. Reconst. Surg.* 21 (1987): 303-305.

Berkowitz, I., and A. Frodi. "Reactions to a Child's Mistake." *Social Psych. Quart.* 42 (1979): 420-425.

Berscheid, E., and E. Walster. *Interpersonal Attraction*. Reading, Mass.: Addison-Wesley, 1987.

Bull, R. "The Psychological Effects of Facial Deformity." *Love and Attraction*. Eds. M. Cook, M. and G. Wilson. Oxford: Pergamon Press, 1979.

Clifford, M., and E. Walster, "The Effect of Physical Attractiveness on Teacher Expectations." *Soc. of Ed.* 46 (1973): 248-258.

Hildebrandt, K.A., and H.E. Fitzgerald. "Adults' Reponses to Infants Varying in Perceived Cuteness." *Behavioral Processes*. 3 (1977): 159-172.

Hildebrandt, K.A., and H.E. Fitzgerald. "Adults; Responses to Infant Sex and Cuteness." *Sex Roles*. 5 (1979): 471-481.

Kershaw, J.D. *Handicapped Children*. 3rd ed. London:Heinemann, 1973.

Kiehle, T., Bramble, W., and J. Mason. "Teacher's Expectations." *J. of Esp. Ed.* 43 (1974): 54-60.

Konigova, R., and I. Pondelicek. "Psychological Aspects of Burns." *Scand. J. Plast. Reconstr. Surg.* 21 (1987): 311-314.

Langlois, J., and C. Stephan. "The Effects of Physical Attractiveness and Ethnicity on Children's Behavioral Attributions and Peer Preferences." *Child. Dev.* 48 (1977): 1694-1698.

Lerner, R.M., and S.A. Karabenick. "Physical Attractiveness, Body Attitudes and Self Concept in Late Adolescents." *J. Youth and Adoles.* 3 (1974): 307-316.

Love, H., and J. Walthall. *A Handbook of Medical, Educational and Psychological Information for Teachers of Physically Handicapped Children.* Springfield, Ill.: Charles C. Thomas, 1977.

MacGregor, M. *Facial Deformities and Plastic Surgery: a Psychosocial Study.* Springfield, Ill.: Charles C. Thomas, 1953.

Moncada, G.A., "The Facially Disfigured Child." *Topics in Early Childhood Special Education.* 6 (1987): 101-114.

Navarre, E.L. "Psychological Maltreatment: the Core Component of Child Abuse." Eds. M. Brassard, R. Germain, and S. Hart. *Psychological Maltreatment of Children and Youth.* New York: Pergamon Press, 1987.

Rumsey, N., R. Bull, and D. Gahagan. "The Effect of Facial Disfigurement on the Behavior of the General Public." *J. Appl. Soc. Psych.* 12 (1982): 137-150.

Solnit, A., and M.H. Stark. "Mourning and the Birth of a Defective Child." Ed. R. Eissler. *Physical Illness and Handicap in Childhood.* New Haven: Yale University Press, 1977.

Thomas, A. and S. Chess. *Temperament and Development.* New York: Brunner, Mazel, 1977.

Udry, J. "The Importance of Being Beautiful: A Reexamination and Racial Comparison." *Am. J. Soc.* 83 (1977): 154-160.

Chapter 4

Arden, C. Bowers. *Clinical Manual of Health Assessment.* St. Louis, Mo.: C.V. Mosby Company.

Potter, Patricia A. *Pocket Nurse Guide to Physical Assessment.* St. Louis, Mo.: C.V. Mosby Company.

Heinz, Feneis. *Pocket Atlas of Human Anatomy.* Stuttgart, New York: Georg Thieme Verlag.

Kapp, Marshall B. *Legal Guide for Medical Office Managers.* Chicago: Pluribus Press.

Davis, Neil M. *Medical Abbreviations.* Huntingdon Valley, Pa.: Neil M. Davis Associates.

The Nursing Theories Conference Group. *Nursing Theories.* Englewood Cliffs, N.J.: Prentice-Hall.

Front Office Management. Alpharetta, Ga.: The Medical Management Institute.

Bernthal, Patricia J. and James D. Spiller, *Understanding the Language of Medicine.* New York: Oxford University Press.

Chabner, Davi-Ellen, *The Language of Medicine.* Philadelphia: W.B. Saunders Company.

Foy, Donald F., and Lawton M. Murray, *Medical Assistants.* St. Louis, Mo.: C. V. Mosby Company.

Redman, Barbara K. *The Process of Patient Education.* St. Louis, Mo.: C. Mosby Publishing Company.

Dorland's Pocket Medical Dictionary. Philadelphia: W. B. Saunders Company.

Clayman, Charles B., M.D., *The American Medical Encyclopedia of Medicine*. New York: Random House.

Chapter 5

Albers, Josef. *Interaction of Color*. New Haven and London: Yale University, 1963.

Allen, Jeanne. *Showing Your Colors*. San Francisco: Chronicle Books, 1986.

Birren, Faber. *Principles of Color*. New York: Van Nostrand Reinhold, 1969.

Kueppers, Harold. *The Basic Law of Color Theory*. New York: Barrons Educational Series, Inc., 1980.

Luscher, Dr. Max, and Ian Scott. *The Luscher Color Test*. New York: Washington Square Press, 1969.

Mueller, Conrad G., and Rudolph Mae. *Light and Vision*. New York: Life Science Library, 1966.

Osborn, Roy. *Lights and Pigments*. New York: Harper and Row Publishers, 1980.

Sharpe, Deborah T. *The Psychology of Color and Design*. Chicago: Nelson-Hall, 1974.

Stoddard, Alexandra. *Alexandra Stoddard's Book of Color*. New York: Bantam Doubleday Dell Publishing Group, 1989.

Chapter 10

For books written on training and suggesting adaptive techniques contact: The Greater Pittsburgh Guild for the Blind, 311 Station St., Bridgeville, PA 15017, and ask for any of the following publications: *Household Arts, Techniques of Daily Living*, or *Sensory Training and Mobility*.

The following books come in braille and large print:

Smith, Margaret M. *If Blindness Strikes, Don't Strike Out*. Published by Charles C. Thomas: available through: Recording from the Blind Inc., or Talking Book Library (Library of Congress),

Josephson, Eric. *The Social Life of Blind People*. New York: American Foundation for the Blind, 1968

Sperber, Al. *Out of Sight*. Boston: Little, Brown and Company.

Chapter 11

Chase, Deborah. *The Medically Based No Nonsense Beauty Book*. New York: Alfred A. Knopf Inc., 1989.

Clayman, Charles. *The American Medical Association Encyclopedia of Medicine*. New York: Random House Publishers, 1989.

Dorland's Pocket Medical Dictionary. 23rd Edition. Philadelphia: W.B. Saunders Company, 1982.

Dorland's Illustrated Medical Dictionary 27th Edition. Philadelphia: W.B. Saunders Company, 1988.

Draelos, Zoe Kececioglu. *Cosmetics in Dermatology*. New York: Churchill Livingstone, 1990.

Dvorine, William. *A Dermatologist's Guide to Home Skin Treatment.* New York: Charles Scribner's Sons Publishing, 1983.

Freudlberg, Frank, and Stephen Emanuel. *Herpes: A Complete Guide to Relief and Reassurance.* Philadelphia: Running Press, 1982.

Frost, Phillip, and Steven Horwitz. *Principles of Cosmetics for the Dermatologist.* Chapter 43. St. Louis, Mo.: C.V. Mosby Company, 1982.

Fulton, James, and Elizabeth Black. *Acne.* New York: Barnes and Noble Books, 1984.

Goodman, Thomas, and Stephanie Young. Smart Face, New York: Prentice Hall Press, 1988.

Grossbart, Ted A., and Carl Sherman. *Skin Deep.* New York: William Morrow and Company, 1986.

Haberman, Fredric, and Denise Fortino. *Your Skin: A Dermatologist's Guide to a Lifetime of Beauty and Health.* New York: Berkley Books.

Leider, Morris, and Morris Rosenblum. (1968) *A Dictionary of Dermatologic Words, Terms and Phrases.* McGraw-Hill Book Co., 1986.

Novick, Nelson. *Super Skin: A Leading Dermatologist's Guide to the Latest Breakthroughs in Skin Care.* New York: Clarkson N. Potter, Inc. Publishers, 1988.

Physicians' Desk Reference. 43rd Edition. Oradell, N.J.: Edward Barnhart Publisher, Medical Economics Company Inc. Publishers, 1989.

Steigleder, Gerd Klaus, and Howard I. Maibach, *Pocket Atlas of Dermatology.* New York: Thieme-Stratton Inc., 1981.

Strassler, Stephen, *Cosmetic Ingredient and Training Manual.* Haddonfield, N.J.: Reviva Labs, Inc. Publishers, 1989.

Chapter 12

Graham, Jean Ann, and Albert M. Kligman, *The Psychology of Cosmetic Treatments.* New York: Praeger, 1985.

Bernstein, Norman R., and Martin Robson. *Comprehensive Approaches to the Burned Person.* New York: Medical Examination Publishing Co., 1983.

Bernstein, Norman R., A.J. Breslau, and J.A. Graham. *Coping Strategies for Burn Survivors and Their Families.* New York: Praeger.

Boswick, John A. *The Surgical Clinics of North America: Burns.* Volume 67-Number 1. Philadelphia: W.B. Saunders Co. 1987.

Coleman, William, Gustavo Colon, and Ronald Davis. *Outpatient Surgery of the Skin.* New York: Medical Examination Publishing Company, 1983.

Gior, Fino. *Modern Electrology: Excess Hair, Its Causes and Treatments* New York: Milady Publishing Company, 1987.

Jackson, Ian, and E.S. Macallan. *Plastic Surgery and Burns Treatment.* William Heinemann Medical Books, 1971.

Marze, Elaine Hodge. *Up From the Ashes.* New York: Vantage Press Inc., 1987.

Ross, Rudolph, and Jack Fisher. *Skin Grafting*. Boston: Little, Brown Publishers, 1979.

Chapter 14

Doan-Noyes, Diane, and Peggy Mellody. *Beauty and Cancer*. Los Angeles: AC Press.

Kater, Suzy. *Looking Up, The Complete Guide for Looking and Feeling Better for the Cancer Patient*. New York: McGraw-Hill Book Co.

Cox-Gedmark, Jan. *Coping with Physical Disability*. Philadelphia: Westminster Press.

The American Medical Encyclopedia. New York: Random House.

Goodman, Thomas, M.D., and Stephanie Young. *Smart Face*. New York: Prentice-Hall Press.

Gjerde, Mary. *Organic Makeup*. Los Angeles: Nash Publishing.

Jeanne Rose's Kitchen Cosmetics. San Francisco: Panjandrum/Aris Books.

Simonton, Matthews-Simonton, and Crieghton. *Getting Well Again*. New York: Bantam Books.

Winter. *A Consumer's Dictionary of Cosmetic Ingredients*. New York: Crown Books.

Brumberg, Elaine. *Save Your Money, Save Your Face*. New York: Facts on File Publications.

Appendix A

Elson, M.L. "The Utilization of Glycolic Acid in Photoaging." *Cosmetic Dermatology*. 5 (1992): 12–15.

Elson, M.L. "Differential Effects of Glycolic Acid and Tretinoin in Acne Vulgaris." *Cosmetic Dermatology* (in press).

Elson, M.L. "Treatment of Photoaging with Combined Therapy." *Journal of Cutaneous Aging and Cosmetic Dermatology* (in press).

Van Scott, E.J., and R.J. Yu. 1989. "Alpha Hydroxy Acids: Procedures for Use in Clinical Practice." *Cutis*. 43 (1989): 222–118.

Van Scott, E.J. and R.J. Yu. "Alpha Hydroxy Acids: Therapeutic Potentials." *Canadian Journal of Dermatology*. 1 (1989): 108–112.

Glossary/Index